T0365726

Medicine on a Larger Scale

In a world of growing health inequity and ecological injustice, how do we revitalize medicine and public health to tackle new problems? This groundbreaking collection draws together case studies of social medicine in the Global South, radically shifting our understanding of social science in healthcare. Looking beyond a narrative originating in nineteenth-century Europe, a team of expert contributors explores a far broader set of roots and branches, with nodes in Sub-Saharan Africa, South America, Oceania, the Middle East, and Asia. This plural approach reframes and decolonizes the study of social medicine, highlighting connections to social justice and health equity, social science and state formation, bottom-up community initiatives, grassroots movements, and an array of revolutionary sensibilities. As a truly global history, this book offers a more usable past to imagine a new politics of social medicine for medical professionals and healthcare workers worldwide. This title is also available as open access on Cambridge Core.

ANNE KVEIM LIE is Professor of Medical History, Department of Community Medicine and Global Health, University of Oslo.

JEREMY A. GREENE is William H. Welch Professor of Medicine and the History of Medicine, Johns Hopkins University School of Medicine.

WARWICK ANDERSON is Janet Dora Hine Professor of Politics, Governance, and Ethics in Health, based in the School of Social and Political Sciences and the Charles Perkins Centre, University of Sydney.

Medicine on a Larger Scale

Global Histories of Social Medicine

Edited by

Anne Kveim Lie
University of Oslo

Jeremy A. Greene
Johns Hopkins University

Warwick Anderson
University of Sydney

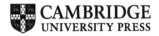

CAMBRIDGE
UNIVERSITY PRESS

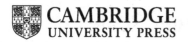

Shaftesbury Road, Cambridge CB2 8EA, United Kingdom

One Liberty Plaza, 20th Floor, New York, NY 10006, USA

477 Williamstown Road, Port Melbourne, VIC 3207, Australia

314–321, 3rd Floor, Plot 3, Splendor Forum, Jasola District Centre,
New Delhi – 110025, India

103 Penang Road, #05–06/07, Visioncrest Commercial, Singapore 238467

Cambridge University Press is part of Cambridge University Press & Assessment,
a department of the University of Cambridge.

We share the University's mission to contribute to society through the pursuit of
education, learning and research at the highest international levels of excellence.

www.cambridge.org
Information on this title: www.cambridge.org/9781009428569

DOI: 10.1017/9781009428514

First published 2025

A catalogue record for this publication is available from the British Library

*A Cataloging-in-Publication data record for this book is available from the
Library of Congress*

ISBN 978-1-009-42856-9 Hardback
ISBN 978-1-009-42855-2 Paperback

Cambridge University Press & Assessment has no responsibility for the persistence
or accuracy of URLs for external or third-party internet websites referred to in this
publication and does not guarantee that any content on such websites is, or will
remain, accurate or appropriate.

For Paul and Per
This book is dedicated to the memory of Paul Farmer and Per Haave, two scholars and practitioners of what global social medicine has been, should be, and could become, who helped to inspire and lend their efforts to the project this book would become but are not here to see its publication. Their generosity, support, and capacious vision is written through every page.

Contents

List of Figures   *page* ix
List of Contributors   x

Introduction: The Many Lives and Afterlives of Social Medicine   1
WARWICK ANDERSON, JEREMY A. GREENE,
AND ANNE KVEIM LIE

1   Decentering Rudolf Virchow: The Making of a Social
    Medicine Pioneer   20
    CARSTEN TIMMERMANN

2   Social Medicine in the Arab World: Colonial Legacies
    and Postcolonial Praxis   40
    JOELLE M. ABI-RACHED AND LIDIA HELOU

3   Latin American Social Medicine, across the Waves   60
    ERIC D. CARTER

4   Imperial Social Medicine in Southeast Asia: The Bandung
    Intergovernmental Conference on Rural Hygiene   81
    LAURENCE MONNAIS AND HANS POLS

5   Social and Socialist: Ideas of Health, Medicine, and Society
    across the Iron Curtain   106
    DORA VARGHA

6   Social Medicine in Social Democracy   122
    ANNE KVEIM LIE AND PER HAAVE

7   American Social Medicine in the Shadow of Socialized Medicine   143
    JEREMY A. GREENE, SCOTT H. PODOLSKY,
    AND DAVID S. JONES

8   A "Counter-Hegemonic" Social Medicine: Leftist Physicians
    during the Latin American Cold War   167
    SEBASTIAN FONSECA

9 The African Roots of Community-Oriented Primary Care   186
   ABIGAIL H. NEELY

10 Barefoot Doctors and Social Medicine in China   201
   XIAOPING FANG

11 From "*Saúde Pública*" to "*Medicina Social*"
   to "*Saúde Coletiva*": The Emergence of a Transepistemic
   Arena in Brazil   218
   KENNETH ROCHEL DE CAMARGO

12 Settler Colonial Social Medicine and Community Health:
   Australasian Adaptations, Reinventions, and Denials   237
   WARWICK ANDERSON, JAMES DUNK, AND CONNIE MUSOLINO

13 Social Medicine beyond Colonial Rule: The Medical Field
   Units of Ghana, 1930–2000   257
   DAVID BANNISTER

14 Changing Avatars of Social Medicine in the Indian
   Subcontinent   278
   RAMA V. BARU

15 Social Medicine, *Otherwise*: Cuban Health(Care)
   as Political Praxis   297
   P. SEAN BROTHERTON

   Afterword: Struggling with and for Social Medicine   318
   ANNE-EMANUELLE BIRN

   Afterword: The Future(s) of Social Medicine   322
   HELENA HANSEN

Index   325

Figures

1.1 Virchow around 1848   *page* 23
1.2 Railway map of Germany in 1849   25
1.3 Carl Wilhelm Hübener, *The Silesian Weavers* (1844)   27
1.4 Barricade in Berlin, 1848   30
1.5 Virchow later in life, in his study, surrounded by skulls
and skeletons   33
1.6 Henry Sigerist in his office   34
2.1 Tawhida Ben Cheikh featured on Tunisia's
new 10 dinar banknote, 2020   52
3.1 Front page of the *Boletín Médico de Chile*   67
3.2 Alliance for Progress public health promotion poster   72
4.1 The main building of the Technical School in Bandung   82
4.2 An envelope issued for the Bandung Conference   83
4.3 Index cards used to facilitate triage by the medical doctor
in charge of a health sector   93
4.4 A *mantri* (health worker) educates a family   95
4.5 Name badge for the delegates to the Bandung Conference   99
4.6 The opening ceremony of the Bandung Conference
on August 3, 1937   102
11.1 Sérgio Arouca and Hésio Cordeiro   228
11.2 Michel Foucault lecturing at the Instituto de Medicina Social   229
13.1 (a)–(d) Community health facilities in rural Ghana, 2018   259
13.2 (a)–(c) Internal documents, organizational structures,
and reports of the Medical Field Units in 1952 and 1961   268
15.1 Cuban and Italian doctors meeting in Turin, Italy, to
combat Covid-19   298
15.2 Abdala Covid-19 vaccine   300
15.3 Cuba solidarity blocked   313

Contributors

JOELLE M. ABI-RACHED is a tenured Associate Professor of Medicine at the American University of Beirut, with a secondary appointment in History and Archaeology, and Associate at the Department of History of Science at Harvard University. She is an interdisciplinary social scientist of medicine, trained as a medical doctor, a philosopher, and a historian of science. Among her publications are *'Aṣfūriyyeh: A History of Madness, Modernity, and War in the Middle East* (MIT Press, 2020) and *Neuro: The New Brain Sciences and the Management of the Mind* (Princeton University Press, 2013) co-authored with Nikolas Rose.

WARWICK ANDERSON is Janet Dora Hine Professor of Politics, Governance, and Ethics in the School of Social and Political Sciences and the Charles Perkins Centre at the University of Sydney. His most recent book is *Spectacles of Waste* (Polity, 2024). In 2023, he was awarded the John Desmond Bernal Prize of the Society for Social Studies of Science.

DAVID BANNISTER is a historian and anthropologist of disease and public health at the Institute for Health and Society, Faculty of Medicine, University of Oslo. His research includes changing conceptions of fairness in health, social histories of state healthcare, social and community medicine, and how healthcare reshapes natural environments.

RAMA V. BARU is Professor Emeritus at the Centre of Social Medicine and Community Health, Jawaharlal Nehru University. Her research focus is on social determinants of health, health policy and comparative health.

ANNE-EMANUELLE BIRN is Professor of Global Development Studies at the University of Toronto. Her books include *Marriage of Convenience: Rockefeller International Health and Revolutionary Mexico* (University of Rochester Press, 2006); *Comrades in Health* (Rutgers University Press, 2013); *Textbook of Global Health* (Oxford University Press, 4th ed., 2017); *Peripheral Nerve: Health and Medicine in Cold War Latin America* (Duke University Press, 2020); and *Going Public: The Unmaking and Remaking of Universal Healthcare* (Cambridge University Press, 2023).

She received the Viseltear Prize for Lifetime Achievement in Public Health History, 2023.

P. SEAN BROTHERTON is Professor and Chair of Anthropology at New York University and the President of the Society for Medical Anthropology. Among his publications are *Revolutionary Medicine: Health and the Body in Post-Soviet Cuba* (Duke University Press, 2012) and *Global Health, Otherwise: Cuba and the Politics of Humanitarianism* (Duke University Press, in press).

KENNETH ROCHEL DE CAMARGO is full Professor at the Hésio Cordeiro Institute of Social Medicine, Rio de Janeiro State University. He is Editor Emeritus of the *American Journal of Public Health*, Senior Editor of *Global Public Health*, and a member of the Editorial Advisory Board of Editora Fiocruz.

ERIC D. CARTER is Edens Professor of Geography and Global Health at Macalester College, Saint Paul, USA. He is the author of *In Pursuit of Health Equity: A History of Latin American Social Medicine* (University of North Carolina Press, 2023).

JAMES DUNK is Research Fellow at the School of Social and Political Sciences, and Co-Director of the Ecological Emotions Research Lab, University of Sydney. A historian and interdisciplinary researcher, his historical studies of mental health, psychology, and planetary health has been published in medical, psychological, and historical journals.

XIAOPING FANG is Associate Professor of Chinese Studies at Monash University. He is the author of *Barefoot Doctors and Western Medicine in China* (University of Rochester Press, 2012) and *China and the Cholera Pandemic: Restructuring Society under Mao* (University of Pittsburgh Press, 2021).

SEBASTIAN FONSECA is Postdoctoral Fellow at the Wellcome Trust-funded "Connecting 3 Worlds," University of Exeter, and a physician with a PhD in Global Health and Social Medicine. He also lectures at the University of Maastricht. His research interests lie at the intersection between the history of medicine, Cold War scholarship, and Science and Technology Studies.

JEREMY A. GREENE is a practicing physician and historian based in Baltimore, MD, whose writing explores the social lives and political stakes of everyday medical technologies and the unfulfilled promise of health equity. He is the founding Director of the Center for Medical Humanities and Social Medicine at Johns Hopkins University and sees patients in a community health center in East Baltimore.

PER HAAVE was Guest Researcher at the Institute of Health and Society, University of Oslo. He published on topics such as the history of psychiatry, eugenics and sterilization, of the Romani people in Norway, and on the history of the "welfare state" as a key concept in Norwegian politics. Sadly, Haave passed away before the completion of this book.

HELENA HANSEN is Professor of Psychiatry and Anthropology at the University of California, Los Angeles, and an addiction psychiatrist and anthropologist. She is also leading a national movement for training clinical practitioners to address social determinants of health which she with Jonathan Metzl have labeled "Structural Competency."

LIDIA HELOU is currently pursuing a PhD in Middle Eastern and Islamic Studies – Culture and Representation – at New York University. She holds a double degree in history and political sciences from the Sorbonne University and a dual master's degree in international and world history from Columbia University and the London School of Economics.

DAVID S. JONES teaches the history of medicine, medical ethics, and social medicine at Harvard University. He trained in psychiatry and the history of science. David's research has ranged from the history of epidemics to heart disease, cardiac therapeutics, air pollution, and the effects of the climate crisis on health.

ANNE KVEIM LIE is Professor of Medical History at the University of Oslo. As a physician–historian, her work has explored the history of infectious disease and pharmaceuticals, antibiotic resistance, and climate change. She works as a physician north of the Polar Circle every summer and volunteers at the Health Centre for undocumented migrants in Oslo.

LAURENCE MONNAIS is Professor of the History of Medicine and Public Health at the University of Lausanne–Lausanne University Hospital. A specialist of the history of medicine in Southeast Asia, she has also worked on the history of public health and mass vaccination in Canada. Her most recent project deals with a global history of measles.

CONNIE MUSOLINO is Research Fellow in Stretton Health Equity at the University of Adelaide. She is an early career researcher with expertise in social science, gender studies and public health. Currently she is examining policies and practices to address health inequalities in Australia.

ABIGAIL H. NEELY is Associate Professor of Geography at Dartmouth College. Her book *Reimagining Social Medicine from the South* (Duke University Press, 2021) rethinks the history of social medicine through African communities. Her current book project examines the failures of post-apartheid South Africa through the epidemic of death amongst the country's youth.

SCOTT H. PODOLSKY is Professor of Global Health and Social Medicine at Harvard Medical School and Director of the Center for the History of Medicine at the Countway Medical Library, Harvard University. He is the author of *The Antibiotic Era: Reform, Resistance, and the Pursuit of a Rational Therapeutics* (Johns Hopkins University Press, 2015).

HANS POLS is Professor at the School of History and Philosophy of Science at the University of Sydney. His research focuses on the history of medicine in the Dutch East Indies and Indonesia as well as on the recent history of psychiatry and mental health services in Indonesia and Australia.

CARSTEN TIMMERMANN is Director of the Centre for the History of Science, Technology and Medicine at the University of Manchester. His research focuses on the history of modern biomedicine. He has published on pharmaceuticals, cancer research and therapy, cardiovascular disease, and the debate over a crisis of medicine in interwar Germany.

DORA VARGHA is Professor of History and Medical Humanities at the University of Exeter, jointly based at Humboldt University in Berlin, with a research focus on global health history from a socialist perspective. She is author of *Polio across the Iron Curtain* (Cambridge University Press, 2018).

Introduction

The Many Lives and Afterlives of Social Medicine

Warwick Anderson, Jeremy A. Greene,
and Anne Kveim Lie[*]

What is social medicine? For many reformers inside and outside the medical profession, the field emerged in the nineteenth century as a means to temper the overzealous scientism of an increasingly narrow biomedical approach to disease and therapeutics. For others, the term itself was a tautology that described the role of social sciences as basic sciences of medicine – for how could health or disease ever be fully understood without including the socio-economic determinants of health and the life worlds of patients and caregivers? Alternatively, for many politicians left, right, and center, "social medicine" soon became an expression of the strengths or possibilities of new state-based approaches to health and healthcare, from Otto von Bismarck's pioneering German social insurance scheme through the proliferation of national health systems in the wake of the Second World War. But for some public health advocates and community activists who sought to locate disease prevention and healthcare beyond the hospital or clinic, often under the rubric of "community health," the older term itself embodied a form of medicalization: another overreach by the medical profession artificially inflating its impact on the health of populations, when economic transformation, grassroots advocacy, and radical social change might prove better at prevention or care.

There is not, and never has been, a single consensual definition of social medicine. During the twentieth century, on every populated continent, across vastly different political spaces, social medicine came to acquire a constellation of meanings. Yet, as the question of what social medicine might be, or might become, exercised the minds of countless reformers in the twentieth century,

[*] For comments on earlier drafts, we would like to thank Eric Carter, James Dunk, Arthur Kleinman, and Charles Rosenberg. Conversations with contributors to this volume greatly influenced our thinking on these matters. We are grateful to the Norwegian Research Council (#283370 Biomedicalization from the Inside Out) and Johns Hopkins University for support (for an initial workshop and for the publication of this book). We would also like to thank the University of Sydney, the Johns Hopkins University, and the Norwegian Research Council (#283370) for funding the Open Access publication of this book. Anderson's research was supported by the Australian Research Council (SR200200920 and DP220100624).

some general areas of agreement can be traced. Generally, the designation implied depreciation, if not rejection, of reductionist and technical attributes of contemporary biomedicine, especially its narrow focus on individual treatment, laboratory research, and molecular explanation. In contrast, social medicine was imagined as an integrative enterprise, an ambitious, often idealized, attempt to reckon with the social, political, and economic determinants of health and disease in our communities – to think beyond the routinism of pills, potions, and other expedients. It drew on emergent social sciences to reshape and deepen understanding of disease patterns, thereby accommodating health and disease within more complex and realistic sociological configurations. Advocates of social medicine thus might propose radical changes to pathogenic social, political, and economic structures, demanding an overhaul of the systemic inequalities and injustices that make us sick – not mere patching-up or deferral or other conventional medical makeshifts. Always elusive, always escaping precise definition and definitive realization, social medicine came to signify reformist and interdisciplinary impulses within the health professions, socioeconomic inquiries in public health, and occasionally even radical political change.[1]

All the same, by the turn of the twenty-first century, most of the medical world had stopped asking questions about social medicine. Long associated with national reform movements and international health organizations, social medicine appeared incongruent with growing neoliberal globalization. Its reach in medical school curricula had receded from a watermark that had never been that high and it was rarely part of the repertoire of "global health" as it developed from the 1990s.[2] And yet, in a world of widening health inequalities,

---

[1] Among many versions of the history of social medicine are George Rosen, "What Is Social Medicine?," *Bulletin of the History of Medicine* 21 (1947): 674–733; Dorothy Porter and Roy Porter, "What Was Social Medicine? An Historiographic Essay," *Journal of Historical Sociology* 1 (1988): 90–106; Dorothy Porter (ed.), *Social Medicine and Medical Sociology in the Twentieth Century* (Amsterdam: Rodopi, 1997); and Dorothy Porter, *Health, Civilization and the State: A History of Public Health from Ancient to Modern Times* (New York, NY: Routledge, 2005).

[2] On global health, see Theodore M. Brown, Marcos Cueto, and Elizabeth Fee, "The World Health Organization and the Transition from 'International' to 'Global' Public Health," *American Journal of Public Health* 96 (2006): 62–72; Anne-Emanuelle Birn, "The Stages of International (Global) Health: Histories of Success or Successes of History?," *Global Public Health* 4 (2009): 50–68; Andrew Lakoff, "Two Regimes of Global Health," *Humanity* 1 (2010): 59–79; Vincanne Adams, "Against Global Health: Arbitrating Science, Non-science, and Nonsense through Health," in Jonathan M. Metzl and A. Kirkland (eds.), *Against Health: How Health Became the New Morality* (New York, NY: New York University Press, 2020), 40–60; João Biehl, "When People Come First: Beyond Technical and Theoretical Quick Fixes in Global Health," in R. Peet, P. Robbins, and M. Watts (eds.), *Global Political Ecology* (London: Routledge, 2010), 114–44; Didier Fassin, "That Obscure Object of Global Health," in Marcia C. Inhorn and E. A. Wentzell (eds.), *Medical Anthropology at the Intersections: Histories, Activisms, and Futures* (Durham, NC: Duke University Press, 2012), 95–115; Paul E. Farmer, Arthur Kleinman, J. Kim, and M. Basilico (eds.), *Reimagining Global Health: An Introduction* (Berkeley: University of

depleted public health services, and narrowly focused "precision" medicine, we perhaps need a renovated and reimagined social medicine – that is, a decanonized and revised social medicine – more than ever. Accordingly, we have gathered together these restorative chapters that show us how we might remake a social medicine fit for addressing our alarming and oppressive times. From multiple sites, often drawing inspiration from beyond Western Europe and North America, the contributors to this volume seek usable histories of social medicine and its various proxies, necessary histories that will enable fresh critiques of elite biomedical reductionism, clinical individualism, and professional abnegation. These stories from the militant interstices of canonical biomedicine in the Global North and from the vanguard of health activism in the Global South open to us a planetary vista of what social medicine might become, should become, in the twenty-first century.

Pluralizing the Histories of Social Medicine

What, then, was social medicine supposed to be?[3] The standard narrative, favored by the influential American historian of medicine and public health George Rosen, among others, traces a genealogy back to a European ancestor, liberal pathologist Rudolf Virchow.[4] Many now know Virchow, if at all, through a single useful quotation, in which he asserted that, "medicine is a social science and politics is nothing else but medicine on a larger scale."[5] Virchow, the story goes, was radicalized as a young physician, soon after graduating from medical school in Berlin, when sent in the 1840s to evaluate a typhus epidemic afflicting the recently occupied Prussian territory of Upper Silesia. In a report that continues to resonate today, Virchow concluded the most important determinants of epidemic emergence were poverty, oppression, and dispossession – which implicated Prussian imperialism. Virchow thus became both a hero of biomedical sciences – helping to found the new discipline of cellular pathology – *and* the iconic figure of the socially engaged physician, leading the liberal political reform movement of 1848 and setting forth a progressive and later dominant, agenda for social medicine. If health professionals learn anything about social medicine these days, they come to understand that this European tradition,

California Press, 2013); Warwick Anderson, "Making Global Health History: The Postcolonial Worldliness of Biomedicine," *Social History of Medicine* 27 (2014): 372–84; and Randall P. Packard, *Global Health: A History of Intervening in Other Peoples' Problems* (Baltimore: Johns Hopkins University Press, 2017).
3   Porter and Porter, "What Was Social Medicine?"
4   Rosen, "What Is Social Medicine?"; Erwin H. Ackerknecht, *Rudolf Virchow: Doctor, Statesman, Anthropologist* (Madison, WI: University of Wisconsin Press, 1953).
5   Leon Eisenberg, "Rudolf Ludwig Karl Virchow, Where Are You Now That We Need You?," *American Journal of Medicine* 77, no. 3 (1984): 524–32.

beginning with Virchow, was transported to new worlds, where it might be taken up and transformed by national savants and colonial elites.

Once rendered portable in the twentieth century, once stabilized at multiple national and colonial sites, this moderately progressive style of social medicine, lacking real revolutionary appetite, settled in for the duration of the Cold War. With earlier support from the League of Nations Health Organization (LNHO) and then the World Health Organization (WHO), most nation states could endorse modest programs in social medicine, in small doses, sometimes in homeopathic dilutions.[6] Participants in the post-Second World War nation-based order built up a tolerance for integrating social science and medicine and sometimes for expanding community health programs, while remaining allergic to any serious structural changes, let alone the overthrow of the capitalist world system. What was left out of this institutionalized social medicine is always at least as interesting as what was left in it. Even so, in out-of-the-way places, and sometimes in North America and Western Europe during this period, scattered marginalized and suppressed scholars and activists could still imagine a more incendiary social medicine, one committed to social and racial justice and to health equity, as demonstrated in contributions to this volume.

We aim here to decenter Virchow and to offer alternatives to the anodyne and patchy liberal or reformist visions of the globalized mode of social medicine attributed to him. There are other social medicines that we seek to make visible, many dating from the social movements of the 1960s and 1970s, often from post-colonial Latin America and decolonizing Africa, usually animated by radical, sometimes Marxist, politics. Importantly, it is this postcolonial insurgency – so often omitted from generic histories of social medicine – that we seek to reveal and revitalize in this volume.

The renewed advocacy for social medicine, as many contributors demonstrate, had deep roots in anticolonial struggles and nationalist aspirations, in rural hygiene schemes, and late-colonial "development" regimes. A potent and varied mixture of liberal humanitarianism, Marxism, feminism, liberation theology, and Indigenous organizing would force its growth from the 1960s onward. The germinal beds for this new social medicine, focused on social justice and health equity, were located in Southern Africa and across

[6] Paul Weindling, "Social Medicine at the League of Nations Health Organisation and the International Labour Office Compared," in Weindling, *International Health Organisations and Movements, 1918–1939* (Cambridge: Cambridge University Press, 1995), 134–53; Iris Borowy, "International Social Medicine between the Wars: Positioning a Volatile Concept," *Hygiea Internationalis* 6, no. 2 (2007): 13–35; Iris Borowy, "Shifting between Biomedical and Social Medicine: International Health Organizations in the 20th Century," *History Compass* 12, no. 6 (2014): 517–30; Iris Borowy and Anne Hardy (eds.), *Of Medicine and Men: Biographies and Ideas in European Social Medicine between the World Wars* (Frankfurt am Main: Peter Lang, 2008); and Marcos Cueto, Theodore M. Brown, and Elizabeth Fee, *The World Health Organization: A History* (Cambridge: Cambridge University Press, 2019).

South America and the Caribbean, where revolutionary possibilities seemed imminent and inevitable. Maoist China contributed community health workers or "barefoot doctors," while India took up Gandhian principles of self-reliance. For more advanced riders of this new revolutionary wave, the old European genealogy of social medicine displayed little allure. Although southern advocates of social medicine were supporting the usual efforts to ally social science and medicine, they tended to go further, emphasizing the need to address through radical measures the social determinants of health, the need, that is, to transform public health through reconstructing economic and political systems. In this way, the category of the "social" itself became the target of intervention, as P. Sean Brotherton argues in Chapter 15. The reactivation of the social in social medicine – and its translation into political economies of health – had profound intellectual consequences, not least the development of social epidemiology, seeded by anti-racist white South African physicians who migrated to the United States. The impact of the new wave of social medicine on health outcomes, however, proved variable and infinitely contestable. Any fervor, such as it was, for radical social medicine from the Global South seemed to dwindle toward the end of the twentieth century.

Even as we try to shift focus away from mythologies of Virchow and those who sought to canonize him, we also should acknowledge some radical possibilities lodged deep in his early work that have long been forgotten. Preoccupied with the sociopolitical visions of twentieth-century social medicine, it is easy to forget that for Virchow and others in the nineteenth century, social medicine meant countering distinctly environmental pathologies. Social inequality and worker exploitation appeared to be expressed through pathogenic local environments. But the environmental concerns of early social medicine eventually were displaced later in the century by social pathologies, frequently mediated by the transmission of germs. Some environmental factors persisted in the epidemiological calculus, of course, particularly in specialties like environmental health, toxicology, industrial hygiene, and disease ecology – but mainstream biomedicine and public health were diverted into a semiautonomous social world, full of behavioral risks and threats.[7] Humans might alter their environments but it seemed their environments rarely hit back. In the 1990s, when a fresh cohort of radical physicians and epidemiologists, many of them trained in social medicine, began to recognize the

---

[7] In the United States in the middle of the twentieth century, some leading figures in social medicine, generally European émigrés, did retain a geographical vision, though often in parallel rather than integrated. See, for example, Henry E. Sigerist, "Problems of Historical-Geographical Pathology," *Bulletin of the History of Medicine* 1 (1933): 10–18; René J. Dubos, *Mirage of Health: Utopias, Progress, and Biological Change* (London, 1959); René J. Dubos, *Man, Medicine, and Environment* (New York, NY: Pall Mall Press, 1968); and Erwin H. Ackerknecht, *History and Geography of the Most Important Diseases* (New York, NY: Hafner, 1965).

impacts on human health of climate change and the degradation of the Earth's life-support systems, they sought a label for the pernicious social and political processes they were describing. Social medicine, long since shorn of its environmental sensibilities, seemed inapt, even irrelevant. Instead, they settled on the name "planetary health."[8] Of course, had they been better attuned to critical and encompassing histories of social medicine, as presented in these chapters, they may have realized that planetary health can be – indeed, should be – social medicine too, only scaled up.

Attending to Multisited Histories of Social Medicine

This collection of chapters brings together a wide assortment of histories of social medicine, most of them written from postcolonial and other critical standpoints, assuming multisited or transnational perspectives. Each chapter foregrounds a different set of politics of social medicine in relation to healthcare professions, the state, and social movements. Taken together, these accounts offer generative intersections and common themes. First, the chapters examine how social medicine can act as a boundary marker or as border-space between healthcare professions, the social sciences, and state bureaucracies. Second, they explore how social medicine works to contest reductionistic approaches of biomedicine from within, while also serving, perhaps perversely, as a site from which to medicalize the wider social world. Third, these chapters collectively highlight the processes by which the field of social medicine could paradoxically be undone by its own success – or, in contrast, thrive while occupying marginal or counterhegemonic positions. The contributors to this volume ask: what is the "social" in social medicine, and what is, or who does, the "medicine" (as opposed to broader conceptions of health) in the well-worn conjunction. When does the yoking together of the social and the medical offer a strong position to intervene in the world and when does amalgamation paradoxically limit the potential impact of its principles?

The first four chapters (by Carsten Timmermann, Chapter 1; Joelle M. Abi-Rached and Lidia Helou, Chapter 2; Eric D. Carter, Chapter 3; Laurence Monnais and Hans Pols, Chapter 4) actively refigure the intellectual legacy of European figures like Rudolf Virchow and Jules Guérin and institutions such as the interwar LNHO, the Rockefeller Foundation, and the postwar WHO, in our understanding of the development of social medicine. These authors seek to reframe this history in broader experiments of inter-imperial contests and through decolonization movements. As Timmermann shows in Chapter 1, the legend of Virchow as an enlightened European whose ideas diffused to the

---

[8] Warwick Anderson and James Dunk, "Planetary Health Histories: Toward New Ecologies of Epidemiology?," *Isis* 113, no. 4 (2022): 767–88.

far reaches of the world misses a more robust production of the field of social medicine at the edges of empires and within the state formations and civil societies of emergent nations in the global South. His chapter works to decenter the hero-myth of Virchow and re-emphasize the colonial relations of his foundational works. Abi-Rached and Helou, Carter, and Monnais and Pols work to refocus – and at least partially decolonize – the heavily Euro-American authoritative history of social medicine, turning attention to engagements in this field from the Middle East, Southeast Asia, and Latin America – toward these obscured and neglected, yet still determinate, alternative histories.

Abi-Rached and Helou trace in Chapter 2 how social medicine moved through Francophone Arabic engagements in the late nineteenth century as a form of social critique and praxis. The formal concept of social medicine in Arabic (*at-ṭibb al-ijtimāʿī*)was never taken up in the medical or popular literatures despite a prolific practical entanglement with implied precepts of social medicine. Abi-Rached and Helou speculate that there are at least two reasons for this: first, the concept is tautological in Arabic. The *ḥakīm* or doctor (which in Arabic literally means "sage," "judicious," or "wise") has throughout history carried a social responsibility, namely serving as a "wise" and trustworthy counselor for both the rulers and the needy. And second, in contrast to France or Germany where social medicine took a life of its own in the early twentieth century, the Arabic world was caught up in a period of revolutionary buoyancy, in which social medicine seemed a relatively minor concern or even a distraction from truly radical change. The term had been translated into Arabic in 1912, a few years before the revolutionary moments that convulsed the Arab world in the aftermath of the First World War, which would lead to the redrawing of national boundaries. If anything, social medicine was implicit in the practical philosophy of caring for the "wretched of the earth": first, in the face of colonial powers, including the Ottomans; then, in the face of authoritarian and patriarchal regimes in the post-independence period. But it rarely took on an autonomous, active presence.

In Chapter 3, Carter traces the broader history of social medicine in Latin America, thus reconnecting two distinct waves of social medicine in a unified narrative. As he shows, first-wave social medicine, whose protagonists included figures such as Salvador Allende (and other members of the Vanguardia Médica) of Chile and Ramón Carrillo in Argentina, expressed ambivalent relations with the esteemed Virchow – or simply disregarded him. These early explicit formations of social medicine gained strength in the interwar period, leaving an indelible imprint on Latin American welfare states by the 1940s. Second-wave social medicine, marked by the more confrontational Marxist analytical frameworks of figures such as Juan César García, Sérgio Arouca, and Asa Cristina Laurell, took shape in the early 1970s, crystallized institutionally in ALAMES (regionally) and ABRASCO (in Brazil). This radical version of social medicine was heavily inflected by social theory, including liberation theology and world-systems/dependency theory, vernacular doctrines from Latin America. Yet, as Carter explains, the apparent hiatus between the first and second waves must also be reconsidered as an important and productive period. Reading both "waves" together can accentuate biographies and itineraries of social medicine thinkers (such as Josué de Castro) that do not "fit" one or another formation, revealing how social medicine evolves in complex reactions to both changes in the health field and developments in geopolitics.

Monnais and Pols in Chapter 4 revisit the Intergovernmental Conference on Rural Hygiene in Bandung, Dutch East Indies (now Indonesia), which took place in August 1937 under the auspices of the LNHO. Widely viewed as foundational for social medicine, driving it to prominence in international public health, this sentinel conference should also be recognized as reflecting regional intercolonial rivalry and ambiguous responses to decolonization movements. Bandung is often recounted as a spot on the trajectory toward internationalism, foregrounding the LNHO and anticipating the WHO, even prefiguring the primary healthcare policy enshrined in the Alma-Ata Declaration of 1978.[9] Monnais and Pols, however, seek to recover the distinctly colonial Southeast Asian context. Set against popular nationalist movements, athwart Depression-era poverty across the region, the recommendations made in Bandung cannot be divorced from colonial actors and anticolonial movements.

Tensions between social medicine and socialist medicine would prove a contentious issue over the course of the twentieth century. Chapters 5–8 – by Dora Vargha; Anne Kveim Lie and Per Haave; Jeremy A. Greene, Scott H. Podolsky, and David S. Jones; and Sebastian Fonseca, respectively – emphasize different conceptualizations of the role of the state in social medicine across Eastern Europe, Scandinavian states, the United States, and Latin America. In Chapter 5, Vargha examines the global influence of the "second world" of the socialist bloc, another marginalized but prolific generator of models of social medicine. She describes how the basic tenets underpinning social medicine gained new purchase in the "Global East" with the rise of state socialism and the emergence of a socialist worldview. New socialist or communist governments were sympathetic to theories postulating social, economic, and environmental determinants of health and disease – as well as open to fresh opportunities to extend the remit of the centralized state. And yet, as Vargha

---

[9] On the significance of the Alma-Ata Declaration and its focus on primary healthcare delivery, see Socrates Litsios, "The Long and Difficult Road to Alma Ata: A Personal Reflection," *International Journal of the Health Services* 32 (2002): 709–32; Marcos Cueto, "The Origins of Primary Health Care and Selective Primary Health Care," *American Journal of Public Health* 94 (2004): 1864–74; Fran Baum, "Health for All Now! Reviving the Spirit of Alma Ata in the Twenty-First Century: An Introduction to the Alma Ata Declaration," *Social Medicine* 2 (2007): 34–41; and Packard, *Global Health*.

shows, there was no single answer to what might constitute socialist medicine. She traces manifold and diverse connections between socialist politics, health policies, and medical practice across Eastern Europe, mapping divergences and overlaps in what became a key point of distinction in Cold War rhetoric, setting apart socialist East and capitalist West.

Kveim Lie and Haave, in Chapter 6, look at the contributions of doctrines of social medicine within the Scandinavian welfare state, an easily romanticized framing of capitalist socialism or socialist capitalism. In Scandinavia, health policies of the welfare state during much of the postwar period were premised on social medicine, which was swiftly established as a core medical specialty. This chapter follows the rise of social medicine within Scandinavia from the interwar period, tracking its ramifications in international health agenda and global health governance, before exploring broader negotiations of social medicine as an academic, activist, and clinical field during the postwar years.

Unlike Scandinavia, the United States quickly turned "socialist medicine" into a red-baiting slur. The inferred proximity between "social" and "socialist" meant that social medicine achieved little institutional stature in the US, leaving it perched on the edges of a few medical schools. Nonetheless, elite American universities did harbor several key figures in global social medicine and the Rockefeller Foundation intermittently preached the mission of social medicine abroad. As Greene, Podolsky, and Jones suggest in Chapter 7, this almost spectral presence poses a challenge for critical scholars: should their historical analysis focus only on renegades who outed themselves as theorists or practitioners of social medicine, or should they cast a broader net to include fellow travelers who identified differently (for example, with social hygiene, preventive medicine, community medicine, and so on) but nonetheless were animated with the spirit of social medicine? The chapter takes a hybrid approach. It reviews celebrated early US theorists of social medicine (such as Henry Sigerist, René Dubos, and George Rosen), showing how their ideas influenced the international health and domestic medical education through entities like the Rockefeller Foundation. At the same time, the authors ask why other key figures working at the intersection of health and the social world, especially Black social theorists like W. E. B. Du Bois, have been excluded from the social medicine vanguard. They trace the growth and fracture of American social medicine as a field that saw itself as liminal – between academic departments and community organizing efforts – thereby hoping to reframe the past, present, and future of the field.

In striking contrast, the history of social medicine in Latin America often takes an assertively Marxist demeanor.[10] Established in 1984, the Latin

---

[10] See also Herbert Waitzkin, C. Iriart, A. Estrada, and S. Lamadrid, "Social Medicine Then and Now: Lessons from Latin America," *American Journal of Public Health* 91 (2001): 1592–601;

American Social Medicine Association (ALAMES) represents the most stable transnational association in the region, examining the social basis of population health through lenses of Marxist historical materialism. Characterized as a "movement" deeply rooted in populist struggles of the region, the impetus for ALAMES's radical social medicine has generally emerged from public universities and scholarly institutes. As Fonseca shows in Chapter 8, not enough is known about the critical engagement between social movements, academic institutions, and the Pan-American Health Organization (PAHO) in this "second wave" revival of social medicine. Fonseca demystifies the relationship between ALAMES and PAHO, unearthing creative tension and generative ruptures around key actors like Ramon Villareal, the editors of *Educación Médica y Salud* (established in 1966, the PAHO's journal on human resources), and the occupants of multiple public higher education and research institutions. The chapter positions radical Latin American social medicine against the widespread ideological suppression enforced during the Cold War.

The broad theme of South–South transmission of models of community health, community medicine, and collective health shaped different trajectories of social medicine from Pholela to Mississippi, China to Mexico, and across South America and Australasia, as detailed in Chapters 9–12. Abigail H. Neely in Chapter 9 recenters the women of Pholela, South Africa, to recapture their role in the genesis and spread of community health practices that later helped to reconstitute social medicine. She traces one of the more easily elided origin points of the goal of delivering primary healthcare for all the world – as ultimately expressed in the Alma-Ata Declaration of 1978 – to a remote rural health center called the Pholela Community Health Centre. There, a new brand of social medicine – Community-Oriented Primary Care (COPC) – was born. While the health center's first medical director, Sidney Kark, would go on to help write the Alma-Ata Declaration, Neely argues that he learned both theory and practice from the community health workers in Pholela. This chapter explores the experiment in social medicine that took place in Pholela from the perspective of the people who lived in the health center's catchment. In so

D. Tajer, "Latin American Social Medicine: Roots, Development during the 1990s, and Current Challenges," *American Journal of Public Health* 93 (2003): 2023–7; Marcos Cueto and Steven Palmer, *Medicine and Public Health in Latin America: A History* (Cambridge: Cambridge University Press, 2014); Anne-Emanuelle Birn and Carles Muntaner, "Latin American Social Medicine across Borders: South–South Cooperation and the Making of Health Solidarity," in Emily E. Vasquez, Amaya G. Perez-Brumer, and Richard Parker (eds.), *Social Inequities and Contemporary Struggles for Collective Health in Latin America* (New York, NY: Routledge, 2020), 41–58; Eric D. Carter and Marcelo Sánchez Delgado, "A Debate over the Link between Salvador Allende, Max Westenhöfer, and Rudolf Virchow: Contributions to the History of Medicine in Chile and Internationally," *História, Ciências, Saúde – Manguinhos* 27 (2020): 899–917; and P. M. Sesia, "Global Voices for (Global) Epistemic Justice: Bringing to the Forefront Latin American Theoretical and Activist Contributions to the Pursuit of the Right to Health," *Health and Human Rights* 25, no. 1 (2023): 137–47.

doing, it reveals both the possibilities and limitations of this distinctive form of social medicine. As COPC traveled from Pholela, the efforts of the African women who lived around the health center became manifest again, at a distance, in places like Mound Bayou, Mississippi, and elsewhere in the developing world. Focusing on Pholela's residents, this story of social medicine not only offers an important corrective to more common accounts concentrating on medical doctors and bureaucratic luminaries – it also forces us to rethink how we understand social medicine and who makes it happen.[11]

Another key proposition of the Alma-Ata Declaration derived from "barefoot doctor" practices in rural China, a flowering of an alternative vision for social medicine, one that might be called transnational medical Maoism. As Xiaoping Fang shows in Chapter 10, social medicine in post-revolutionary China highlighted the legacies, good and bad, of growing commitment to international health, in which China was both recipient and contributor. Chinese social medicine amalgamated influences from semi-colonial Western hygiene and public health officers, many of them representatives of the Rockefeller Foundation, nationalist physicians, and rural health experts from the LNHO, along with later Soviet advocates of socialist medicine. But China contributed a unique method of tackling social determinants of health and the relationship between medicine and social justice. Fang follows the domestic production and international export of this "barefoot doctor" model at the height of the Cultural Revolution. For the Chinese government, the barefoot doctor system justified its radical transformation of society and publicized its political legitimacy. For the international health community, barefoot doctors became exemplars of how developing countries should deal with infectious diseases and provide primary healthcare. Fang's chapter analyzes the political assumptions and institutional structures that facilitated implementation of the barefoot doctor scheme. He also observes the residual structural inequalities within government administration that may have limited benefits of this form of social medicine – a mode of intervention actively romanticized and promoted around the world. With a sense of changing practice and meaning over time, Fang explores how barefoot doctors meant different things to different audiences, inside and outside of China, during the late twentieth century.

---

[11] See also Shula Marks, "South Africa's Early Experiment in Social Medicine: Its Pioneers and Politics," *American Journal of Public Health* 87 (1997): 452–9; Theodore M. Brown and Elizabeth Fee, "Sidney Kark and John Cassel: Social Medicine Pioneers and South African Émigrés," *American Journal of Public Health* 92 (2002): 1744–5; Mervyn Susser, "A Personal History: Social Medicine in a South African Setting, 1952–5. Part 1: The Shape of Ideas Forged in the Second World War," *Journal of Epidemiology and Community Health* 60 (2006): 554–7; Mervyn Susser, "A Personal History: Social Medicine in a South African Setting, 1952–5. Part 2: Social Medicine As a Calling: Ups, Downs, and Politics in Alexandra Township," *Journal of Epidemiology and Community Health* 60 (2006): 662–8.

In Chapter 11, Kenneth Rochel de Camargo delineates the autochthonous emergence of Brazilian social medicine at the intersection of academic and state institutions in Rio de Janeiro and Sao Paulo, which crystallized in a movement for "collective health" (*saúde coletiva*). Brazil boasts a long tradition in public health, with roots in the colonial period, when the first medical schools were established, reinforced in later nationalist self-assertion. The recent history of the field was deeply intertwined with the struggle to re-democratize the country after the military coup in 1964. As part of a broad social coalition, the *Movimento da Reforma Sanitária* mobilized left-leaning public health physicians connected to Latin American social medicine, who became instrumental in designing Brazil's National Health System, the Sistema Único de Saúde (SUS), after the restoration of democracy. The creation of the Instituto de Medicina Social (IMS) in 1974 at the Universidade do Estado do Rio de Janeiro (Rio de Janeiro State University) gave additional force to these developments. The professors and researchers at IMS advanced a body of theory as well as galvanizing government action. As Camargo shows, the IMS emerged as a prime mover in Brazilian social medicine and a motivating force in directing domestic and international aid work in the Lusophone world.

Chapter 12 takes a longer view on social medicine from the antipodes, revealing possibilities for integration of the field with community health and community medicine and with environmental and planetary imaginaries. After the Second World War, social medicine manifested in Australia largely through proxies and surrogates, which included tropical medicine (in the north of the continent), Aboriginal health, colonial health (in Papua and New Guinea and parts of the Pacific), pediatrics, geriatrics, and some non-institutional aspects of psychiatry. As Warwick Anderson, James Dunk, and Connie Musolino explain, these fields often emphasized socioeconomic drivers of disease emergence as well as social or political solutions to population health problems. Aspects of social medicine enthralled physicians on the right and the left in Australia, all of them afire with enthusiasm for further state intervention and white population management. From the 1970s, however, radical politicians and public health leaders began to support nationwide projects in "community health," influenced by strong campaigns for women's health, workers' health, sexual health, Indigenous health (based on the Black Panther health movement), and colonial health clinics – as well as by similar schemes in Britain, North America, and Southern Africa. The goal was to "develop" communities through interdisciplinary centers (including social workers, nurses, mental health workers, and sometimes medical practitioners), embedded in and engaging with local structures and leadership. These centers practiced a mixture of disease prevention, counseling, and conventional therapeutic intervention. As Anderson, Dunk, and Musolino detail, "community health" largely displaced "social medicine," with its unfashionable undertones of medical dominance, even though community health would often function more as a surrogate than a substitute. What was lost in translation – and what was gained – is a focus of this chapter.

The closing chapters of the book, Chapters 13–15, examine the durability of social medicine programs in West Africa, South Asia, and the Caribbean amidst the boom-and-bust cycles of supportive and indifferent governmental regimes and the transnational networks that sustained and were sustained by forms of social medicine from the South. In Chapter 13, David Bannister offers a West African case study in the planning and practice of social medicine in relation to community health. The Medical Field Units (MFU) of Ghana were created by remnant personnel of vertical disease campaigns (against trypanosomiasis and yaws), by a small number of late-colonial activist medical officers working on the rural periphery, who framed the MFU purpose explicitly as promotion of social welfare and countering structural determinants of poor health. The MFU were subsequently embraced and expanded by Ghana's first independent government from 1957, as it became clear that this approach to health provision had been highly successful at reaching populations on the economic and political peripheries. As Ghana went through an economically and politically unstable period following the military overthrow of the first independent government in 1966 (there were seven different governments between 1966 and 1981), Medical Field Units continued to operate successfully as parts of an autonomous medical service, with an independent budget. This chapter is based on research in archives in Ghana and Geneva and on oral histories of urban and rural communities, as well as interviews with current and retired health workers who served from the 1960s to the present.

Social medicine in South Asia is often regarded as the product of European and American ideas, expressed most vividly through the Bhore Committee set up in 1943, which included international experts like John Ryle, Henry Sigerist, and John Grant. Certainly, after independence, the committee's recommendations broadly influenced design of the Indian health services. However, the investment required for a strong state-supported healthcare system was lacking: over subsequent decades, the idea of social medicine waned in the political realm and in professional imagination. Curative medicine became ever more compelling, defining conventional health services and public health. Such is the standard narrative, anyhow. Yet, as Rama V. Baru argues in Chapter 14, the formation of social medicine in India has only one foot in Bhore. The circulation of ideas of critical social medicine from China, Latin America, and Africa gained influence on social and political movements in India, demonstrated in the many community health projects established during the late 1960s and 1970s. Insights from transnational social medicine annealed with vernacular medical theories and practices, including Gandhian speculations, allowing the construction of a specifically Indian form of social medicine, one which often bypassed a failing state, engaging instead with self-government initiatives and with Indigenous knowledge systems. Baru's chapter knits together these diverse strands to make visible the complex textures of social medicine in the Indian subcontinent.

Finally, in Chapter 15, P. Sean Brotherton explores another famous transnational node of social medicine: Cuba's post-revolutionary exportation of healthcare ideologies and practices. The Cuban Revolution of 1959 was an anti-imperialist uprising committed to agrarian reform and ending racial and gender discrimination, the predatory capitalism of economic exploitation and expendability, rampant structural inequality, and widespread corruption. This amalgam constituted diverse and contradictory political projects, incorporating and building on fragments of hopes, fears, desires, frustrations, and anti-colonial struggles, indexing longer historical trajectories within different populations in Latin America and beyond. Brotherton shows how biomedicine in this context was conscripted to serve a project of social medicine and reparative social justice. Since the early 1960s, Cuba's approach to primary healthcare has elicited heated debate on the dimensions of the country's biopolitical project, leading to questions about the resilience of biomedicine, which might continue to transform, even distort, revolutionary potential. This chapter, however, points to the actual plasticity of biomedicine to draw attention to its possible transformation into a diagnostic and therapeutic system of social justice. In other words, the reparative capacity of biomedicine can be molded and transformed to ameliorate the enduring material and embodied legacies of colonialism, now magnified through global capitalism. Cuba's biomedical focus on human health and, by extension, approaches to care, are two sides of the same coin, configured as therapeutic and affective labor, but also a political technology invested in creating the conditions for individuals, groups, and populations to flourish – thus fashioning a new social medicine.

Our collection of chapters concludes with the Afterwords by Anne-Emanuelle Birn, on the links between social medicine and social movements, and by Helena Hansen, on the need to build a usable past for the interdisciplinary fields of social medicine in order to work collectively toward viable futures.

Sentinels Found and Others Deservedly Lost

This is not simply a historical text. The histories assembled here make critical contributions to the pasts and presents of public health, medicine, and caregiving, emphasizing the influences of radical social movements on healthcare, illuminating processes of medical globalization, and above all, charting new paths for medical professionals and healthcare workers worldwide. As clinician-historians dedicated to training health professionals, the editors know only too well that even uttering the conjunction of "social" and "medicine" can still elicit skepticism, and sometimes outright hostility, among colleagues and students. The contributors to this volume venture further than ever before into this enemy territory, seeking to give form and substance to the various social and political specters generatively haunting contemporary biomedicine. In so doing, we hope the multiple figurations of social medicine sketched here will soon come to be embraced rather than feared or repulsed.

In one book, we can offer only a glimpse of the protean manifestations of global social medicine; we cannot encompass them all.[12] We imagine this collection as prompt to further exploration of manifold, endlessly inventive, social medicines around the world. Some omissions are inadvertent, indicating scotomas in current scholarship that may soon, we hope, be remedied. Other gaps are deliberate: we chose not to reiterate the common stories of social medicine in twentieth-century Western Europe, the usual homages to Virchow and other public health luminaries, since these accounts are well known and readily available.

We also decided not to dwell, in the chapters that follow, on the alliances in Western Europe and many settler-colonial societies in the 1930s between social medicine and eugenics and fascism. In those interwar years, many medical agitators on the right proposed greater state responsibility for the health of national populations – implicitly white populations. Since our focus is on the neglected affirmative and constructive aspects of social medicine, we spend less time on its dark sides but we should not try to evade them either – if only to demonstrate that what seems progressive to one generation might look fraught to successors.

To be sure, the alliances before Second World War of social medicine and solidifying state bureaucracies did sometimes incline medical reformers toward fascism and eugenics – encouraging them to lean toward forms of racial nationalism. The evidence for these tendencies is perhaps strongest in Western Europe between the World Wars but as contributions to this volume indicate, eugenic yearnings might be detected too in settler states in the Americas and Australasia. Eugenics, of course, was expressed in a variety of modes, from forced sterilization to advocacy of better child and maternal health and nutrition. Ostensibly, eugenics shared with social medicine the yearning for improvements in the health of populations, generally "white" populations.[13]

---

[12] We do not focus, for example, on the relations of mental health and social medicine but see Anne Kveim Lie and Jeremy Greene, "Introduction to the Special Issue: Psychiatry as Social Medicine," *Culture, Medicine, and Psychiatry* 45 (2021): 333–42; and Anne E. Becker, Giuseppe Raviola, and Arthur Kleinman, "Introduction: How Mental Health Matters," *Daedalus* 152 (2023): 8–23.

[13] Paul Weindling, *Health, Race, and German Politics between National Unification and Nazism, 1870–1945* (Cambridge: Cambridge University Press, 1989); Gunnar Broberg and

But this past affiliation should sharply be distinguished from our contemporary visions of social medicine.

A monitory character, worth considering briefly here, was Alfred Grotjahn, a German physician who combined belief in social etiologies of health and disease with promotion of eugenics.[14] His influential textbook, *Social Pathology* (1912), argued for the importance of social and economic factors in disease causation, an approach he called "social hygiene," drawing on demography and social statistics. Grotjahn believed investments in health education and social support, to reduce disease and debility, should naturally be harnessed to "reproductive hygiene," which would limit proliferation of inferior or degenerate types or weed them out if prevention had failed. Like many others in the field of social medicine at the time, he was particularly concerned with the supposedly low-grade urban white poor, filling up the expanding cities of Europe. Unlike later Nazi emulators, he did not regard Jews, other races, and homosexuals as obvious targets of his eugenic vision of social medicine.[15] Nonetheless, Grotjahn's career, like that of so many votaries of social medicine between the wars, provides an object lesson in how even the most "progressive" ideals can go wrong – and in how careful we should be in identifying intellectual antecedents.

Future Global Social Medicines

For more than one hundred years, physicians, healthcare workers, and political activists organizing around social medicine have sought to reveal the social and economic dimensions of sickness and well-being – and to advocate in the name of health for fundamental structural changes in our societies and economic systems. Yet the development of global health programs since the 1990s, often focusing on modular biosecurity interventions and epidemic technical preparedness, marked a shift away from such broad structural concerns

Nils Roll-Hansen, *Eugenics and the Welfare State: Sterilization Policy in Denmark, Sweden, Norway and Finland* (East Lansing, MI: Michigan State University Press, 1996); Lene Koch, "The Meaning of Eugenics: Reflections on the Government of Genetic Knowledge in the Past and the Present," *Science in Context* 17, no. 3 (2004), doi.org/10.1017/S0269889704000158; and Philippa Levine and Alison Bashford (eds.), *Oxford Handbook of the History of Eugenics* (Oxford: Oxford University Press, 2010). Paul Weindling and Dorothy Porter have argued that the connection of social medicine to eugenics necessarily led to health being a matter for expert advisors and qualified bureaucrats, rather than for political parties, at the expense of democratic principles of accountability and representational politics. The Scandinavian introduction of the sterilization laws did not fit this pattern.

[14] On Grotjahn's early practice as a physician, see Paul Weindling, "Medical Practice in Imperial Berlin: The Casebook of Alfred Grotjahn," *Bulletin of the History of Medicine* 61, no. 3 (1987): 391–410.

[15] Robert N. Proctor, *Racial Hygiene: Medicine under the Nazis* (Cambridge, MA: Harvard University Press, 1988); and Weindling, *Health, Race, and German Politics*.

and political imperatives – accordingly, this new global health, for all its flashy metrics and techniques, has done little to correct the world's growing health inequalities. Hence the need to turn again to diverse histories of social medicine, the rich traditions of progressive activism in healthcare, to learn how we might apply ourselves to current challenges. "A fundamental rethinking of the social role of medicine is required," we are told.[16] In recent years, we failed "to acknowledge the historical debates and struggles that have shaped understandings of the societal determinants of health."[17] Medicine's increasingly narrow and precise focus on molecular biology distracts us from "the large-scale social forces that give rise to human disease and affect its distribution around the globe."[18] As Paul E. Farmer, a rare proponent of social medicine within global health, put it: we suffer from "a tendency to ask only biological questions about what are in fact *biosocial* phenomena."[19] In contrast, social medicine represents "a shared domain of social and medical sciences that offers critical analytic and methodological tools to elucidate who gets sick, why, and what to do about it."[20] It therefore is time for "a revitalization of the field of social medicine as a way to affirm a health agenda that promotes human rights and social justice."[21] For those concerned with human health in a politically unjust and ecologically degraded world, understanding the diverse histories and potentialities of social medicine has never been more urgent.

Contemporary scrutiny of social determinants of health, necessary as it is, does not alone substitute for the political substance and historical depth of social medicine. In 2005, the WHO launched its commission on the social determinants of health, hoping to analyze and attend to growing health inequalities resulting from neoliberal capitalist globalization. The report, *Closing the Gap in a Generation* (2008), effectively assembled evidence relating disease patterns to constellations of economic, social, and political injustices. It urged

[16] Matthew R. Anderson, Lanny Smith, and Victor W. Seidel, "What Is Social Medicine?," *Monthly Review* 56, no. 8 (2005): 27–34, at 34.

[17] Anne-Emanuelle Birn, "Making It Politic(al): Closing the Gap in a Generation: Health Equity through Action on the Social Determinants of Health," *Social Medicine* 4, 3 (2009): 166–82, at 169.

[18] Scott D. Stonington and Seth M. Holmes, "Social Medicine in the Twenty-First Century," *PLoS Medicine* 3, 10, e-445 (2006), doi.org/10.1371/journal.pmed.0030445.

[19] Paul E. Farmer, Bruce Nizeye, Sara Stulac, and Salmaan Keshavjee, "Structural Violence and Clinical Medicine," *PLoS Medicine*, 3, 10, e-449 (2006), original emphasis.

[20] Seth M. Holmes, Jeremy A. Greene, and Scott D. Stonington, "Locating Global Health in Social Medicine," *Global Public Health* 9, no. 5 (2014): 475–80, at 476. Similar arguments are made in Dorothy Porter, "How Did Social Medicine Evolve, and Where Is It Heading?," *PLoS Medicine* 3, 10, e-399 (2006), doi.org/10.1371/journal.pmed.0030399; and Vincanne Adams, Dominique Behague, Carlo Caduff, Ilana Löwy, and Francisco Ortega, "Re-imagining Global Health through Social Medicine," *Global Public Health* 14, 10 (2019): 1383–400.

[21] Michelle Pentecost, Vincanne Adams, Rama Baru, Carlo Caduff, Jeremy A. Greene, Helena Hansen, David S. Jones, Junko Kitanaka, and Francisco Ortega, "Revitalising Global Social Medicine," *The Lancet* (May 28, 2021), doi.org/10.1016/S0140-6736(21)01003-5.

the international health sector to address inequalities in health – yet stepped back from any fundamental political critiques and any radical proposals for systemic change.[22] According to Anne-Emanuelle Birn, the prevailing discourse on social determinants of health evades critical engagement with the underlying structural causes of inequality and injustice. To do so would require deeper historical understanding of political activism in social medicine.[23] Advocates of social medicine from the Global South like Elis Borde and Mario Hernandez also complain that gestures toward the social determinants of health "remain vague, decontextualized and essentially individual, conveying an idea of social 'risk' factors that affect individuals according to their position in the social hierarchy." They demand a more comprehensive critique of the pathologies of power relations under global capitalism – as offered in social medicines past and present. It is necessary, they argue, "to engage seriously with hitherto invisibilized approaches and research traditions," such as social medicine, if we want a radical transformation of our noxious socio-economic system.[24]

Through reading the chapters assembled here, it will become evident that wide-ranging social medicine in the past has drawn on diverse arrays of specialized knowledge. It has constituted a means to escape the strictures of standard biomedicine. Thus, social medicine has derived, in different times and places, from medical visionaries in alliance with other health workers, social scientists, leftist politicians, feminists, Indigenous activists, and progressive social movements. Such collectives have assaulted biomedical citadels from motley institutional sites, whether in dissenting professional groups, marginalized departments in medical schools, infiltrated health bureaucracies, or community health centers. Although often national in aspiration, advocates of social medicine have looked internationally for models and lessons, creating informal intellectual networks that span the globe. Some of the followers of social medicine have demanded fundamental structural change in their societies; others have concentrated on expanding healthcare access; others again, on developing multidisciplinary community health programs. Some have focused on researching and teaching the social determinants of health; or applying sociological insight to clinical practice. Recently, a few disappointed veterans of social medicine have tried to reintegrate ecological conceptions of health

---

[22] Commission on the Social Determinants of Health, *Closing the Gap in a Generation: Health Equity through Action on the Social Determinants of Health* (Geneva: World Health Organization, 2008). See also David Mechanic, "Rediscovering the Social Determinants of Health," *Health Affairs* 19 (2000): 269–76.

[23] Birn, "Making It Politic(al)." See also Vicente Navarro, "What We Mean by Social Determinants of Health," *Global Health Promotion* 16 (2009): 5–16; and Fran Baum, "Cracking the Nut of Health Equity: Top-Down and Bottom-Up Pressure for Action on the Social Determinants of Health," *Promotion and Education* 14 (2007): 90–5.

[24] Elis Borde and Mario Hernández, "Revisiting the Social Determinants of Health Agenda from the Global South," *Global Public Health* 14 (2019): 847–62, at 852, 858.

and disease into social and political frameworks. What unites these disparate figures is the conviction that health and disease are more than assortments of molecules, more than an assemblage of particles sometimes in comity, sometimes awry.

The contributors to this volume believe that in a world of widening global health inequalities, depleted public health services, and narrowly focused precision medicine, we need a revived social medicine more than ever. It is time to resuscitate critical social medicine, to return it to life on a planetary scale. Accordingly, we have gathered here these chapters that show us how we might remake a social medicine fit for addressing our alarming and oppressive times. From multiple sites, the contributors to this volume seek usable histories of social medicine and its various proxies, necessary histories that will enable fresh critiques of elite biomedical reductionism, clinical individualism, and professional passivity.

1   Decentering Rudolf Virchow
The Making of a Social Medicine Pioneer

Carsten Timmermann

The aim of this chapter is to understand the role that the German pathologist and physical anthropologist Rudolf Virchow has come to play, as a historical figure, in the emergence of social medicine as a recognizable set of ideas and practices. The purpose of this exercise is not so much to challenge common assumptions about the value of Virchow's observations and concepts but rather to contextualize both Virchow's endeavors and their interpretations by practitioners and historians. We may want to look at this, I suggest, as a case study that helps us to make sense of the role of a celebrated historical figure in an emerging field of practice.

Virchow's status as a pioneer of social medicine is closely associated with his report on the typhus epidemic in the Prussian province of Upper Silesia in early 1848 and his often cited statement that "Medicine is a social science, and politics nothing but medicine at a larger scale," which appeared later in the same year in an article published in a journal he edited, *Die Medicinische Reform*, on how Virchow believed the state should ensure healthcare was provided to the poor.[1] Virchow's pioneer status has often been taken for granted, so much so that he and his students are almost automatically assumed to have directly shaped national traditions in social medicine, even when and where, on closer examination, no direct links can be found.[2]

I argue in this chapter that while Virchow's observations and programmatic writings have been useful for positioning the ideas and practices we associate with social medicine and establish the notion that social medicine has a long tradition, his central place in the historiography of the field is a product of contingencies. The historical figure of Rudolf Virchow has been appropriated

---

[1] Rudolf Virchow, "Der Armenarzt," *Die medicinische Reform*, no. 18 (November 3, 1848): 125; see also J. P. Mackenbach, "Politics Is Nothing but Medicine at a Larger Scale: Reflections on Public Health's Biggest Idea," *Journal of Epidemiology and Community Health* 63, no. 3 (March 2009): 181–4, doi.org/10.1136/jech.2008.077032.
[2] See, for example, Eric D. Carter and Marcelo Sánchez Delgado, "A Debate over the Link between Salvador Allende, Max Westenhöfer, and Rudolf Virchow: Contributions to the History of Social Medicine in Chile and Internationally," *História, Ciências, Saúde-Manguinhos* 27, no. 3 (September 2020): 899–917, doi.org/10.1590/s0104-59702020000400011.

and injected into the narrative that dominates the historiography of social medicine, with the implicit purpose of providing the new discipline with a distinguished pedigree and specifically because his early concepts and observations provided useful signposts, in combination with his standing as a great medical scholar who made his name above all as a pathologist and anthropologist. Virchow was a key champion of biomedicine in late nineteenth-century Germany. By biomedicine here, I mean scientific medicine taught at universities, embracing hands-on research, dedicated to materialism and empiricism, and firmly rooted in pathological anatomy and the new experimental physiology pioneered by men such as Johannes Müller, one of Virchow's mentors, or François Magendie in France.

Virchow's conceptual legacy in this area is most closely associated with cellular pathology, the proposal that the structural and functional unit of all life was the cell, and that physiological and pathological processes could be most effectively studied and most conclusively understood at the cellular level. Cellular pathology provided an outstandingly productive framework for a wide range of biomedical research programs and, arguably, is still one of the central doctrines of biomedicine. Later in life, Virchow focused his scholarly efforts on institutionalizing anthropology as a scientific pursuit, encompassing what we today term "physical anthropology," as well as ethnography and archaeology. In this context, he was a key promoter, for example, of the activities of Heinrich Schliemann, the "discoverer" of the ancient city of Troy. Throughout his career, Virchow also dedicated much of his time to politics, as a champion of reform, and, as will be discussed in more detail below, temporarily revolution. He was a member of legislative assemblies at municipal, regional, and national levels and held a number of administrative roles, mostly related to public health.

Social medicine for the purposes of this chapter is best understood as a unifying methodological and theoretical framework underpinning preventive medicine and public health, but also as a fundamental reinterpretation of what medicine should aim for and what the object of intervention should be: the social body rather than individual bodies. As such, it is important to interpret social medicine not as a timeless concept but as a historically situated phenomenon that emerged from a specific context in the mid twentieth century in North America and Britain but with major input from émigré scholars from German-speaking Central Europe.[3] I will argue that Virchow did not develop a concept of social medicine, as is often assumed, but that he was written into the genealogy of the new concept by those who had an investment in this concept and the ways in which it linked North America to Europe, namely the historian of medicine, public health official, and scholar of public health,

[3] See also Greene, Jones, and Podolsky, Chapter 7 in this volume.

George Rosen and some of his associates. In doing so, they initiated a partial shift in the perception of Virchow, reversing the timeline of Virchow's biography, from pathological anatomist and physical anthropologist to political radical, by emphasizing activities and writings early in Virchow's career. Virchow's celebrated statement resonated with the self-understanding of early to mid twentieth-century public health practitioners (and theorists) who prioritized addressing the roots of public health problems in health policy over technical interventions.

I will be approaching this chapter from two directions. First, I will look at Virchow's journey to Upper Silesia in 1848 and his experiences in the revolutionary upheavals of that year in an attempt to understand what Virchow imagined when he thought of politics as medicine on a larger scale.[4] Given the enmeshedness of the typhus fact-finding expedition, which has become emblematic in the historiography of social medicine, with Virchow's role as a revolutionary, and his early programmatic writings on medical and public health reform, I argue that the contingencies shaping this particular nexus deserve a closer look. I will then examine the historiography of social medicine, seeking to understand how and why the historical figure of Rudolf Virchow has come to assume such a central place in this historiography. I will very briefly compare appropriations of Virchow in different traditions of social medicine. I argue that historians of medicine especially, such as Henry Sigerist and George Rosen, who were trained in German-speaking Europe and who campaigned for social medicine as an academic discipline in the US, played a crucial role in this story. George Rosen's writings are cited centrally by most authors seeking to situate social medicine historically. I argue that Rosen's representation of Virchow was much more important for modern, post-Second World War understandings of social medicine than the man himself. Rosen employed Virchow because this allowed him to trace the roots of these understandings back to a period which is generally viewed as the time when the foundations of modern biomedicine were established and thus gave the fledgling discipline more gravitas, depth, breadth, and coherence than it may otherwise have been perceived to have.

[4] All Virchow biographies cover the trip to Upper Silesia and discuss his report but some do so relatively briefly. In Goschler's substantial and insightful 2002 biography of Virchow, this episode takes up about 30 out of 400 pages; see Constantin Goschler, *Rudolf Virchow: Mediziner, Anthropologie, Politiker* (Köln: Böhlau, 2002). Schipperges dedicates 4 pages of his slimmer book on Virchow to these events; see Heinrich Schipperges, *Rudolf Virchow* (Reinbek: Rowohlt, 1994); Ackerknecht's classic book is organized around themes and he deals with Virchow's public health writings and his political activities under separate headings; see Erwin H. Ackerknecht, *Rudolf Virchow: Doctor, Statesman, Anthropologist* (Madison, WI: University of Wisconsin Press, 1953). Only in Winter's slim Virchow biography, published in the GDR, are Virchow's activities in 1848 discussed as a turning point; see Kurt Winter, *Rudolf Virchow* (Leipzig: Teubner, 1976).

Revolution and Typhus in Silesia

By all accounts, including his own, the ambitious young physician and medical academic Rudolf Virchow (Figure 1.1) was disgusted by what he encountered in Upper Silesia in 1848. It was the beginning of a year that was an important turning point in the history of Prussia and the other states and principalities that made up the German Confederation: a year of political and social upheaval and revolution, a peculiar mix of uncertainty, hope, and excitement.

The year was also a turning point in Virchow's life and career. He was twenty-six years old, and freshly appointed to the office of Prosector at the Charité Hospital in Berlin. He had completed his doctoral dissertation in 1843 with the influential physiologist and anatomist Johannes Müller. In 1846, he had passed the state examination that qualified him to practice as a physician. In 1847, he had completed the second dissertation (Habilitation) that gave him the right to teach university students – a key step toward a professorial career. He had also, with a friend, launched a journal, the *Archiv für patholo- gische Anatomie und Physiologie und für klinische Medizin* (later known as *Virchows Archiv* and a key outlet for biomedical research in Germany,

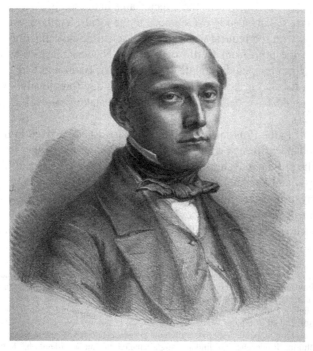

Figure 1.1 Virchow around 1848. Courtesy of the National Library of Medicine.

still in existence). In 1848, however, along with most other intellectuals in Berlin and other cities of the German Confederation, he devoted much time to being a revolutionary. He joined the Berlin barricades and various assemblies and committees dedicated to making the revolution deliver sustainable change. He also launched a second, short-lived journal with another friend, the psychiatrist Rudolf Leubuscher, *Die Medicinische Reform*, which was the main publishing outlet for Virchow's political thoughts. The first issue of *Medicinische Reform* was published on July 10, 1848 and the last on June 29, 1849.[5]

The outbreak in Upper Silesia of what Virchow referred to as "hunger typhus" (*Hungertyphus*) had started to receive considerable attention in the capital Berlin by early 1848 and not only among reform-minded physicians. The newspapers were reporting the outbreak and rumors were circulating about it, along with there being appeals for help for the victims. The Prussian minister in charge of Culture, Education, and Medical Matters, however, had received no reliable reports from local officials and, after some delay, the government grew concerned about the potential consequences of the epidemic (and presumably the rumors). The minister commissioned one of Virchow's senior colleagues at the Charité, the professor of pediatrics, Stephan Friedrich Barez, with a fact-finding visit to the affected area in the southeastern corner of the state of Prussia and also to offer advice to the locals. Virchow was invited to join Barez, with the request to undertake a scientific investigation into the outbreak. On the train from Berlin on the new Niederschlesisch-Märkische Eisenbahn, a line completed a couple of years earlier, Barez and Virchow were able to reach Breslau in Lower Silesia in a single day (previously, by stagecoach, this would have been an arduous journey, taking a week or longer; see Figure 1.2).[6]

They set off in the Prussian capital on February 20 and arrived in the town of Ratibor in Upper Silesia on February 22. They visited a few other towns and villages in the province: Rybnik, Radlin and Loslau, Gleikowitz and Smollna, Sohrau, Pless, and Lonkau. Barez traveled back to Berlin on February 29. Virchow stayed in Sohrau until March 7, very comfortably, at the castle of Count Hochberg, a local aristocrat and large landowner, whom Virchow praised as a generous host.[7] He spent some time observing the work in a hospital set up

[5] A facsimile edition of the journal was published in 1983 by the East German Akademie-Verlag: Rudolf Virchow and Rudolf Leubuscher, *Die Medicinische Reform*, ed. Christa Kirsten and Kurt Zeisler, Dokumente der Wissenschaftsgeschichte (Berlin: Akademie-Verlag, 1983).
[6] Letter to his father, February 20, 1848, Rudolf Virchow, *Briefe an seine Eltern, 1839 bis 1864*, ed. Marie Rabl, 2nd ed. (Leipzig: W. Engelmann, 1907), 123–4.
[7] "Die Diners des Grafen, bei denden namentlich die ausgesuchtetesten Weine u. frische Gemüse (Spargel, Kohlrabi, Radieschen) zu finden waren, behagten uns ausserordentlich," Letter to his Father, February 29, 1848, Virchow, Briefe an seine Eltern, 127–9.

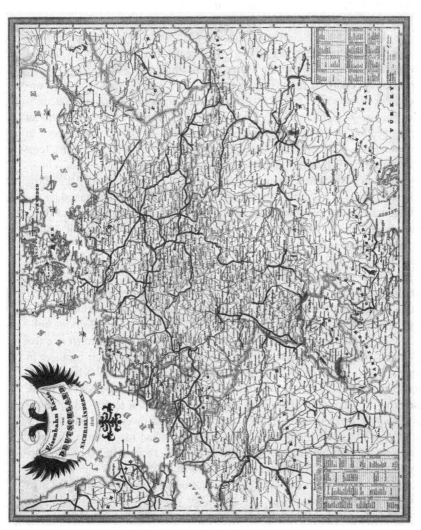

Figure 1.2 Railway map of Germany in 1849. Upper Silesia is located on the right, along the railway line to Krakow. Wikimedia Commons.

specifically to look after victims of the epidemic. On March 10, he also arrived back in Berlin. He would have liked to stay longer, he writes, but had an even stronger urge to participate in unfolding revolutionary developments in Berlin. News of a popular uprising in Paris and the proclamation of the Second French Republic had reached the Prussian capital on February 27 and was reported by the liberal *Vossische Zeitung* on February 28, followed by news of uprisings in a number of southern German states. On March 6, a large people's assembly was held in Tiergarten, not far from the Brandenburg Gate – the beginning of what came to be known as the March Revolution in Prussia.

Virchow's report on his visit to Upper Silesia, 182 pages long, was published later in the same year. It is a report on a substantial piece of epidemiological fieldwork (which is surprising, given the brevity of the visit), with an opening section on the land and its people, a section on endemic conditions in the area and the story of the typhus outbreak under investigation, a third, long section on clinical observations and a discussion of possible causes, and a final, fourth part on possible interventions.[8] So what did Virchow actually find, how did he make sense of it, how was his perception of the epidemic shaped by the contingencies of the revolutionary developments, and how, in turn, did these experiences shape his outlook as a medical reformer, advocate of public health, and health policy maker?

Especially striking are Virchow's descriptions of the people of Upper Silesia. On the one hand, he explicitly acknowledges that the ethnically Polish, Catholic population were victims of 700 years of colonialization by Protestant Prussia, an exploitative and utterly incompetent administration controlled by large land owners, and centuries of spiritual enslavement by Catholic religious leaders. Virchow writes: "700 years have not been sufficient to free the inhabitants [of Upper Silesia] of their Polish habitus, which their brothers in Pomerania and Prussia have lost completely. However, they have been sufficient to destroy their consciousness, to corrupt their language, and to break their spirit."[9] A growing population (from 42,303 in 1834 to 59,320 in 1847) was living in overcrowded, damp, and unhygienic dwellings, which they shared with livestock (Figure 1.3). The authorities had made some attempts to supplement their increasingly poor diet following several failed potato harvests but in ways that did not make sense to Virchow. On the other hand, his descriptions suggest that he was disgusted not only by the conditions but also by the people themselves.

The habits of the Silesians, Virchow observes, were utterly uncivilized: they did not wash and the crusts of dirt on their bodies were only

---

[8] Rudolf Virchow, *Mittheilungen ueber die in Oberschlesien herrschende Typhus-Epidemie* (Berlin: G. Reimer, 1848), 4, at: https://mdz-nbn-resolving.de/urn:nbn:de:bvb:12-bsb10475227-6.
[9] Virchow, Mittheilungen, 10.

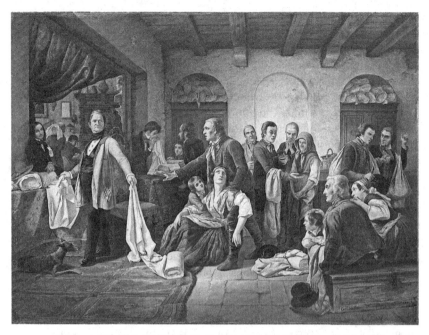

Figure 1.3 Carl Wilhelm Hübener, *The Silesian Weavers* (1844). This painting illustrates a growing awareness in Germany of the fate of poor Silesian workers and the social question more generally. Collection of the Museum Kunstpalast, Düsseldorf, via Getty Images.

occasionally washed away by the rain; vermin such as lice were "permanent guests" on their bodies.[10] They were "dedicated to the consumption of liquor in the most extreme manner."[11] Also, they were subservient like dogs, Virchow writes, and totally disinclined to engage in any intellectual or physical effort, thoroughly lazy, in ways that was bound to trigger disgust rather than pity in any free human being with a good work ethic.[12] The Polish inhabitants of Upper Silesia were the "Other" to the young, liberal, hardworking intellectual visiting from Berlin to investigate the causes of the typhus epidemic. However, he made clear that he blamed the exploitative structures for the deplorable characteristics displayed by the locals, signaling a belief in human improvement that quite clearly had its roots in Enlightenment values. He appeared to appeal to enlightenment as the key to a solution.

[10] Virchow, Mittheilungen, 11.   [11] Virchow, Mittheilungen, 13.
[12] Virchow, Mittheilungen, 11.

The epidemic of typhus Virchow was asked to investigate had started in summer 1847. The victims developed an increasingly high fever, accompanied by extreme fatigue, headache, sometimes loss of hearing and delirium, aching limbs and sharp pain in the feet, fast pulse and often a cough, and a characteristic skin rush. Between the ninth and fourteenth day, this was followed either by (slow) convalescence or a crisis and death. Incidence and mortality figures communicated to him by various officials and local physicians varied. In a community in Ratibor County, for example, according to the numbers reported to him, just under 9 percent of the population were ill and out of these, just over 40 percent died. During a meeting of doctors in the county of Rybnik, organized when Virchow was visiting, some estimated that mortality was as high as one in three. Others assumed 10–20 percent mortality. Virchow concluded that the exact mortality was uncertain, the available data were not reliable enough. Gender, age, or ethnic origin seemed to make no difference – the disease could affect anyone. Virchow undertook four post-mortem examinations and included detailed accounts of his findings in his report, reflected on reports of other autopsies, and reviewed a wide range of literature on typhus and related conditions, going back to Hippocrates and including much recent writing from England and Ireland.

The key question was the following: was the typhus observed in 1847 and 1848 qualitatively different from endemic typhus? Some assumed that the typhus was passed on through a contagion, others suggested that it was caused by miasma, perhaps a product of fermentation, in environmental conditions not particularly good for human health. Virchow conceded that the poor conditions would have made the Silesians increasingly susceptible to any miasma that may have been emerging in their damp and moldy dwellings. But ultimately we had to assume, based on what he had seen and read, that the epidemic and the famine were caused by the same conditions. In a letter to his father, he stated clearly that he did not believe that the hunger caused the typhus but that it promoted the spread of the disease.[13] As typhus was endemic in the region, the cause had to be endemic and the hunger was just a contributing factor making people more susceptible. The real cause, Virchow concluded, was a miasma, a product of chemical decomposition, which led to an epidemic under certain weather conditions and was made worse by the circumstances in which the people were living. The miasma poisoned the blood of typhus patients and, in turn, caused the pathological changes Virchow and others had observed in post-mortem examinations.

Virchow also reported on the measures taken to gain control of the epidemic between the time of his visit and the time of publication: relatively simple measures focusing on providing those affected by the typhus with clean

---

[13] Letter to his Father, February 24, 1848, Virchow, *Briefe an seine Eltern*, 124–7.

surroundings and food and when absolutely necessary, a hospital bed. There was some emphasis on controlling cost and on reporting, and indeed, by the summer, incidence declined dramatically. However, as typhus incidence was declining, other conditions such as intermittent fever returned. How could one prevent future epidemics? Virchow had drawn his conclusions from what he witnessed in Upper Silesia when he returned to Berlin. His conclusions could be summarized in three words, he wrote: "full, unrestricted democracy."[14] It is not easy to reconcile this conclusion with the visceral disgust Virchow appears to have felt when dealing with the sick Upper Silesians. Nevertheless, the last twenty-five pages of the report are a call for revolution. The famous Prussian bureaucracy could not save the people of Upper Silesia, Virchow argued. Only democracy could bring about the structural change needed to liberate and educate them. And Virchow was determined, he declared, to help bring about such a revolution.

Back in Berlin, Virchow dedicated much of his time and energy to the revolution. He took part in assemblies from the very day of his return onward, and as the Prussian king mobilized the army and clashes in the streets of Berlin grew violent, within less than a week of his return, Virchow was joining the barricades on the corner of Friedrichstrasse and Taubenstrasse, fighting against the King's Regiment from Stettin. As he reports in a letter to his father, the soldiers had canons, the revolutionaries only twelve guns. Virchow himself had a pistol. Despite the overwhelming firepower of the army, the revolutionaries held many barricades and erected more. Many were wounded or killed and buildings were damaged. The army withdrew and the king promised concessions (Figure 1.4).

On March 24, Virchow wrote to his father, enthusiastically, that the revolution had been completely victorious.[15] He successfully ran for election to the electoral college for the new national parliament in his district and joined a number of committees and assemblies, while working on the report on Upper Silesia. By summer, on a typical day, he was attending one or two committee meetings, assemblies or club meetings in the afternoons and evenings, after finishing his teaching and work as a prosector in the morning. Politically he located himself on the "extreme left," even if he did not always agree with the means, he wrote, that the left used to achieve their aims.[16] With some of his physician friends he started to draw up plans for a radical reform of medicine. The reflections on what such a reform might entail provided the context for the much cited statement on medicine as a social science.

[14] Virchow, *Mittheilungen*, 163.
[15] Letter to his Father, March 24, 1848, Virchow, *Briefe an seine Eltern*, 139–41.
[16] Letter to his Father, September 29, 1848, Virchow, *Briefe an seine Eltern*, 156–61.

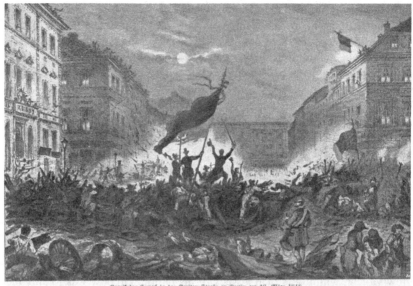

Figure 1.4 Barricade in Berlin, 1848. Par Bettman Collection, via Getty Images.

As a committee member of the Society for Obstetrics, which was chaired by his friend and future father-in-law, Carl Mayer, Virchow acted as a delegate in a series of meetings, many of which he chaired, dedicated to medical renewal – envisaged by Virchow and his friends as a root-and-branch reform of the health system. In July 1848, with his friend, the psychiatrist Rudolf Leubuscher, he launched a journal dedicated to these matters, *Die Medicinische Reform*.[17] The main reasons for the end of the journal, less than one year later, were financial problems, along with frustration over the failure of the revolution in general and specifically with a view to Virchow's ideas for medical renewal. What did Virchow envisage?

Virchow positioned himself as a democrat and a socialist but the ideal society he had in mind is perhaps best characterized as a paternalist technocracy, with medical doctors in key positions as experts, guided above all by their understanding of the natural sciences. This resonates with his distrust, even disgust for the poor in Upper Silesia. Virchow envisaged a privileged role for

[17] Virchow and Leubuscher, *Die Medicinische Reform*; Peter Schneck, "Die Editionsgeschichte der Wochenschrift *Die medicinische Reform* (1848/49) und der Briefwechsel Rudolf Virchows mit seinem Verleger Georg Reimer," *NTM International Journal of History and Ethics of Natural Sciences, Technology and Medicine* 15, no. 3 (August 1, 2007): 179–97, doi. org/10.1007/s00048-006-0244-8.

medicine in the running of the state.[18] The protection of people's health was going to be central to the reformed state. With his ideas for medical reform, he drew on proposals by his friend, the physician Salomon Neumann, who suggested that government had a duty to assure the health of its citizens. Healthy bodies were the only property that the poor controlled. As the government had a duty to protect property, protecting the health of the poor had to be recognized as a key duty of government and, thus, an important goal for medical reform. Neumann called for the right to health to be declared a human right.[19]

Virchow suggested that doctors were "the natural advocates of the poor" and that social questions should come "predominantly under their jurisdiction."[20] He envisaged that an association of all medical doctors should be put in charge of all matters related to health. Doctors were going to be exclusively guided by reason. Virchow's ideas were rooted in a strong and persistent Enlightenment belief in the primacy of reason and the transformative power of the natural sciences for all areas of life, which he shared with other students of the physiologist Johannes Müller, such as Hermann Helmholtz or Emil Du Bois-Reymond.[21] Guided by reason under the leadership of doctors who were applying their anthropological knowledge, the social question would be solved.

Virchow had to adjust his expectations, it seems, when he found himself confronted with the tediousness of practical politics and the lack of support from his medical colleagues. Many did not share his commitments, were reluctant to dedicate themselves to working for medical reform in associations and revolutionary meetings, and did not agree with his idea of compulsory membership in an association of doctors. They did not even subscribe to the *Medicinische Reform* in sufficient numbers to make the journal financially viable.

His visions conflicted with the ideas of other revolutionaries also in another crucial aspect: a solution of the social question to Virchow did not imply the emancipation of workers and the poor. The solution of the social question to him implied the disappearance of the mob (*der Pöbel*), not the involvement of the mob in practical politics. It is plausible to assume that his disgust with the wretched typhus patients in Upper Silesia was related to his perception of

---

[18] Goschler, *Rudolf Virchow*, 76.

[19] Salomon Neumann, *Die öffentliche Gesundheitspflege und das Eigenthum: Kritisches und Positives mit Bezug auf die preußische Medizinalverfassungs-Frage* (Berlin: Rieß, 1847), at: www.digitale-sammlungen.de/de/view/bsb10013762; Goschler, *Rudolf Virchow*, 76–7; Günter Regneri, *Salomon Neumann: Sozialmediziner-Statistiker, Stadtverordneter*, Jüdische Miniaturen 107 (Berlin: Hentrich & Hentrich, 2011).

[20] Rudolf Virchow, "Was die 'medicinische Reform' will," *Die medicinische Reform*, no. 1 (July 10, 1848): 2.

[21] Laura Otis, *Müller's Lab* (Oxford and New York, NY: Oxford University Press, 2007); Gabriel Ward Finkelstein, *Emil Du Bois-Reymond: Neuroscience, Self, and Society in Nineteenth-Century Germany* (Cambridge, MA: The MIT Press, 2014).

the revolutionary mob in Berlin. His report from Upper Silesia did not include patients' perspectives and Virchow's vision of medical reform did not assume that patients and other non-experts were going to be involved in decision-making processes around health and medicine.[22]

Afterlife: The Making of a Social Medicine Pioneer

While he self-identified as a left-wing Democrat, Virchow's politics was patriarchal, based on the assumption that doctors knew better. The embrace of social science was ambition rather than reality. While the young pathologist had supporters in the Prussian administration and was much respected, his involvement in the revolutionary activities of 1848 and 1849 did lead to sanctions. Virchow was not sacked from his positions but his pay was cut and he lost the apartment that originally came with the position of prosector. In May of 1949, he was offered a chair appointment at the University of Würzburg. He accepted, moved, got married, and stopped identifying as a revolutionary.

Virchow's biographers agree that the Würzburg phase was when Virchow established his reputation as Germany's leading pathologist. Schipperges characterizes Virchow's time there as "seven fat years."[23] He continued to edit the *Archiv*, turning it into a key journal for the new scientific approach to medicine that he championed, and from 1854 he published his influential *Handbuch der speciellen Pathologie and Therapie*. In 1855, the term "cellular pathology" appeared in print for the first time, providing the foundation of a new concept for making sense of health and illness, which shapes our thinking about cancer and other conditions until the present day.

In 1856, Virchow returned to Berlin with a chair appointment. In the following year, he was elected as a member of the Berlin city council, which was the start of his career as a politician. In 1861, he was elected to the Prussian Parliament as leader of the German Progress Party (Fortschrittspartei). From 1880 to 1893, he was also a member of the national parliament, the Reichstag. Throughout his career, he was a member of a variety of committees and working parties, and in Berlin he played an important role as a sanitary reformer, campaigning for and overseeing the construction of a new water and sewage system for the city.

An increasingly influential medical academic and politician, Virchow did not renounce his writings in *Medicinische Reform*. While acknowledging that he no longer agreed with every word, he republished key texts from this journal in 1879.[24] Schipperges argues that his programmatic desire to develop

---

[22] Goschler, *Rudolf Virchow*, 81, citing Weindling (1984).
[23] Schipperges, *Rudolf Virchow*, 23.
[24] Schneck, "Die Editionsgeschichte der Wochenschrift *Die medicinische Reform*."

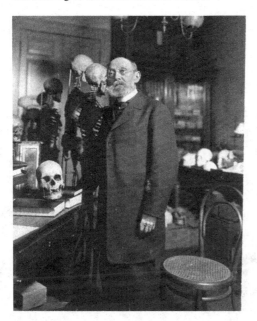

Figure 1.5 Virchow later in life, in his study, surrounded by skulls and skeletons. Courtesy of the National Library of Medicine.

a humane politics based on natural science remains a central motivation of Virchow's actions. Politics was medicine on a large scale and scientifically trained doctors the ideal politicians. The main focus of his scholarship by then, however, was on pathology and anthropology (Figure 1.5). As champion for the natural sciences, he was also a regular participant and speaker on the great scientific controversies of the time at the meetings of the Gesellschaft deutscher Naturforscher und Ärzte (Society of German Natural Scientists and Physicians). Given Virchow's great political ambitions, however, Schipperges suggests that his practical impact was relatively limited.[25]

Immediately following his death in 1902, Virchow was celebrated above all as a pathologist, a physical anthropologist, and a politician. His conceptual interest in social and economic factors as causes of disease was reevaluated, in light of a widespread perception in German-speaking Europe, in the interwar period, that medicine was in crisis.[26] Commentators on the political right tended to view Virchow as part of the problem: the fragmentation that they thought

[25] Schipperges, *Rudolf Virchow*, 113–20.
[26] Carsten Timmermann, "Constitutional Medicine, Neoromanticism, and the Politics of Antimechanism in Interwar Germany," *Bulletin of the History of Medicine* 75, no. 4 (2001): 717–39, doi.org/10.1353/bhm.2001.0198.

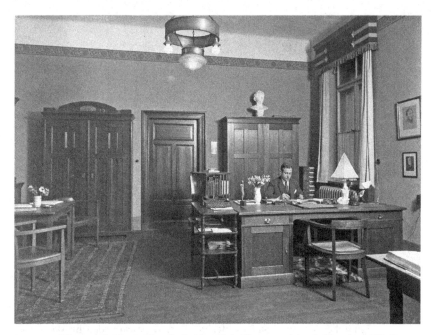

Figure 1.6 Henry Sigerist in his office. Photograph by S. Hoenisch. Wellcome Collection.

was characteristic of modern, scientific medicine. Those on the left, in contrast, viewed his social engagement and especially his declared commitment to medicine as a social science as a pioneering contribution to a potential solution.

In order to appreciate George Rosen's role in reinterpreting Virchow, it is helpful to look at biographical accounts prior to Rosen's two programmatic articles in the late 1940s and perhaps particularly the chapter on Virchow in Henry Sigerist's *Great Doctors*, published in German in 1932 and in English translation in 1933.[27] Sigerist grew increasingly interested in sociological questions and approaches during his time as director of the Leipzig Institute of the History of Medicine, from 1920 onward (Figure 1.6).[28] However, in *Great Doctors*, first published in English in 1933, Sigerist presents Virchow as the key protagonist of a new medicine based on natural science, not the study of social conditions. While he dedicates a couple of pages to Upper Silesia, a

[27] Henry E. Sigerist, *Great Doctors: A Biographical History of Medicine* (London: Allen and Unwin, 1933).

[28] Milton I. Roemer, Leslie A. Falk, and Theodore M. Brown, "Sociological Vision and Pedagogic Mission: Henry Sigerist's Medical Sociology," in Elizabeth Fee and Theodore M. Brown (eds.), *Making Medical History: The Life and Times of Henry E. Sigerist* (Baltimore: Johns Hopkins University Press, 1997), 315–32.

long quote from the end of Virchow's report, and his participation in the revolution, there is no notion of Virchow as a founder of social medicine. Most space is dedicated to cellular pathology and the increasingly central role of the pathological institute and the laboratory for the new scientific medicine. The focus on laboratory medicine, however, was what in the eyes of many early twentieth-century critics caused the crisis of medicine.[29]

This is presented very differently in George Rosen's 1947 essay in the *Bulletin of the History of Medicine*, where Rosen attempts a "genetic analysis" of the concept of social medicine, characterized by Fee and Morman as "rambling," while "would-be seminal."[30] Fee and Morman suggest, convincingly in my view, that the purpose of the paper was "to provide social medicine with a long and distinguished tradition and thus help strengthen the currents of social medical thought within contemporary medicine."[31]

Rosen starts his exploration of the historical origins of the concept of social medicine with Virchow, or to be precise: with the faint praise that Virchow's report on the typhoid fever epidemic in Upper Silesia received from the bacteriologist Emil von Behring in 1893. Bacteriology, of course, was synonymous with laboratory medicine. Von Behring presented Virchow's understanding of the outbreak as caused by "a complex of social and economic factors" as outdated because he believed that bacteriology made all of these complex considerations unnecessary. In the early decades of the twentieth century, however, as Andrew Mendelsohn has shown, it became clear that this was not the case. Epidemics had become complex once again, feeding into the general sense of crisis.[32]

Citing Virchow's statement that, "Medicine is a social science, and politics nothing but medicine on a grand scale," Rosen then uses Virchow (along with his associates Salomon Neumann and Rudolf Leubuscher) to develop a programmatic concept of social medicine, which was integrally linked to democratic principles and the assumption that the state should assume a proactive role in the maintenance of public health.[33] The concept of social medicine that Rosen attributed to Virchow, Neumann, and Leubuscher was founded on three central principles: (1) that "the health of the people is a matter of direct

---

[29] Sigerist, *Great Doctors*.

[30] Elizabeth Fee and Edward T. Morman, "Doing History, Making Revolution: The Aspirations of Henry E. Sigerist and George Rosen," in Dorothy Porter and Roy Porter (eds.), *Doctors, Politics and Society: Historical Essays* (Amsterdam & Atlanta: Rodopi, 1993), 291; George Rosen, "What Is Social Medicine? A Genetic Analysis of the Concept," *Bulletin of the History of Medicine* 21, no. 5 (1947): 674–733.

[31] Fee and Morman, "Doing History, Making Revolution," 292.

[32] Andrew Mendelsohn, "From Eradication to Equilibrium: How Epidemics Became Complex after World War I," in George M. Weisz and Christopher Lawrence (eds.), *Greater than the Parts: Holism in Biomedicine, 1920–1950* (Oxford: Oxford University Press, 1998), 303–31.

[33] Rosen, "What Is Social Medicine?," 676.

social concern," (2) that "social and economic conditions have an important effect on health and disease, and that these relations must be subjected to scientific investigation," and (3) that "steps must be taken to promote health and combat disease, and that the measures involved in such action must be social as well as medical."[34] As a central motivation for Virchow's support for revolution, democracy, and social medicine, Rosen cites a letter by Virchow to his father, in which Virchow declared that he was "no longer a partial man, but a whole one, and that [his] medical creed merge[d] with [his] political and social creed," thus indirectly suggesting that the embrace of social medicine may also be a solution to the fragmentation of scientific medicine in the early to mid twentieth century.[35]

Why did Rosen turn to Virchow in search for historical support for his concept of social medicine? Rosen, born in 1910, was the son of Jewish immigrants to the US. After graduating from Peter Stuyvesant High School and the College of the City of New York, he found himself excluded from Medical School due to access restrictions for Jewish students. In 1930, he enrolled at the University of Berlin, along with two Jewish American companions. In 1933, he approached the new Director of the Berlin Institute of the History of Medicine, Paul Diepgen, about an MD dissertation topic.[36] Diepgen encouraged him to contact Henry Sigerist, who by then had moved to Baltimore. Sigerist suggested he wrote on the European reception of the work of William Beaumont, a nineteenth-century American physician and physiologist. After Rosen's return to the US, he met Sigerist in person at a symposium on the history of industrial and occupational disease held at the New York Academy of Medicine in 1936. This was the beginning of Rosen's informal but close affiliation with the members of the Johns Hopkins Institute for the History of Medicine.[37]

Rosen's engagement with both the history of medicine and public health activism and administration is key to understanding his motivation for developing a new social approach to medicine and unpacking the genealogy of the ideas that may have informed this approach. Unable to find a full-time post in the history of medicine, Rosen took the civil service examinations and in 1941 joined the New York City Department of Health as a physician in the Bureau of Tuberculosis. He also enrolled as a graduate student in the

[34] Rosen, "What Is Social Medicine?," 678–82.
[35] Letter to his Father, May 1, 1848, Virchow, *Briefe an seine Eltern*, 141–5.
[36] On the history of medicine in Germany in the interwar period, see the title essay in Owsei Temkin, *The Double Face of Janus, and Other Essays in the History of Medicine* (Baltimore and London: Johns Hopkins University Press, 1977).
[37] Saul Benison, "George Rosen: An Appreciation," *Journal of the History of Medicine and Allied Sciences* 33, no. 3 (1978): 245–53; Arthur J. Viseltear, "The George Rosen–Henry E. Sigerist Correspondence," *Journal of the History of Medicine and Allied Sciences* 33, no. 3 (1978): 281–313.

Sociology Department in the Graduate Faculty of Political Science, History, and Philosophy at Columbia University, studying with Robert Lynd, Robert Merton, and Robert McIver and focusing on medical sociology. In 1943, Rosen's *History of Miners' Diseases* was published, which correlated the growth of knowledge on these diseases with the social and economic conditions that Rosen believed played a major role in causing them. He was awarded his Doctorate in Sociology in 1944 and in 1946 returned to public health work in the NYC Health Department, while at the same time engaging in formal studies at the School of Public Health at Columbia University, where he was awarded his Master of Public Health degree in 1947.[38] Rosen practiced what he wanted us to assume Virchow preached: he approached medicine as a social science, in the service of public health.

The immediate pretext to Rosen's two articles introducing his ideas around social medicine and establishing Virchow as one of its pioneers, appears to have been an initiative of the Milbank Memorial Fund, which held its annual roundtable meeting at the New York Academy of Medicine in 1947. The New York Academy of Medicine, on the occasion of the Academy's centennial celebration, held what they announced, confusingly for a reader in the early twenty-first century, as an "Institute for Social Medicine," which in effect was a symposium.[39] Rosen was asked to speak on the development of the concept of social medicine, covering the 100-year period from 1848 to 1948. In a letter to Sigerist, he reflected that:

in looking over this paper, which by the way will appear in the January 1948 Milbank Quarterly, as well as the one I read last March at the Academy meeting, and the one at the Cleveland meeting it struck me that they actually form an outline for a history of the Idea of Social Medicine, of the theory of social medicine from the eighteenth century to the present.[40]

Rosen's approach may have been informed by the crisis debate in German medicine in the early twentieth century, but he wrote the essay in 1948, when it was already obvious that a different, much more comprehensive approach to welfare than had ever before been seen, was being embraced in many European countries. The year 1948 was when the National Health Service was launched in Britain and Rosen mentions the foundational Beveridge Report approvingly. The paper also includes a critique of the apparent reluctance of medical and political elites, especially in the English-speaking world, to

---

[38] Benison, "George Rosen"; Viseltear, "The George Rosen–Henry E. Sigerist Correspondence."

[39] Elizabeth H. Jackson, "Review of *Social Medicine: Its Derivations and Objectives*, by Iago Galdston," Milbank Memorial Fund Quarterly 27, no. 3 (1949): 344–7, doi.org/10.2307/3348078.

[40] Reproduced in Viseltear, "The George Rosen–Henry E. Sigerist Correspondence," 292; the papers referred to here are Rosen, "What Is Social Medicine?"; and George Rosen, "The Place of History in Medical Education," *Bulletin of the History of Medicine* 22, no. 5 (1948): 594–629.

whole-heartedly embrace the proactive pursuit of public health as part of a comprehensive concept of social medicine and as a central remit of a modern welfare state.

Conclusion: Virchow and Social Medicine

Virchow's famous statement predated Bismarck's social insurance reforms and thus the beginnings of the welfare state by four decades. In fact, while he presents Virchow as the pioneer, Rosen looks to the ideas around social hygiene, developed by the likes of Alfred Grotjahn, as a model for his concept of social medicine. Grotjahn did not have his ideas from Virchow. Grotjahn, who qualified as a doctor in 1894 and then worked as a general practitioner in Berlin, actually received training in the social sciences when he attended the seminars of the *Nationalökonom* Gustav Schmoller at the University of Berlin.[41] While certainly not a revolutionary, Grotjahn was one of very few professors in German medicine in the early twentieth century who openly supported social democracy. He was a member of the Social Democratic Party and a member of the Reichstag for a few years in the early 1920s.

Where does this leave us with our attempt to reassess Virchow's role? Virchow found that the democratic ideal of the sovereignty of the people could not easily be reconciled with the primacy of reason that he envisaged for the future of Prussian politics following the March Revolution of 1848, based on the application of natural science and overseen by physicians pursuing the same ideals that he embraced. The revolutionary impulse may have led him to dismiss the frequently praised Prussian bureaucracy and hail democracy as key solution to the problems he witnessed in Upper Silesia but the democracy he was calling for was not universal; he was envisaging a republic of experts, which would necessarily lead to the disappearance of "the mob."

When I was thinking about how to square Virchow's commitment to democracy and socialism with his disgust with the poor and the ways in which they lived in Upper Silesia, I started to wonder if it might help to turn to the postcolonial historiography of medicine for a different perspective than that taken in most traditional accounts assessing Virchow's role in the history of social medicine.[42] Reading Virchow's account of his brief expedition to Upper Silesia in the context of his experiences during the Revolution suggests

---

[41] Paul Weindling, "Medical Practice in Imperial Berlin: The Casebook of Alfred Grotjahn," *Bulletin of the History of Medicine* 61, no. 3 (1987): 391–410; S. Milton Rabson, "Alfred Grotjahn, Founder of Social Hygiene," *Bulletin of the New York Academy of Medicine* 12, no. 2 (February 1936): 43–58; on Schmoller, see Erik Grimmer-Solem, *The Rise of Historical Economics and Social Reform in Germany, 1864–1894* (Oxford: Clarendon Press, 2003).

[42] Warwick Anderson, "Where Is the Postcolonial History of Medicine?," *Bulletin of the History of Medicine* 72, no. 3 (1998): 522–30.

that we do not need to look for colonies to find the patterns that characterized colonial medicine: an othered population on the margins of society, living and working in poor conditions, governed by an elite whose members were representatives of the metropolis, who may show compassion but feel little kinship with the locals. Virchow deplored these conditions but merely wanted to replace the rule of the backward old elite with the rule of enlightened, progressive experts. This is not an approach that George Rosen would have endorsed in 1947.

By shifting emphasis away from Virchow's status as the father of cellular pathology and champion of (physical) anthropology and by presenting him as a pioneer of the kind of social medicine that Rosen championed (and embodied) in the mid twentieth century, we may want to argue that Rosen decentered Virchow. Authors, especially in the Americas, drawing on Rosen's vision of social medicine, followed his lead.[43]

[43] Carter and Delgado, "A Debate."

2 Social Medicine in the Arab World
Colonial Legacies and Postcolonial Praxis

Joelle M. Abi-Rached and Lidia Helou[*]

This chapter outlines a genealogy of the concept of "social medicine" in Arabic. We argue that despite widespread practical engagement with its principles, the term *at-ṭibb al-ijtimāʿī* (social medicine) has not gained significant traction in either the medical or popular literatures in the Arab world. We propose two main reasons for this. First, the term is somewhat tautological in Arabic. Historically, the figure of the *ḥakīm* – meaning "sage," "judicious," or "wise" – has always embodied a social responsibility, serving as a trusted advisor to both rulers and the needy. Second, unlike in France or Germany, where social medicine developed into a distinct academic field, physicians in the Arab world have approached it more as a practical endeavor than a theoretical one. The term "social medicine" first appeared in Arabic in 1912, shortly before popular revolutions convulsed the Arab world in the aftermath of the First World War and the redrawing of national boundaries. In essence, social medicine has functioned as a practical philosophy of care for the "wretched of the earth" – to borrow Jacques Roumain's (1945) evocative phrase – purged of its colonial justification originally attached to it by the French doctor, Jules Guérin, as this chapter will illustrate.

We examine two early and rare reflective essays on the concept of social medicine written by Shibli Shumayyil and Amin A. Khairallah, medical doctors trained at the American University of Beirut (AUB) nearly four decades apart. Although their analyses of what social medicine is and should be differ radically, both seem to share a holistic and idealistic vision of medicine as a remedy not only for the limitations of clinical medicine but also for the social ills and diseases afflicting their societies. Amid the worsening impoverishment in the Arab world and the growing misery wrought by colonialism, authoritarianism, war, and social strife throughout the twentieth century, many doctors emerged as outspoken advocates for the poor, marginalized, and oppressed.

[*] We thank Samar Mikati, Dalia Nouh, and Nabila Shehabeddine at the Archives and Special Collections of the American University of Beirut for their assistance in identifying one of the sources for this chapter.

This chapter examines several illustrative examples of social medicine as both social critique and praxis, focusing on the revolutionary work of prominent early physician-activists from Tunisia, Sudan, and Egypt.

These revolutionary social medical doctors, as we describe them, represent a group of physicians united by their language, cycles of exile and return, and transregional influences. Unlike European theoreticians of social medicine, they engaged with deeper layers of social critique, protest, and anti-colonial struggles. They often went beyond merely expressing "social medicine as social critique," instead embodying – and even performing – both ideas in their daily lives. In doing so, these practitioners exemplified the meaning originally attributed to social medicine by the French doctor Jules Guérin following the 1848 French Revolution. This interpretation was later reimagined by the Levantine physician Shumayyil at the turn of the twentieth century during a period of intellectual renewal that lasted until the First World War. Far from being hagiographical, these biographical accounts offer a portrait of a practical engagement with social medicine, while also serving to connect histories that have remained isolated – and often silenced – by the legacy of colonial archiving. Ultimately, the chapter argues that, in the Arabic-speaking world, social medicine signifies the practice of medicine as politics by other means.

Social Medicine As Subservient to the Colonial Project

Jules Guérin (1801–86), a French surgeon-orthopedist of Belgian origin, might seem an unlikely figure in the genesis of the concept of social medicine or its later iterations. This apparent incongruity prompted Ligia Maria Vieira da Silva to investigate Guérin's motivation.[1] She argues that Guérin was an opportunist. His paper on "*médecine sociale*" (social medicine), published on March 11, 1848, in the influential *Gazette médicale de Paris*, was an outlier, given that his professional focus was almost entirely on orthopedic surgery. Moreover, despite claims to the contrary, Vieira da Silva found no evidence of a "movement" coalescing around this new concept. She also characterizes Guérin as a "last-minute Republican," an opportunist who aligned himself with the revolutionary fervor of 1848, despite having previously supported the Orléanist monarchy.[2] For all of these reasons, Vieira da Silva concludes that Guérin was a careerist, motivated by a desire to secure a position in the new political regime following the revolution.

While useful, this is a somewhat oversimplified critique. To start with, orthopedic surgery was not yet an established specialty. It was in the process of

---

[1] Ligia Maria Vieira da Silva, "Jules Guérin and Social Medicine in 1848," *Journal of Medical Biography* (May 18, 2022): 1–7, doi.org/10.1177/09677720221100211.
[2] Vieira da Silva, "Jules Guérin," 6.

being institutionalized and Guérin was, at least in the French context, considered to be one of its pioneers.[3] Hence, like many physicians at the time, including Shibli Shumayyil whom we will mention shortly, Guérin was involved and engaged in various questions and issues that preoccupied his generation; questions that had to do with the relationship between science and medicine, medicine and society, as well as medicine and the state. We will see shortly how this latter concern led him to a specific definition of social medicine. More relevant perhaps for us is the fact that Guérin was an innovator in medical thinking; his medical thesis was after all about "medical observation."[4] And in that regard even if he did not make a career in what would come to be known as social medicine, Guérin was an astute, if sly, "observer" of new ways of thinking about medicine, especially at a time of revolution and social upheaval. Indeed, Guérin is remembered not only for a number of medical aphorisms in French, but also for having revamped an influential medical periodical at the time, the *Gazette de santé*, which he renamed *Gazette médicale de Paris* and started editing from 1930 onward, also publishing in it mainly, but not only, on orthopedic surgery.[5] Accordingly, that his specialty is not relevant to the subject matter is insufficient for delegitimizing him as a key figure in the genealogy of social medicine.

Nevertheless, Vieira da Silva is correct in highlighting the distinct way in which Guérin defined social medicine, a definition quite different from what it came to mean much later in the twentieth century, namely the social determinants of health. However, she does not address the transformation his neologism introduced. Georges Canguilhem observed that, in the eighteenth century, health ceased to be understood primarily as a moral constitution. Instead, reframed through vital statistics, it became linked to the health of the nation, measured by economic performance and military strength.[6] Michel Foucault, building on this interpretation from his teacher, viewed social medicine as a prime example of the politicization of life – a phenomenon he termed "biopolitics." For Foucault, biopolitics represents a liberal state technology aimed at "normalizing life" through its medicalization and governance.[7] But is this what Guérin intended by social medicine?

Emmanuel Renault shows how Foucault in fact missed the nuances of what social medicine meant in the context of the 1848 French Revolution and how

[3] For more see, Grégory Quin, "Jules Guérin : Brève Biographie d'un Acteur de l'institutionnalisation de l'orthopédie (1830–1850)," *Gesnerus* 67, nos. 3–4 (2009): 237–55.

[4] Jules Guérin, "Essai sur l'observation en médecine et particulièrement de l'observation dans l'état actuel de cette science," MD, University of Paris, 1826.

[5] Quin, "Jules Guérin." Grégory Quin, "Jules Guérin : Brève biographie d'un acteur de l'institutionnalisation de l'orthopédie (1830–1850)."

[6] Georges Canguilhem, *Études d'histoire et de philosophie des sciences* (Paris: J. Vrin, 1994), 403.

[7] Emmanuel Renault, "Biopolitique, médecine sociale et critique du libéralisme," *Multitudes* 34, no. 3 (2008): 195–6, doi.org/10.3917/mult.034.0195.

Foucault's rendering of social medicine is too sweeping, reductionist, and convenient for his overarching thesis.[8] Indeed, Guérin gave two specific and intertwined meanings to social medicine that complicate the hegemonic biopolitical interpretation.[9] The first one is closer to what we would call a "sociology of medicine," with its examination of the social causes of mortality and morbidity. The second meaning is closer to what Charles Rosenberg calls a "political vision" of social medicine.[10] More specifically, Guérin talks about the "humanitarian" dimension of medicine.[11] For him, not only is medicine a form of "priesthood" (*sacerdoce*), but is also a means to achieve social justice.[12] It should ultimately aim at uplifting nations from poverty and improving the social conditions of the working classes through practical "solutions" to social problems.[13]

Moreover, Guérin distinguished "social medicine" (*médecine sociale*) from both "political medicine" (*médecine politique*) and "scientific medicine" (*médecine scientifique*).[14] By social medicine, he meant the various ways in which medicine interacts with society free from any ideology or dogma. He explicitly contrasted this with "socialist medicine" (*médecine socialiste*), which he saw as a specific approach to medicine aligned with socialist principles.[15] In contrast, social medicine, as Guérin envisioned it, was meant to transcend political partisanship and remain detached from any normative or prescriptive frameworks. This perspective aligns with Guérin's positivism, influenced by Auguste Comte and Victor Cousin.[16] For Guérin, medicine's privileged position – its access to the inner depths of society (*les entrailles de la société*) – made it uniquely suited to enable social reform and societal transformation (*regénération sociale*).[17] This is why medicine was inherently at the service of society. Consequently, it behooved medical doctors – in fact, the entire medical establishment – to diagnose and address the pressing social problems of their time. Social medicine, therefore, was a means of attending to the health of a nation in a broad sense by identifying its "social pathologies"

---

[8] Renault, "Biopolitique, médecine sociale et critique du libéralisme," 195–200.

[9] Renault, "Biopolitique, médecine sociale et critique du libéralisme," 201–2.

[10] Charles E. Rosenberg, "Erwin H. Ackerknecht, Social Medicine, and the History of Medicine," *Bulletin of the History of Medicine* 81, no. 3 (2007): 511.

[11] Jules Guérin, "Médecine sociale: Au corps médical de France," *Gazette médicale de Paris* (March 11, 1848): 184.

[12] Guérin, "Au corps médical de France," 184.

[13] Guérin, "Au corps médical de France," 183 and 184.

[14] Guérin, "Au corps médical de France," 184; Jules Guérin, "Médecine sociale: La médecine sociale et la médecine politique," *Gazette médicale de Paris*, no. 13bis (March 25, 1848): 231.

[15] Jules Guérin, "Médecine sociale: La médecine sociale et la médecine socialiste," *Gazette médicale de Paris*, no. 12 (March 18, 1848): 203.

[16] Quin, "Jules Guérin," 240.

[17] Guérin, "Au corps médical de France," 183; Guérin, "La médecine sociale et la médecine politique," 231.

(*pathologies sociales*), promoting the principles of "social hygiene" (*hygiènes sociales*), and prescribing "social therapeutics" (*thérapeutiques sociales*).[18]

In contrast to social medicine, which had higher ideals, "political medicine" was an arm of the state apparatus. Curiously, while social medicine did not embrace any particular philosophy or ideology, it "serve[d] them all."[19] This is problematic for two reasons. First, is that it could obviously serve an oppressive or unjust regime. And second, "society" for Guérin meant at the very least French society, not some universal society that included all nations and peoples. Interestingly, Guérin uses Algeria (which was formally annexed as a French colony in 1834) to illustrate the difference between political and social medicine. From the vantage point of political medicine, Guérin argues, the colonization of Algeria should have been abandoned, as vital statistics clearly demonstrated the deadly toll the harsh climate took on acclimating colonial troops. In contrast, social medicine aimed to identify and address the challenges faced by settlers and colonists, ensuring the success of the colonial enterprise.[20] For Guérin, this task of social medicine –making colonialism viable and sustainable, was unproblematic, as he believed it contributed to the "moral and physical improvement of societies writ large."[21] But whose societies was he referring to? As it turns out, he was speaking exclusively of (and to) the societies of the so-called civilized world.

While Renault limits his analysis of Guérin's definition of social medicine to its role in complicating Foucault's concept of biopolitics, much more can be said about Guérin's uncritical stance on empire, his failure to recognize the humanity (and hence rights) of colonized peoples, and the role of colonialism in generating new health inequalities and inequities. Colonialism not only neglected the health of indigenous populations but also exacerbated their preexisting health conditions through exploitation and enslavement.[22] At the same time, this lack of critique is a paradox of this revolutionary moment; it is vertically revolutionary but lacks horizontal reach. For Guérin, colonialism was uncontroversial, indeed taken for granted, after all social medicine was a means to make the colonial conquest possible at any cost even if the empirical evidence pointed to the contrary, which is somewhat contradictory for an alleged positivist. Regardless, it is clear that social medicine was imperialist in its scope, with the "general interest" of the French nation, in Rousseauan terms, positioned as the highest good to be achieved – not a universal morality

[18] Guérin, "La médecine sociale et la médecine socialiste," 203.
[19] Guérin, "La médecine sociale et la médecine socialiste," 203.
[20] Guérin, "Médecine sociale: La médecine sociale et la médecine politique," 231.
[21] Guérin, "Médecine sociale: La médecine sociale et la médecine politique," 231.
[22] Yin Paradies, "Colonisation, Racism and Indigenous Health," *Journal of Population Research* 33, no. 1 (March 1, 2016): 83–96, doi.org/10.1007/s12546-016-9159-y.

or even a broader humanitarian concern. In this framework, the "human" was the "civilized," while everyone else was excluded.

Curiously, the medical doctors we examine next do not address the colonial justification of social medicine. Instead, they reinterpret its principles to advocate for the emancipation of all peoples from all forms of oppression and injustice.

Social Medicine As Clinical Sociology

Two early references make use of the term "social medicine" in Arabic (*at-tibb al-ijtimāʿī*) in radically different ways. The first is by Shibli Shumayyil, a medical doctor, intellectual, and social reformer, and the second by Amin A. Khairallah, a surgeon, educator, and professor of medicine. Both were products of a new medical school established in Beirut in 1867, a year after the founding of the Syrian Protestant College by Protestant American missionaries (later renamed the American University of Beirut in 1920) and where medicine was originally taught in Arabic until 1880.[23]

Shumayyil (1850–1917), who was perhaps among the first medical doctors to have used the concept of social medicine in Arabic, graduated in 1871 and had additional clinical training in Paris and Istanbul.[24] His medical and humanitarian work with earthquake survivors in 1870 (while still a medical student), his efforts among Egyptian *fellahin* (peasants) during a deadly cholera epidemic, and his later work with the urban poor in Cairo, along with his staunch support of female medical doctors, all shaped his social medicine approach through praxis.[25] This stands in stark contrast to Guérin, who, as we saw earlier, championed political participation while remaining somewhat socially conservative.

A popularizer of medical and scientific ideas, Shumayyil pioneered new medical journals, such as *ash-Shifāʾ* (Healing), which started publishing in 1886 (until 1891) and, *al-Mustakbal* (The Future), launched in 1914 with the Egyptian journalist and modernizer, Salāma Mūsā, to build a new progressive society based on modern science.[26] This period of intellectual and cultural effervescence characterized what came to be known as the *Nahḍa* movement

---

[23] For more, see Joelle M. Abi-Rached, *ʿAsfūriyyeh: A History of Madness, Modernity, and War in the Middle East* (Cambridge, MA: MIT Press, 2020), 50–6.

[24] Georges Haroun, *Šiblī Šumayyil: Une pensée évolutionniste Arabe à l'époque d'an-Nahḍa* (Beirut: Librairie Orientale, 1985), 23, 24, and 44; Susan Laila Ziadeh, "A Radical in His Time: The Thought of Shibli Shumayyil and Arab Intellectual Discourse (1882–1917)," PhD, University of Michigan, 1991; Abi-Rached, ʿAsfūriyyeh, 44–8.

[25] Haroun, *Šiblī Šumayyil*, 46, 50, 56, 82, and 84.

[26] P. C. Sadgrove, "Shumayyil, Shiblī," in *Encyclopaedia of Islam, Second Edition* (Brill, 2012), https://referenceworks.brillonline.com/entries/encyclopaedia-of-islam-2/shumayyil-shibli-SIM_6988?s.num=406&s.start=400.

(usually translated as "renaissance," "reawakening," or "renewal"). Shumayyil
was a key member of that movement, promoting secular and "rational" ideas
to challenge what he viewed as regressive and superstitious forces that kept
the region under Ottoman tyranny, sociopolitical stagnation, and intellectual
lethargy. His socialist thinking was influenced by figures such as Ibn Khaldun
and Gamal Al-Din Al-Afghani, the latter being both an anti-imperialist and an
anti-monarchist.[27]

For Georges Haroun, author of one of Shumayyil's rare biographies, the
"grand merit" of this Levantine doctor was his ability to extract from European
evolutionary theories a system of social reforms.[28] His innovations included
one of the first mentions in the Ottoman world of the question of laborers'
rights and status, along with a defense of socialism's viability as a system and
its translation into Arabic as *"ijtima'iyya"* instead of the commonly used word
"ishtirakiyya," to denote a more direct sense of "association" as expressed in
biological phenomena of subsistence, making social and living bodies objects
of the same laws.[29] This is why we also speculate below that Shumayyil is perhaps the first to have coined the term social medicine in Arabic with this biosocial sense of *"ijtima'iyya"* implied in the concept. As underlined by Jean Lecerf,
even Shumayyil's scientific work was imbued with socialist thinking and social
Darwinism.[30] In this sense, Shumayyil was both avant-gardist and a man of
his time, convinced that the best way to achieve social justice was through the
adoption of evolutionary theory as a principle of social life.[31] But he was also
a progressive thinker who proposed a carceral reform under Ottoman rule and
pleaded for a justice informed by advances in science and medicine.[32]

When it came to social medicine, his views were equally idiosyncratic
but attuned to the spirit of his time. In a short book that compiles his "opinions" (*ārā'*) on man, disease, society, and politics with a rather general title,
The Opinions of Doctor Shibli Shumayyil (*Ārā' al-Duktūr Shiblī Shumayyil*),[33]
Shumayyil used social medicine in the sense of "medical sociology," not as we
understand it today, as a sociological analysis of medicine (through its institutions, actors, practices, assumptions, etc.) but the other way around, as a medical or clinical analysis of society, that is to say, a discipline or approach that
purports to analyze society with surgical precision and clinical astuteness, diag-
nosing its maladies as well as proposing a cure to the ailing social body (*al-
jism al-ijtimā'ī*).[34] In that way, and without mentioning either Guérin or Rudolf

---

[27] Haroun, *Šiblī Šumayyil*, 66.   [28] Haroun, *Šiblī Šumayyil*, 10.
[29] Haroun, *Šiblī Šumayyil*, 118, 220–1, 243, and 244.
[30] Jean Lecerf, "Šibli Šumayyil : Métaphysicien et Moraliste Contemporain," *Bulletin d'études
orientales* 1 (1931): 157 and 158.
[31] Haroun, *Šiblī Šumayyil*, 236.   [32] Haroun, *Šiblī Šumayyil*, 251.
[33] Shiblī Shumayyil, *Ārā' al-Duktūr Shiblī Shumayyil* (Cairo: Maṭba'at al-Ma'ārif, 1912).
[34] Shumayyil, *Ārā' al-Duktūr Shiblī Shumayyil*, 23–8 and 26.

Virchow (1821–1902) who would expand on the original concept of social medicine, Shumayyil shared with them the same premise of social medicine as a physiological science of society. Indeed, for Virchow, "if medicine is the science of the healthy as well as of the ill human being (which is what it ought to be), what other science is better suited to propose laws as the basis of the social structure, in order to make effective those which are inherent in man himself."[35]

Shumayyil's holistic yet physiological or clinical approach to society aligned with the broader project of the Nahḍa, which unapologetically – if at times stridently – critiqued its own society while advocating for a prescriptive, progressive, secular, and one can say positivistic science of state and society. In this context, social medicine became a powerful trope for social critique.[36] And as we will see with the revolutionary social medical practitioners discussed later, social medicine evolved into a trope or signifier for social protest. If for Guérin, social medicine was meant to critique the state's instrumentalist use of medicine, for Shumayyil it served as a critical tool for understanding sociopolitical malaise.

And while Shumayyil can be regarded as the instigator – or even translator – of the concept of social medicine in the Arabic-speaking world, he was also a sympathizer of Lord Cromer, the British colonial ruler of Egypt, revealing himself to be a man of many contradictions.[37]

Social Medicine As Social Science

Like Shumayyil, Amin A. Khairallah (1889–c. 1955) was a medical doctor who graduated from the American University of Beirut. Trained as a surgeon, he served on the AUB faculty from 1933 until his death and was a member of the local committee overseeing the Lebanon Hospital for Mental and Nervous Disorders, commonly known as ʿAsfūriyyeh – the only modern psychiatric hospital in the Levant between Cairo and Constantinople.[38] A highly accomplished physician, Khairallah published extensively on medicine, medical history, and medical ethics.[39] Notably, he authored the first article in Arabic that

---

[35] Genevieve Miller, "*Disease, Life, and Man, Selected Essays* by Rudolf Virchow, Lelland J. Rather," *Isis* 52, no. 3 (1961): 436–6, at: www.jstor.org/stable/228095.

[36] Abi-Rached,ʿAsfūriyyeh, 24.   [37] Haroun, *Šiblī Šumayyil*, 233.

[38] "Medical News," *British Medical Journal* (December 30, 1950): 1503; Mounir (Munir) E. Nassar, *Clinical Medicine Research History at the American University of Beirut, Faculty of Medicine 1920–1974* (Bloomington, IN: WestBow Press, 2014); Abi-Rached, ʿAsfūriyyeh.

[39] Some of his works include: Amin A. Khairallah, *A Brief Medical Bible: Ethics in Medicine* (Beirut: American University of Beirut, 1953); Amin A. Khairallah, *Outline of Arabic Contributions to Medicine and the Allied Sciences* (Beirut: The American Press, 1946); Amin A. Khairallah, "A Century of American Medicine in Syria," *Annals of Medical History* 1, no. 5 (September 1939): 460–70; Amin A. Khairallah, "Medicine's Debt to Syria," *Annals of Medical History* 3, no. 2 (March 1941): 140–7; Amin A. Khairallah, "Arabic Contributions to Anatomy and Surgery," *Annals of Medical History* 4, no. 5 (September 1942): 409–15.

tackled social medicine as it came to be understood in the mid-twentieth century as the study of social determinants of health inequalities.

In an article published in 1950 in *al-Abḥath* (a periodical published by AUB since 1948) on the "Importance of Social Medicine and Its Aims" (*Ahamiyyat at-Ṭibb al-Ijtimāʿī wa-Ahdāfah*) Khairallah laid out a roadmap of what social medicine entails.[40] Unlike the Hippocratic tradition, which emphasized the physical environment as a cause of pathology, Khairallah viewed social medicine as the missing link between the individual and society highlighting its role in addressing widespread ignorance about the causes of mortality and morbidity. Interestingly, he contrasted social medicine with "bedside medicine" (*at-ṭibb al-sarīrī*) or "clinical medicine" which focuses more on the individual.[41] Echoing Guérin (though without mentioning him), Khairallah argued that social medicine is concerned with society or the group (*al-jamāʿa*) rather than the individual.[42] Social medicine's emergence, as Khairallah outlines, coincided with several key developments. First, the failure of clinical medicine to address the wider causes of health and disease.[43] Second, changes in medical education accompanied by efforts to make healthcare more affordable and cost-effective.[44] Third, the aging of the population and the consequent shift toward chronic diseases, which demand a broader understanding of pathology with a focus on prevention.[45] Fourth, the recognition of the inextricable link between pathology and human relationships (*ʿalāqāt an-nāss al-ijtimāʿiyya*).[46] Fifth, an improved understanding of the role the mind plays in the pathogenesis of many diseases.[47]

Here Khairallah aligns with Shumayyil's interpretation of social medicine though without citing him, by drawing a parallel between what he terms "individual pathology" (*al-pathūlūgiya al-fardiyya*) and "social pathology" (*al-pathūlūgiya al-ijtimāʿiyya*). He writes: "Just as *individual pathology* relates to the science of clinical medicine, we can also look at *social pathology* as it relates to social medicine. It does not matter that this relationship takes place in the office of a sociologist, health engineer, statistician, epidemiologist, or in other social sciences."[48] Finally, he cites increased urbanization and

---

[40] Amin A. Khairallah, "*Ahamiyyat at-Ṭibb al-Ijtimāʿī wa-Ahdāfah*" (Importance of Social Medicine and Its Goals), *al-Abhath* (June 3, 1950): 205–15.
[41] Khairallah, "*Ahamiyyat at-Ṭibb al-Ijtimāʿī wa-Ahdāfah*," 205.
[42] Khairallah, "*Ahamiyyat at-Ṭibb al-Ijtimāʿī wa-Ahdafah*," 211–12.
[43] Khairallah, "*Ahamiyyat at-Ṭibb al-Ijtimāʿī wa-Ahdafah*," 208.
[44] Khairallah, "*Ahamiyyat at-Ṭibb al-Ijtimāʿī wa-Ahdafah*," 210.
[45] Khairallah, "*Ahamiyyat at-Ṭibb al-Ijtimāʿī wa-Ahdafah*," 211.
[46] Khairallah, "*Ahamiyyat at-Ṭibb al-Ijtimāʿī wa-Ahdafah*," 212.
[47] Khairallah, "Ahamiyyat at-Ṭibb al-Ijtimāʿī wa-Ahdafah," 213.
[48] Emphasis added. Khairallah, "*Ahamiyyat at-Ṭibb al-Ijtimāʿī wa-Ahdafah*," 212–13.

industrialization as major drivers of what could be described as a shift toward social medicine.[49]

For Khairallah, health is more than just the absence of disease – an idea that had only been formally articulated two years earlier in the 1948 charter of the newly established World Health Organization. He shows how social medicine is far-reaching, encompassing every aspect of the social, environmental, and economic life that can affect the health of individuals and communities. Rather than a movement, Khairallah presents social medicine as an approach to health and disease that is holistic, preventative, and inherently long-term in its aims, in contrast to the more immediate focus of clinical medicine. He defines social medicine as akin to a comprehensive approach to "public health" (as-ṣoḥḥa al-ʿāmma).[50] Interestingly, he expands on Shumayyil's definition of social medicine as merely medical sociology by emphasizing that social medicine requires a broad knowledge of all the social sciences.[51]

He concludes with a pseudo-Marxist appeal for the emancipation of humanity through an understanding of the social and material conditions underlying the pathologies of modernity, pleading for the recourse to social medicine as a means to "liberate the human spirit from ignorance and superstition, and reform our institutions for the benefit and comfort of the human race."[52]

Revolutionary Social Medical Doctors

Given the limited scope of this chapter, we have selected a few doctors whom we think exemplify our characterization of "social medicine as social praxis." This approach corresponds to what Guérin referred to as "humanitarian medicine" but inflected with the reformist ideals envisioned by Shumayyil. Instead of theorizing social medicine from the comforts of their ivory towers, the revolutionary doctors discussed here put social medicine to the test through action and practice. They embodied and enacted what social medicine means or should mean by speaking on behalf of the poor, oppressed women, and the marginalized. Their goal was not only to challenge what they saw as regressive social norms and practices but also to resist the colonial-settler apparatus and its various postcolonial iterations, including the authoritarian and patriarchal regimes they had to confront in their respective countries. Remarkably, some of the early revolutionary doctors were women and feminists.

---

[49] Khairallah, "Ahamiyyat at-Ṭibb al-Ijtimāʿī wa-Ahdafah," 214.
[50] Khairallah, "Ahamiyyat at-Ṭibb al-Ijtimāʿī wa-Ahdafah," 207.
[51] Khairallah, "Ahamiyyat at-Ṭibb al-Ijtimāʿī wa-Ahdafah," 213.
[52] Khairallah, "Ahamiyyat at-Ṭibb al-Ijtimāʿī wa-Ahdāfah," 215.

Tawhida Ben Cheikh (1909–2010)

Tawhida Ben Cheikh was born in 1909 into a bourgeois and politically active family from Ras Jebel in Tunisia, which was a French protectorate since 1881.[53] Ben Cheikh began her education at the school for girls on Rue Pacha before joining a French lycée where Étienne Burnet, a French doctor and director of the Pasteur Institute in Tunis, as well as his wife, met the young student and recommended her for medical studies in Paris.[54] In 1928, Ben Cheikh became the first female holder of a baccalaureate certificate in Tunisia and, faced with the absence of medical schools there (none were established until after independence in 1956), she traveled to Paris to pursue medical studies.[55] Shaped by both hyperlocal and diasporic experiences from the start, Ben Cheikh's years as a student in Paris were marked by political activism through her involvement in the "115" (the Association of Muslim and North African Students, which was "apolitical" in name but staunchly anti-colonial in practice).[56]

In 1936, Ben Cheikh returned to Tunis as the first female Tunisian doctor (and the only one for several years), knowing that, as a Tunisian woman, she could not practice medicine in a public hospital.[57] This, however, did not stop her from establishing her private practice at 42 Rue Bab Menara, which would later become a stronghold for women's emancipation movements and a hub for gynecological research.[58] By navigating and challenging both legal constraints and patriarchal norms, Ben Cheikh carved out a space that accommodated her medical practice while fostering her political activism. Situating her clinic in the heart of the city disrupted the dichotomy between marginality and centrality vis-à-vis women's health, creating a space where social critique was not only articulated but also embodied through the very presence of a female doctor resonating throughout the Tunisian capital.

---

[53] "Tunisie : Dix choses à savoir sur Tawhida Ben Cheikh, première femme médecin du Monde Arabe," *Jeune Afrique*, accessed June 24, 2023, at: www.jeuneafrique.com/918320/politique/tunisie-dix-choses-a-savoir-sur-tawhida-ben-cheikh-premiere-femme-medecin-du-monde-arabe.

[54] Dorra Mahfoudh Draoui and Amel Mahfoudh, "Mobilisations des femmes et mouvement féministe en Tunisie," *Nouvelles questions féministes* 33, no. 2 (2014): 15, doi.org/10.3917/nqf.332.0014; Balqīs Yūsuf Badrī and Aili Mari Tripp, *Women's Activism in Africa: Struggles for Rights and Representation* (London: Zed Books Ltd, 2017), 65.

[55] Jane D. Tchaicha and Khédija Arfaoui, *The Tunisian Women's Rights Movement: From Nascent Activism to Influential Power-Broking* (London: Routledge, Taylor and Francis Group, 2017), 43.

[56] Frédéric Brun, Sylvia Marcon, and Benoit Monange, "Itinéraire d'un scientifique engagé, entretien avec Mohamed Larbi Bouguerra, propos recueillis par Frédéric Brun, Sylvia Marcon, Benoit Monange," *Écologie et politique* 54, no. 1 (2017): 149–50; Mahfoudh Draoui and Mahfoudh, "Mobilisations des femmes et mouvement féministe en Tunisie," 15.

[57] Tchaicha and Arfaoui, *The Tunisian Women's Rights Movement*, 43; Badrī and Tripp, *Women's Activism in Africa*, 65.

[58] "Tunisie: Dix choses à savoir."

Strikingly, many Tunisian men refused to let their female family members get auscultated by men and in the absence of female doctors, women's health conditions often went untreated or even undiagnosed.[59] Ben Cheikh's medical practice, along with her recognition by local feminists and activists, marked a significant disruption in a male-dominated space, generating an unavoidable female presence and signaled the beginning of a more proactive medical feminism and gendered social protest.

Indeed, her revolutionary voice echoed well beyond her clinical work. Besides being a pioneer physician, Ben Cheikh was also the editor-in-chief of the monthly *Leila* (1936–41), the first francophone feminist magazine in Tunisia, which sought to introduce and promote a feminist discourse to North African women. Under Ben Cheikh's direction starting in 1937, the magazine adopted an anti-colonial stance aligned with feminist ideology initiating an intersectionality *avant la lettre*.[60] In this spirit, Ben Cheikh publicly condemned and testified about the crimes of torture and murder committed by French Army General Pierre Garbay in 1952 against Tunisian women and activists.[61] Like many of the medical practitioners featured in this chapter, she served on the executive committees of several medico-social organizations, including the Red Crescent and the Muslim Union of Tunisian Women.[62] Another remarkable aspect of Ben Cheikh's practical social medicine ethos was her commitment to protecting and economically empowering unmarried pregnant women who sought care at the Aziza Othmana Hospital, where she had directed the Gynecology Department since 1964.[63]

In line with her practice, Ben Cheikh's most significant legacy was the establishment of the first birth-control clinic in Tunisia at the Charles Nicolle Hospital in 1963.[64] This initiative paved the way for the opening of the Montfleury clinic in 1970, the first facility of the Tunisian Association for Family Planning.[65] Throughout her career, Ben Cheikh led significant political efforts against anti-abortion laws and in 1968, she co-founded the Tunisian

---

[59] Fatima Sadiqi (ed.), *Women Writing Africa: The Northern Region* (New York, NY: The Feminist Press at The City University of New York, 2009), 63.

[60] Tchaicha and Arfaoui, *The Tunisian Women's Rights Movement*, 27; Hafedh Boujmil, *Leïla: Revue illustrée de la femme, 1936–1941* (Tunis: Éditions Nirvana, 2007), 47.

[61] Fatima Sadiqi, *Women's Movements in Post-"Arab Spring" North Africa* (New York, NY: Palgrave Macmillan, 2016), 203.

[62] Sadiqi, *Women's Movements in Post-"Arab Spring" North Africa*, 203; "Tunisie: Dix choses à savoir"; Khédija Arfaoui, "Bchira Ben Mrad: A Pioneer Feminist (1913–1993)," *International Journal of Research* 8, no. 8 (2020): 311, doi.org/10.29121/granthaalayah.v8.i8.2020.1058.

[63] Sadiqi, *Women's Movements in Post-"Arab Spring" North Africa*, 201.

[64] Sadiqi, *Women's Movements in Post-"Arab Spring" North Africa*, 201.

[65] Tchaicha and Arfaoui, *The Tunisian Women's Rights Movement*, 43; Sadiqi, *Women's Movements in Post-"Arab Spring" North Africa*, 201.

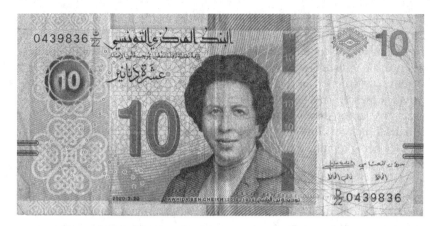

Figure 2.1 Tawhida Ben Cheikh featured on Tunisia's new 10 dinar banknote, 2020. Photo by the authors, courtesy of the Central Bank of Tunisia.

Family Planning Association, which played a pivotal role in securing Tunisian women's right to abortion in 1965 (Figure 2.1).[66]

Her achievements reverberated across the region in both Arabophone and Francophone milieux with a feminist medicine embedded in a *silsila* (a lineage) of women who wrote and acted for a more equitable Arab world. From Nazik Abid in Syria and Lebanon to Houda Chaarawi who inspired a nationalist movement in Egypt, Arabic-writing and speaking feminists transcended borders, transforming local struggles into cross-regional movements.[67] The cyclical movements of travel and return further defined Ben Cheikh's commitment to social medicine. Her engagement in such circles undoubtedly sharpened her critique of both gender inequality and colonial oppression.

A major conference in 1937 celebrating Ben Cheikh's work and achievements on behalf of Tunisian women resonated throughout the country, inspiring the emergence of feminist associations across Tunisia.[68] Her efforts positioned women's health as a central issue and challenged perceptions of women's status as peripheral. In 1957, Tunisia became the first Arab country to grant women the right to vote, a milestone achieved in part thanks to the

---

[66] Warren C. Robinson and John A. Ross, *The Global Family Planning Revolution: Three Decades of Population Policies and Programs* (Washington, DC: World Bank, 2007), 64; Mahfoudh Draoui and Mahfoudh, "Mobilisations des femmes et mouvement féministe en Tunisie," 17; J. Ben Brahem, "Le gouvernement tunisien s'efforce de développer le planning familial et les pratiques du contrôle des naissances," *Le Monde*, November 3, 1965.

[67] Mahfoudh Draoui and Mahfoudh, "Mobilisations des femmes et mouvement féministe en Tunisie," 16.

[68] Arfaoui, "Bchira Ben Mrad," 313.

efforts and courage of women like Ben Cheikh, who leveraged the influence of her medical practice to drive progressive change.

Abdel Halim Mohamed Halim (1910–2009)

After the Mahdist War ended in 1899 and condominium rule by Egypt and Great Britain (effectively controlled by Britain) was established over Sudan, the British authorities sought Western-educated medical practitioners fluent in both Arabic and English. Unlike Egyptian doctors, whose strong nationalist sentiments posed a potential threat to British rule, "Syrians" emerged as a better option.[69] Under British supervision and control, Syrian and Sudanese medical professionals worked closely together, with British doctors often relying on the experience and knowledge of Syrian physicians such as Yusef Derwish and Nesib Baz, Sudan's references on sleeping sickness.[70]

The question of training Sudanese physicians arose later, with the establishment of the Kitchener School of Medicine in Khartoum in 1924. Named in memory of Lord Kitchener, the Governor-General of Sudan from 1898 to 1900, the school was partly intended to prevent the politicization of Sudanese students studying abroad.[71] Ironically, the British authorities did not anticipate that their own school of medicine would produce fierce critics of their colonial rule, including physician-activists like Abdel Halim Mohamed Halim, one of Kitchener's first medical graduates.[72]

Halim was born in 1910 in Omdurman, British-controlled Sudan, into a family of scholars, religious leaders, and figures of Mahdist authority.[73] After attending a religious school, he joined Gordon Memorial College (founded in 1902) in 1924 and the Kitchener School of Medicine in 1929, from which he graduated in 1933.[74] Nicknamed "the wise sheikh" by scholar Mansour Khalid, "father of medicine" by the cohorts of Sudanese medical professionals he trained, Halim went down in history for his many "firsts," as highlighted by his friend and student Omar Fadl: first Sudanese member and fellow of the Royal College of Physicians, first chairman of the Sudanese Medical Association, and

---

[69] Heather Bell, *Frontiers of Medicine in the Anglo-Egyptian Sudan, 1899–1940* (Oxford: Clarendon Press, 2004), 43 and 44.

[70] Alexander Cruickshank, *Itchy Feet – A Doctor's Tale* (Ilfracombe: Stockwell, 1991), 39; Bell, *Frontiers of Medicine*, 41 and 42. "Syrian" is used generically to refer to the lands of what are today modern Lebanon and Syria.

[71] Report, Kitchener School of Medicine 1924–1925, 10 in Bell, *Frontiers of Medicine*, 32, 43–4, and 52.

[72] Bell, *Frontiers of Medicine*, 52.

[73] Farouk Fadl, "Abdel Halim Mohammed Abdel Halim," *British Medical Journal* 338 (June 13, 2009): 1446, doi.org/10.1136/bmj.b2311.

[74] Fadl, "Abdel Halim Mohammed Abdel Halim," 1446; Tarik AKA Elhadd, "Abdel Halim Mohamed Halim," Royal College of Physicians Museum, 2009, at: https://history.rcplondon.ac.uk/inspiring-physicians/abdel-halim-mohamed-halim.

first Sudanese senior physician in the British colonial Sudan medical service.[75] Moreover, the man who would become Mayor of Khartoum, Director of the Khartoum teaching hospital, Chancellor of Khartoum University, and president of several sports committees, also spearheaded the creation of crucial medical services in Sudan, irremediably changing the country's medical landscape and relation to medicine.[76]

As for his politics, Halim is described not as a politician per se but rather as a doctor with a political pen.[77] His political activity started in the mid 1920s, upon his entry into Gordon College and the creation of "Al-Fajr" (Dawn), a literary club of "mutual learning" before morphing into a hub for nationalist and literary enlightenment.[78]

Nourished by the spirit of the brief yet instrumental Sudanese Revolution of 1924 and inspired by the writings of Egyptian scholars such as Muhammad Abduh and Taha Hussein, the members of Al-Fajr launched an eponymous magazine in 1934, describing it as "the literary embodiment of the Sudanese younger generation."[79] Halim's magnum opus, *Mawt el-Duniyā* (Death of the World) co-authored with a fellow member of Al-Fajr, Mohamed Ahmad Mahjub, narrated the emergence of the movement and magazine, incorporating autobiographical elements, poetic tournures, and nationalistic ethos, granting its political message a lasting resonance.[80] In both writing and practice, the "wise sheikh" articulated a clear vision for Sudanese medical care and anti-colonial resistance, extensively critiquing the 1936 Anglo-Egyptian Agreement Treaty in the pages of *Al-Fajr* and *Mawt el-Duniyā*, condemning the Treaty for obstructing the Sudanese people's political will and their right for self-determination.[81] To support his political ambitions, Halim built a structure of care imbued with the tenets of social medicine. He cofounded the Graduate Students Conference in 1938, which called for both wider access to education and a more politically active student body, ultimately setting in

---

[75] Elhadd, "Abdel Halim Mohamed Halim"; Omer Fadl, "Obituary: Abdel Halim," *The Guardian*, July 23, 2009, at: www.theguardian.com/theguardian/2009/jul/23/abdel-halim-obituary; Elizabeth Douglas, "Remembering Abdel Halim Mohamed Halim," Royal College of Physicians Museum, September 24, 2021, at: https://history.rcplondon.ac.uk/blog/remembering-abdel-halim-mohamed-halim; Fadl, "Obituary: Abdel Halim."

[76] Elhadd, "Abdel Halim Mohamed Halim."

[77] Fadwa Abdel Rahman Ali Taha, "Dawr ʿAbdel-Halīm Muhamad as-Siyāsī" (The Political Role of Mohamed Abdel El Halim)," at: Hashmab.net, accessed June 26, 2023, at: www.hashmab .net/page1211.html.

[78] Yousif Omer Babiker, "The Al-Fajr Movement and Its Place in Modern Sudanese Literature," PhD, University of Edinburgh, 1979, 64.

[79] Babiker, "The Al-Fajr Movement," 54; Heather J. Sharkey, "Reappraising *The History of Arabic Culture in the Sudan* by the Egyptian Scholar 'Abd al-Majid 'Abidin," *Cahiers d'études africaines* 60, no. 240 (4) (2020): 812, at: www.jstor.org/stable/27126499.

[80] Sharkey, "Reappraising *The History of Arabic Culture in the Sudan*," 814.

[81] Ali Taha, "Dawr ʿAbdel-Halīm Muhamad as-Siyāsī"; Babiker, "The Al-Fajr Movement," 125.

motion the movement for Sudan's independence (in 1956) and the creation of political parties that persisted after independence.[82] While steering away from partisan politics in favor of his medical practice, Halim took a leading role in drafting the political memorandum that sought autonomy from British rule in 1942.[83]

This, however, did not mean that Halim stopped being politically active after independence. By intertwining medicine and politics in both writing and praxis, he, along with other Sudanese doctors, played a central role in the resistance movement against the dictatorship of General Ibrahim Abboud (who ruled from 1958 to 1964). This was achieved both because of and in spite of his position as a senior civil servant.[84] In fact, Farouk Fadl's obituary of Halim noted that "doctors were always at the forefront of movements that resisted dictatorship and injustice in Sudan," likely referencing Halim's participation in the interim five-member ruling council formed after Abboud's fall in 1964. This council included other notable physicians, such as psychiatrist El-Tigani El-Mahi and obstetrician El-Mabarak El-Fadil Shaddad.[85]

The interlacing of medical and revolutionary praxis in Sudan, exemplified by Halim's career, provided a foundation for anticolonial critique not only among Sudanese medical practitioners but also among many others living under British rule. Among them was physician Selim Bey Yusuf Atiyah, the father of writer Edward Atiyah, who moved to Sudan in 1898. Another notable figure was the francophone Syrian doctor Malhamé who turned his clinic in Khartoum into a hub of anti-imperialist critique in response to the racism of his British superiors.[86] Similarly, the Lebanese Nicola Maalouf who came to Sudan as a medical officer to the Anglo-Egyptian Army became the confidant of both the Mirghani and the Mahdi clans while marking the Sudanese topography through the inauguration of a "Maalouf tramway station" near his clinic in Khartoum.[87] In this regard, Edward Atiyah's autobiography offers fascinating glimpses into Sudanese medical life, featuring a certain "Dr. Selim" – a proud Darwinist and likely reader of Shumayyil – who left the Syrian Protestant College to join the military hospital in Omdurman around 1899.[88] All of these

---

[82] Ali Taha, "Dawr 'Abdel-Halīm Muhamad as-Siyāsī"; Elhadd, "Abdel Halim Mohamed Halim"; Fadl, "Obituary: Abdel Halim."

[83] Elhadd, "Abdel Halim Mohamed Halim"; Fadl, "Abdel Halim Mohammed Abdel Halim," 1446.

[84] Elhadd, "Abdel Halim Mohamed Halim."

[85] Fadl, "Abdel Halim Mohammed Abdel Halim," 1446.

[86] Edward Atiyah, *An Arab Tells His Story* (London: John Murray, 1946), 149–50; Bell, *Frontiers of Medicine in the Anglo-Egyptian Sudan*, 46–47.

[87] Norma Malouf Kefouri, "A Piece of the History of Sudan – A Tale of Two Families: Norma Malouf Kefouri at TEDx Sobawomen," TEDx Talks, December 20, 2013, at: www.youtube.com/watch?v=E6jPjE9UISw&t=86s.

[88] Atiyah, *An Arab Tells His Story*, 44 and 66.

medical lives had no choice but to cross paths with politics and to acknowledge the imperfection of their politicized science.

Nawal El-Saadawi (1931–2021)

Around the time when Ben Cheikh's return from Paris was being celebrated, Nawal El-Saadawi was born in 1931 into a poor family in Kafr Tahla, Egypt.[89] Describing herself as "a novelist first, a novelist second, a novelist third," El-Saadawi channeled her medically informed activism through the powerful and accessible medium of the novel, using storytelling as a vehicle of social medicine, as social critique or, in her case, social critique as social medicine.[90] A survivor of female genital mutilation (FGM), El-Saadawi's fight for gender equality began early in her life and later extended into the medical field, fulfilling her father's wish for her to pursue a medical career.[91]

Graduating in 1955 from the University of Cairo, El-Saadawi's education confronted her with her own condition as a woman and as a survivor of FGM, irrevocably shaping her voice as a defender of women's health and political integrity, unsilencing what had long been shrouded in guilt and taboo.[92]

Medicine carved El-Saadawi's mind and literary work, helping her become a writer of the truth with "facts and fiction [being] inseparable, like body and mind."[93] Surgery was a life-transforming experience. It broke the fear of the unknown and unleashed an inner independence, allowing her "to talk about all the parts of the body like poets talk of the beating of the heart."[94] Empowered by her education but mocked by her colleagues for "having achieved none of the five goals of the profession: a clinic, a car, a house, a farm, and a bride (or bridegroom)," El-Saadawi had to create a social medicine that would irremediably tie her pen to the scalpel.[95]

The Egyptian psychiatrist's medical practice, particularly among the rural poor, deeply influenced her writing and inspired her internationally acclaimed 1973 novel *Woman at Point Zero*. By blending fiction with reality, and

[89] First published as "Feminism in Egypt: A Conversation with Nawal El Saadawi," an interview with Sarah Graham-Brown, *MERIP Report* 95, March–April 1981, in Nawal El Saadawi, *The Essential Nawal El Saadawi: A Reader*, ed. Adele S. Newson Horst, Zed Essential Feminists (London and New York, NY: Zed; Palgrave Macmillan, 2010), 316.

[90] Homa Khaleeli, "Nawal El Saadawi: Egypt's Radical Feminist," *The Guardian*, April 15, 2010, at: www.theguardian.com/lifeandstyle/2010/apr/15/nawal-el-saadawi-egyptian-feminist.

[91] Khaleeli, "Nawal El Saadawi"; Amira Nowaira, "Foreword" to "Writing and Freedom," in Sadiqi (ed.), *Women Writing Africa*, 285–93; El Saadawi, *The Essential Nawal El Saadawi*, ix.

[92] Nowaira, "Foreword" to "Writing and Freedom," 285.

[93] El Saadawi, *The Essential Nawal El Saadawi*, 9.

[94] El Saadawi, *Death of an Ex-Minister*, trans. Shirley Eber in El Saadawi, *The Essential Nawal El Saadawi*, 221.

[95] El Saadawi, "Writing and Freedom," trans. Amira Nowaira in Sadiqi (ed.), *Women Writing Africa*, 292.

intertwining medicine with politics, El-Saadawi crafted a feminist icon in the novel based on the life of an inmate she had encountered at Al-Qanatir Prison during her research on neurosis in Egyptian women.[96] Through her work, El-Saadawi brought medical literature and narrative medicine to the forefront of her fight for gender equality.

Her sociomedical battles were fierce, costing her the position of editor-in-chief at the Egyptian magazine *Health* in 1972, as well as her roles as Director General of Public Health at the Ministry of Health and Assistant General Secretary of the Medical Association in Egypt.[97] "This was one more consequence of the path," she had chosen "as a feminist author and novelist whose ideas were viewed unfavorably by the authorities."[98] In September 1981, she was arrested by the Egyptian police along with other "Marxists, Nasserites, Islamic scholars, Coptic priests, and feminists."[99] El-Saadawi's three months in prison inspired her *Memoirs from the Women's Prison*, written in her cell on a roll of toilet paper using an eyebrow pencil.[100] Retaliations against El-Saadawi initiated a long cycle of exile and return, mirrored both in her novels and in her life, highlighting the risks of social critique when expressed by a "woman of dark skin."[101] Forced to leave Egypt under Hosni Mubarak's regime, she moved to the United States but returned to Cairo in 1996. In 2004, she made headlines by presenting her candidacy for the Egyptian presidency.[102]

As a prophetess of individuality who defied the conventions of patriarchal lineage, El-Saadawi rejected patronymics, whether from husbands or philosophers, asserting that she did not "carry the names of other people."[103] And while El-Saadawi can undoubtedly be regarded as a revolutionary, she herself offered a critical perspective on the role: "Women should be politically powerful inside a revolution. Otherwise, they may be used by the revolution as tools, as cheap labor, cheap fighters – to die first and be liberated last."[104] Far from

---

[96] El Saadawi, "Preface," in *Woman at Point Zero*, trans. Sherif Hetata (London: Zed Books, 2015), ix.

[97] El Saadawi, *The Essential Nawal El Saadawi*, x; Nowaira, "Foreword" to "Writing and Freedom," 285.

[98] El Saadawi, "Preface," in *Woman at Point Zero*, ix.

[99] El Saadawi, "Preface," in *Woman at Point Zero*, xi; Nowaira, "Foreword" to "Writing and Freedom," in Sadiqi (ed.), *Women Writing Africa*, 286.

[100] Khaleeli, "Nawal El Saadawi."

[101] Khaleeli, "Nawal El Saadawi"; El-Saadawi, "Writing and Freedom," 289.

[102] Ramzi Saiti, "Paradise, Heaven, and Other Oppressive Spaces: A Critical Examination of the Life and Works of Nawal El-Saadawi," *Journal of Arabic Literature* 25, no. 2 (1994): 158, 159, doi.org/10.1163/157006494x00059; Miriam Cooke, "Foreword," in *Woman at Point Zero*, viii.

[103] An interview with the Belgian philosopher Lieven De Cauter, initiator of the Brussels Tribunal on the war in Iraq, at which El Saadawi was a witness. Brussels, February 16, 2007, in El Saadawi, *The Essential Nawal El Saadawi*, 324, 325.

[104] El Saadawi, *The Essential Nawal El Saadawi*, 320.

being merely symbolic, El-Saadawi's social medicine fueled decades of social revolution and critical inquiry.

Concluding Thoughts

This chapter has shown how social medicine functioned both as a clinical analysis of society, aimed at reforming it, and as a tool for protesting the deteriorated health and wealth of colonized, subjugated, and oppressed peoples. We traced the genealogy of social medicine in Arabic and provided several examples of its early practice as social protest and praxis in the twentieth century. Initially directed against various imperial and colonial endeavors in the Arab world, this approach to social medicine later evolved to challenge and resist patriarchal and autocratic regimes.

Since then, the engagement of these "revolutionary social medical doctors," as we have described them, has morphed into numerous movements, associations, and organizations dedicated to advancing social medicine as a form of politics by other means. In a region where homosexuality remains criminalized, sexual health clinics have emerged in the Arab world as acts and sites of resistance, protest, social critique, and advocacy. These clinics operate amid persistent state persecution, stigmatization, and homophobia.[105] Another notable example is the Sudanese Professionals Association, which includes medical doctors and initially campaigned for improved socioeconomic conditions under Omar al-Bashir. The association played a pivotal role in the 2019 protest movement that ousted the longtime autocrat.[106] A month later in Algeria, young doctors joined the Hirak movement as a way to resist an entrenched and corrupt ruling political class.[107] That same year, during the protests in Lebanon, a group of doctors and nurses calling themselves "The White Coats" (al-Qumṣān al-Baiḍā') publicly condemned the serious human rights violations against unarmed protestors who were being shot at indiscriminately (many lost their eyes and incurred serious injuries to the head and heart) in a country already plagued by limited social protections.[108]

---

[105] Leona Zahlan, Nicole Khauli, and Brigitte Khoury, "Sexual Health Services in the Arab Region: Availability, Access, and Utilisation," *Global Public Health* 15, no. 4 (April 2020): 485–96, doi.org/10.1080/17441692.2019.1682029.

[106] Reem Abbas, "How an Illegal Sudanese Union Became the Biggest Threat to Omar Al Bashir's 29-Year Reign," *The National*, January 28, 2019, at: www.thenationalnews.com/world/africa/how-an-illegal-sudanese-union-became-the-biggest-threat-to-omar-al-bashir-s-29-year-reign-1.819159.

[107] Mohamed Mebtoul, *Libertés dignité algérianité: Avant et pendant le « Hirak* (Paris: L'Harmattan, 2019).

[108] Press conference of the "White Coats" doctors on the violations against the demonstrators, Alghad TV, August 14, 2020, at: www.youtube.com/watch?v=v7unXOtgRT4.

A recurring theme in this brief genealogical exercise is the invisibility of the Arab world in the historiographical scholarship on social medicine and the apparent disregard for the health and well-being of over 456 million inhabitants. This neglect persists despite Richard Horton, the editor-in-chief of the influential medical journal *The Lancet*, initiating a bold reflection on "Health in the Arab World,"[109] spurred by the 2011 Arab uprisings. As we saw in Guérin's original articulation and framing of social medicine, indigenous Algerians were excluded from an approach ostensibly designed to aid in the acclimatization of French colonists. At the same time, medical activism has historically served as a powerful tool for political resistance, enabling empowerment and creating spaces of social critique. From the Algerian National Liberation Movement to the Black Panthers and the HIV/AIDS pandemic,[110] and today amid the systematic destruction of Gaza's healthcare infrastructure,[111] health is widely recognized as a basic human right worth fighting and dying for. It also serves as a form of resistance against occupation, injustice, discrimination, racism, and oppression. However, the systematic targeting of healthcare workers and facilities by contemporary regimes in the region (be it in war-torn Syria or in the occupied Palestinian territories) is also becoming increasingly normalized. This trend underscores how medical professionals continue to be a sociopolitical force to reckon with, even in the face of violence and repression.

---

[109] Huda Zurayk et al., "The Making of the *Lancet* Series on Health in the Arab World," *The Lancet* (British Edition) 383, no. 9915 (2014): 393–5, doi.org/10.1016/S0140-6736(13)62370-3.

[110] Adam Schatz, *The Rebel's Clinic: The Revolutionary Lives of Frantz Fanon* (New York, NY: Farrar, Straus and Giroux, 2024), 365.

[111] Joelle M. Abi-Rached, "The War on Hospitals," *Boston Review*, December 20, 2023, at: www.bostonreview.net/articles/the-war-on-hospitals/.

3   Latin American Social Medicine,
         across the Waves

Eric D. Carter

The recent Covid-19 pandemic has prompted renewed appraisals of what makes health systems work – how did different countries cope with the challenges of the pandemic? For Latin America, the overall picture is still inconclusive. In the more pessimistic analyses, countries of the region were ill-prepared for pandemic response and lacked sophisticated social safety nets. The ferocious early wave of Covid-19 in Ecuador, the record-high mortality in Peru, or political divisions over pandemic response in Brazil all seem to substantiate this negative take on Latin America's resilience to health crisis. Such a perspective shares some ground with Marcos Cueto and Steven Palmer's historically informed notion of a "culture of survival" in the region, meaning that "most health interventions directed by states have not sought to resolve recurrent and fundamental problems that, in the final analysis, have to do with the conditions of life."[1]

A more optimistic reading of the situation is that the health and safety of the average person in Latin America is now more highly valued and protected than ever. Across Latin America, there is a broad consensus that health is a human right and that well-functioning health systems may serve as a compensating mechanism for the inequalities that typify many Latin American societies.[2] Some governments performed admirably during the pandemic, not just in places that might be viewed as anomalously efficient (Costa Rica, Uruguay) but also in countries like Ecuador, which, only a year after experiencing the early terrors of the pandemic, rolled out one of the fastest vaccination campaigns in history. In countries where the pandemic response has been disastrous, it is usually because political leaders have gone against the advice of their health experts; the capacity for a more humane, consistent and effective response exists, but may be underutilized. From this vantage point, the

---

[1] Marcos Cueto and Steven Palmer, *Medicine and Public Health in Latin America: A History* (New York, NY: Cambridge University Press, 2015), 7.

[2] Paola M. Sesia, "Global Voices for Global (Epistemic) Justice: Bringing to the Forefront Latin American Theoretical and Activist Contributions to the Pursuit of the Right to Health," *Health and Human Rights* 25 (2023): 140–1.

pandemic demonstrates Cueto and Palmer's contrasting concept, "health in adversity," which "seeks to register the sanitary gains that have been achieved, despite the discourses and practices of hegemonic power, in terms of the adaptations born of questioning, resisting, and proposing alternatives." This view emphasizes the "work of many health professionals, activists, and popular leaders who have developed holistic projects and tried to modify the vicious cycle of poverty–authoritarianism–disease in favor of a more inclusive society and public health."[3]

The spirit of "health in adversity" is embodied in Latin American social medicine, an academic and political movement that, while often working at the margins, has made an outsized impact on health across the region. Many Latin American countries have been able to build robust health systems and raise living standards under conditions of adversity. This change – some might call it progress – did not come overnight, and without tremendous ingenuity, sacrifice, and collective effort. This progress, I would argue, could not have happened without social medicine's efforts to promote health equity.

Latin American social medicine (LASM) is a field that helped produce broad-based public health improvements across the region in the twentieth century. However, the deep historical roots, institutional bases, political influence, and public health achievements of LASM have received scant attention, even with rising interest in the subject among scholars and public health practitioners.[4] In this chapter, I seek to understand the ideological roots of social medicine, how institutional and interpersonal networks supported the diffusion and development of social medicine in Latin America, and how ideas in social medicine translated into social policy. I analyze the shortcomings of previous treatments of the history of social medicine in Latin America and elsewhere, and explain the outline of a useful new narrative of the movement.[5]

First-wave social medicine grew out of the scientific hygiene movement, gained strength in the interwar period, and left its imprint on Latin American welfare states by the 1940s. Second-wave social medicine, marked by more explicitly leftist analytical frameworks, took shape in the early 1970s and crystallized institutionally in the Latin American Social Medicine Association (ALAMES) (regionally) and Brazilian Association of Collective Health

---

[3] Cueto and Palmer, *Medicine and Public Health*, 7–8.
[4] Scott Stonington and Seth M. Holmes, "Social Medicine in the Twenty-First Century," *PLoS Med* 3, no. 10 (2006), Doi: 10.1371/journal.pmed.0030445; Dorothy Porter, "How Did Social Medicine Evolve, and Where Is It Heading?," *PLoS Med* 3, no. 10 (2006), Doi: 10.5860/rusq.53n2.119; Jaime Gofin, "On 'A Practice of Social Medicine' by Sidney and Emily Kark," *Social Medicine* 1, no. 2 (2006): 107–15; Nancy King, *The Social Medicine Reader: Patients, Doctors, and Illness*, 2nd ed. (Durham, NC: Duke University Press, 2005).
[5] For a fuller exploration of this history, see Eric D. Carter, *In Pursuit of Health Equity: A History of Latin American Social Medicine* (Chapel Hill, NC: University of North Carolina Press, 2023).

(ABRASCO) (in Brazil). It is certainly possible to treat these waves as separate and unconnected, given some important differences in theoretical foundations and political praxis. However, I argue that a dialectical process links these two waves into a single history. Early social medicine demands, once institutionalized in welfare states and the international health-and-development apparatus, led to complacency and ineffective bureaucratic routines, which in turn sparked critical reflection, agitation for change, and a new wave of social medicine activism. Disaffected technocrats, often in exile from authoritarian regimes, became the essential nucleus for a second wave of Latin American social medicine. From its rebirth in unorthodox academic networks, LASM would become institutionalized in university programs and help spark national health systems reforms, first in Brazil and eventually in an array of leftist "Pink Tide" governments of the 2000s.

The Contested Historiography of Social Medicine

Social medicine has sometimes been a slippery subject in the historiography of public health and medicine in Latin America. There are three mostly separate scholarly conversations about LASM, crafting different narratives for slightly different audiences: treatments by academic historians of the first wave of social medicine in the region, roughly around the 1920s to the 1940s; an interdisciplinary exploration of the more recent wave of social medicine, starting in the 1970s; and the stories told by LASM insiders and their allies in the North American academy, which paints a portrait of an LASM movement with deep historical roots in European revolutionary socialism going back to the middle of the 1800s.

The mainstream historiography of public health, medicine, and the welfare state in Latin America recognizes a vibrant social medicine movement in the early twentieth century. Case studies from Peru, Mexico, Costa Rica, and Chile suggest that interest in social medicine emerged around the same time in many countries, prompting policy discussions that often led to more robust national systems of social insurance or socialized medicine.[6] Historical accounts of other fields, like eugenics, puericulture, and hygiene, point to overlaps or dialogues with social medicine. In this line of historical research, the connections between national-scale social medicine movements are

---

[6] Ana María Kapelusz-Poppi, "Rural Health and State Construction in Post-revolutionary Mexico: The Nicolaita Project for Rural Medical Services," *The Americas* 58, no. 2 (2001): 261–83; María Eliana Labra, "Medicina social en Chile: Propuestas y debates (1920–1950)," *Cuadernos Médico Sociales (Chile)* 44, no. 4 (2004): 207–19; Marcos Cueto, "Social Medicine in the Andes, 1920–1950," in Esteban Rodríguez Ocaña (ed.), *The Politics of the Healthy Life: An International Perspective* (Sheffield: EAHMH Publications, 2002), 181–96; Steven Palmer, *From Popular Medicine to Medical Populism: Doctors, Healers, and Public Power in Costa Rica, 1800–1940* (Durham, NC: Duke University Press, 2003).

often unspecified. But international institutions (such as the International Labor Organization [ILO] or the League of Nations Health Office [LNHO]) and social policy entrepreneurs (like René Sand of Belgium), are frequently cited for disseminating social medicine ideas from Western Europe to Latin America.[7]

A separate line of research seeks to account for the origins of a second wave of Latin American social medicine, starting around the early 1970s and into the present day. Here, the work of Brazilian scholars stands out for explorations of the country's collective health (*saúde coletiva*) movement, its institutionalization in university programs and civil society organizations, and its influence on milestone reforms to the Brazilian health system in the 1980s (see de Camargo, Chapter 11 in this volume).[8] Other scholars have helped reconstruct the often clandestine international networks that connected social medicine thinkers and practitioners together in the 1970s and early 1980s, when authoritarian governments suppressed leftist thought and forced many health professionals into exile.[9] Participants in second-wave LASM organizations like ALAMES have also contributed accounts of social medicine's origins, including colonial-era antecedents.[10] And historians are now piecing together a more comprehensive history of this era (see Fonseca, Chapter 8 in this volume).

However, the most prominent historical narrative of LASM traces its origins back to the foundational figure of Rudolf Virchow. This pioneering Prussian-German pathologist was active politically in his early career, and his diagnosis of the roots of a typhus epidemic in Upper Silesia in 1848 anticipates the "biosocial" lens of integrative fields like social medicine and social epidemiology (see Timmermann, Chapter 1 in this volume). This standard history of social medicine, with origins in the revolutionary year of 1848, was first crafted by a group of politically progressive European and US historians in the 1930s and 1940s. Henry Sigerist, George Rosen, and Edwin Ackerknecht, in particular, first constructed the image of Virchow as the founder of social medicine, over

---

[7] Eric D. Carter, "Social Medicine and International Expert Networks in Latin America, 1930–1945," *Global Public Health* 14, nos. 6–7 (2019): 791–802.

[8] Everardo Duarte Nunes, "La salud colectiva en Brasil: Analizando el proceso de institucionalización," *Salud Colectiva* 12, no. 3 (2016): 347–60; Sarah Escorel, *Reviravolta na saúde: origem e articulação do movimento sanitário* (Rio de Janeiro: Editora Fiocruz, 1999); Nísia Trindade Lima, José Paranaguá de Santana, and Carlos Henrique Assuncao Paiva (eds.), *Saúde coletiva: a Abrasco em 35 anos de história* (Rio de Janeiro: Editora Fiocruz, 2015).

[9] Diego Galeano, Lucia Trotta, and Hugo Spinelli, "Juan César García and the Latin American Social Medicine Movement: Notes on a Life Trajectory," *Salud Colectiva* 7, no. 3 (2011): 285–315; Hugo Spinelli, Juan Martín Librandi, and Juan Pablo Zabala, "Los Cuadernos Médico Sociales de Rosario y las revistas de la medicina social latinoamericana entre las décadas de 1970 y 1980," *História, Ciências, Saúde-Manguinhos* 24 (2017): 877–95.

[10] Francisco Rojas Ochoa and Miguel Márquez (eds.), *ALAMES en la memoria: selección de lecturas* (La Habana: Editorial Caminos, 2009); Jaime Breilh, *Eugenio Espejo: la otra memoria* (Cuenca: Universidad de Cuenca, 2001).

and above his long-recognized contributions as a pioneer in cellular pathology.[11] Later Sigerist's work was taken up by figures like Milton Roemer, Milton Terris, Vicente Navarro, Gustavo Molina Guzmán, Elizabeth Fee, Nancy Krieger, and Paul Farmer, who represent a vocal leftist-progressive front against business-as-usual in the health field. Virchow's name is often invoked as a symbol of social medicine's transformative potential and revolutionary credentials, as in a 2021 *New York Times* commentary by epidemiologist Jay S. Kaufman.[12]

The genealogical connection between LASM and the founding father figure of Rudolf Virchow became a received narrative through the work of the US sociologist-physician Howard Waitzkin. In a series of articles and books published in the early 2000s, Waitzkin contended that Virchow's student in Germany, Max Westenhöfer, became a mentor to a young Salvador Allende in Chile of the 1930s and inspired his political activism, in the health sector and beyond.[13] This narrative is alluring because of its uncanny historical continuity, with a thread connecting early leftist revolutionaries of Europe to the first wave of social medicine in Latin America, and, over the long arc of Allende's political career, to later promises of socialist governance and its sudden end in the violence of dictatorship – which, in turn, gave rise to the neoliberal development model against which second-wave social medicine has built its identity. Waitzkin's narrative has been widely cited, and often much simplified, in sympathetic accounts of LASM in the Anglophone academic world.[14]

As I have detailed elsewhere (with Marcelo Sánchez Delgado), this version of the history of Latin American social medicine, especially those claims of Virchow's or Westenhöfer's influence on early Latin American social medicine, demands reconsideration.[15] The main problem is that during social medicine's first wave in Latin America, before historians like Sigerist began to

---

[11] Dorothy Porter, "How Did Social Medicine Evolve, and Where Is It Heading?"*PLoS Med* 3, no. 10 (2006): 1667; Dorothy Porter and Roy Porter, "What Was Social Medicine? An Historiographical Essay," *Journal of Historical Sociology* 1, no. 1 (1988): 90–109; Elizabeth Fee, "Henry E. Sigerist: From the Social Production of Disease to Medical Management and Scientific Socialism," *Milbank Quarterly* 67 (1989): 127–50.

[12] Jay S. Kaufman, "Science Alone Can't Heal a Sick Society," *New York Times*, September 10, 2021.

[13] For example, Howard Waitzkin, "Commentary: Salvador Allende and the Birth of Latin American Social Medicine," *International Journal of Epidemiology* 34, no. 4 (August 12005): 739–41. For more details of this historiographic debate, see Eric D. Carter and Marcelo Sánchez Delgado, "Una discusión sobre el vínculo entre Salvador Allende, Max Westenhöfer y Rudolf Virchow: aportes a la historia de la medicina social chilena e internacional," *História, Ciências, Saúde – Manguinhos* 27 (2020): 899–917.

[14] For example, Christopher Hartmann, "Postneoliberal Public Health Care Reforms: Neoliberalism, Social Medicine, and Persistent Health Inequalities in Latin America," *American Journal of Public Health* 106, no. 12 (2016): 2145; Adam Gaffney, *To Heal Humankind: The Right to Health in History* (New York, NY: Routledge, 2018), 67; Porter, "How Did Social Medicine Evolve?," 1668.

[15] Carter and Sánchez Delgado, "Una discusión."

revive the memory of Virchow, he was considered a pioneering biomedical researcher but seldom, if ever, invoked as a forerunner of social medicine. The association between Westenhöfer and Allende is tenuous, if it existed at all, and they did not align ideologically, given that Westenhöfer supported the Third Reich and Allende was resolutely anti-fascist. Additionally, circulation of social medicine ideas, in Chile and across Latin America, clearly predate Allende's medical and political career, although he did become a major figure in Chilean social medicine in the 1930s, as explained below.

More generally, histories of LASM written by committed members of the movement today overlook inconveniently non-leftist social medicine figures of the early twentieth century (such as Carlos Paz Soldán of Peru, Eduardo Cruz-Coke in Chile, or Ramón Carrillo in Argentina); raise up symbolic movement avatars like Che Guevara, who was actually uninvolved in social medicine networks during his lifetime; erase vibrant ideological debates within the movement; and neglect the reasons for social medicine's mid-century ebb before its revival around 1970. By exploring the contributions of a range of actors, taking seriously the genealogy of ideas and ideology, critically evaluating European origin stories, and being attentive to broader political, geopolitical, and scientific contexts, I present a new perspective on the history of LASM.

The First Wave: From Hygiene to Socialized Medicine

Social medicine's first wave emerged from broader discourses on the so-called social question, a confrontation with the changes resulting from rapid capitalist modernization in some Latin American countries. Situated between traditional, conservative elites, on the one hand, and the more radical proposals of movements like anarchism, anarcho-syndicalism, and socialism, the positivist intellectuals drawn to the social question settled largely for a middle way: gradual political reform to channel the demands of the working class, along with social policies meant to improve living standards and mitigate the worst excesses of capitalist development. Under the sway of Comtean positivism, Latin American health reformers saw society as malleable and manageable through the application of scientific knowledge. Reformers also drew occasionally on the notion of "social justice" from Catholic social doctrine, which was essentially the church's doctrinal reckoning with the social question. Major ideological formations of the era – socialism, anarchism, liberalism – do not map neatly on to different types of social medicine. Rather, we find that social medicine blended, eclectically, ideas that may seem ideologically incompatible, as Dorothy Porter suggested.[16]

---

[16] Porter and Porter, "What Was Social Medicine?," 93; Carter and Sánchez Delgado, "Una discusión," 913.

Social medicine's advocates were also fully immersed in the tenets of *higienismo*, the hygiene movement. In a sense, social medicine was a potent expression of the hygiene movement's conviction that society's ills could be managed with the analytical tools of medical science backed by strong states. As Foucault argued in his 1970s essay "The Birth of Social Medicine," the field was not "anti-medicine" but rather it intensified the medicalization of social problems, as developmental states became concerned with the environmental conditions of cities and the productivity of human capital.[17] Social medicine extended the domain of hygienism, as infectious disease epidemics began to wane while chronic, entrenched problems, from alcoholism to malnutrition to child mortality, became more visible. In Latin America, social medicine as an elevated form of *higienismo* was personified in experts like Carlos Enrique Paz Soldán in Peru, Germinal Rodriguez and Ramón Carrillo in Argentina, or Luis Morquio in Uruguay, who often worked in narrower domains like puericulture, sexual hygiene, occupational medicine, nutrition, and rural medicine. They thrived in an era of Latin American "political doctors," liberal scientific modernizers with an often-highhanded view on the working class.

Nowhere in Latin America were medical professionals so engaged politically as in Chile, where social medicine was prominent during an eventful, sometimes turbulent period in the country's political history. Around the end of the First World War, anarchists (or libertarian socialists), such as physician and writer Juan Gandulfo, questioned the necessity of the state and sought to help the working class emancipate itself through grassroots consciousness-raising and health promotion. Progressive physicians, who channeled Gandulfo's radical energy more than his policy ideas, attempted to organize as Chile's first medical labor union, the Sindicato de Médicos, founded in 1924 in the anarcho-syndicalist hotbed of Valparaíso. This union was short-lived but other medical labor organizing followed, in the form of the Vanguardia Médica (Medical Vanguard), aligned with the Chilean Socialist Party, which laid the foundations for the AMECH, the Chilean Medical Association (Figure 3.1). Doctors organized primarily to defend their professional interests and prerogatives within a new social insurance system – the Caja del Seguro Obrero, or CSO – and to avoid being reduced to "mere functionaries" within a large government bureaucracy. But labor organizing in medicine became fractious since there were many competing objectives: maintaining professional autonomy, regulating the practice of medicine, protecting workplace conditions, engaging the political system directly (in elections and legislation), and improving health conditions for all Chileans.

[17] Michel Foucault, "Nacimiento de la medicina social," *Revista Centroamericana de Ciencias de la Salud*, 6 (1977): 91.

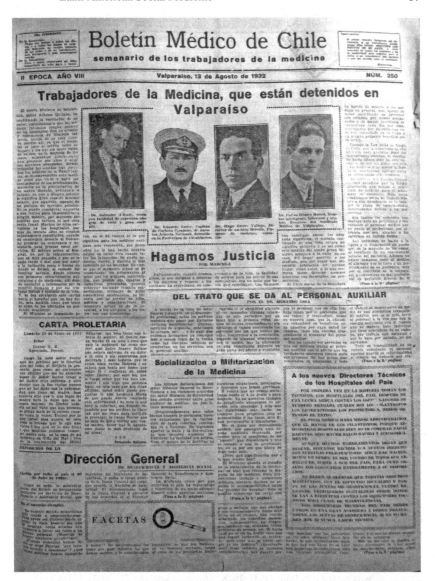

Figure 3.1 Front page of the *Boletín Médico de Chile*, the voice of the Vanguardia Médica, August 13, 1932. This story reports the detention of Salvador Allende (then 24 years old, at left) and other left-wing figures, including doctors and health workers, during a chaotic period known as the "Socialist Republic of Chile."

68	Eric D. Carter

While the social medicine movement was accelerated by leftist political figures, it was not an exclusively socialist project. Salvador Allende, who would prove to be the most famous member of the Vanguardia Médica, attempted to align social medicine with the goals of his Socialist Party. Like Gandulfo, the anarchist doctor, Allende's political career began with organizing students at the University of Chile, coordinating with labor unions and other groups to hold anti-government protests and general strikes. Meanwhile, in a parallel stream within social medicine, a group of relatively conservative doctors influenced by Catholic social doctrine, led by Eduardo Cruz-Coke, worked to improve health conditions through such measures as the Law of Preventive Medicine and the establishment of the National Council on Nutrition. From 1937 to 1942, first Cruz-Coke and then Allende took turns as ministers of health under different governments, using this power effectively to strengthen health policy.[18] Soon after starting his term as Minister of Health, Allende wrote the report *La realidad médico-social chilena*, which later attracted the attention of Waitzkin and other chroniclers of social medicine's history.[19] While Allende and Cruz-Coke maintained amicable relations despite their political rivalry, leftist and conservative factions divided at the birth of AMECH, partly due to Allende's insistence on placing the legalization of abortion on the agenda at the association's first conference, in 1936, sparking a boycott by a group of doctors affiliated with the Catholic University of Chile, including Cruz-Coke.[20]

The ideological diversity within Chilean social medicine helps to explain why, when the legislation that would eventually create Chile's National Health Service (the SNS, or Servicio Nacional de Salud) was introduced to the national congress in 1950, many years after it was first proposed, representatives of almost every political party stood up to claim, legitimately, a role in constructing this national health system.[21] Despite often contentious disagreements, the parties converged in giving priority to social justice, the development of human capital, and the socialization of medicine. From the 1920s to the 1950s, Chilean social medicine was a fluid field of policy experiment, where participants drew inspiration from a hodgepodge of internationally available health policy options and worked to adapt them to their evaluation of Chilean realities. At the same time, as Maria Eliana Labra has argued, existing policy

---

[18] Carlos Huneeus Madge and María Paz Lanas, "Ciencia política e historia. Eduardo Cruz-Coke y el estado de bienestar en Chile: 1937–1938," *Historia (Santiago)* 35 (2002): 151–86.

[19] Waitzkin, "Commentary"; Claudio Schuftan, "Una verdadera joya en los anales de la medicina social: el legado del joven Allende," *Medicina Social* 1, no. 3 (2006): pp. 73–5.

[20] Andrea Del Campo, "El debate médico sobre el aborto en Chile en la década de 1930," in María Soledad Zarate (ed.), *Por la salud del cuerpo: historia y políticas sanitarias en Chile* (Santiago: Ediciones Universidad Alberto Hurtado, 2008), 131–88.

[21] Maria Angélica Illanes, '*En el nombre del pueblo, del estado y de la ciencia': historia social de la salud pública, Chile 1880–1973* (Santiago: Ministerio de Salud, [1993] 2010), 316.

structures, especially the CSO, imposed a path-dependency that bounded the scope of reform proposals.[22]

During this period, networks to support a stable international epistemic community in social medicine were weakly developed. Instead, there was a mix of influences from abroad to support national-level projects of health reform. Although there was no programmatic diffusion of social medicine thought from Europe to Latin America, it is true that the Geneva-based LNHO and ILO offered policy models like social insurance and some support for research into pressing public health issues, like malnutrition and infant mortality. European and North American expertise in such areas was often sought out and welcomed; for example, Allende would draw extensively from a 1935 survey of nutritional conditions in Chile, carried out by two European experts sponsored by the LNHO.[23] Though numerically insignificant and politically marginal at the time, the Latin American left wing – the Apristas and José Carlos Mariátegui of Peru, libertarian socialists, anarchists, and vanguard intellectuals – influenced social medicine, though the interests and preoccupations of medical doctors frequently failed to harmonize with those of the labor movement more broadly.[24] Sometimes there were cross-national policy transfers – as with Costa Rica's "Caja" system of social insurance, which used the Chilean CSO as a blueprint – but mostly social medicine failed to coalesce in sustained institutional form across Latin America.

The Chilean experience from the 1920s to the creation of the SNS in the early 1950s demonstrates an irony of the politics of social medicine: namely, successful strengthening of the state's health institutions tends to undermine social medicine's role as a critical and integrative intellectual field. The Vanguardia Médica saw disease and illness as the end result of a web of causal factors, a fraying of the social fabric that lay mostly outside the domain of medicine. This exercise in causal analysis took political doctors beyond the space of the clinic – either in their mind's eye or in their daily practices – into the slums, the *conventillos*, the rural shanties, and the northern mining towns. Confidence in the new SNS shifted attention to the narrower territory of the health system. The creation of the SNS was a success story for first-wave social medicine, but the old spark of subversive and revolutionary possibilities in social medicine mostly disappeared, supplanted by the concerns and routines of a new generation of health technocrats.

---

[22] Labra, "Medicina Social en Chile," 219.

[23] Carlo Dragoni and Etienne Burnet, "L'alimentation populaire au Chili," *Revista Chilena de Higiene y Medicina Preventiva* 1, no. 10–12 (1938): 407–611.

[24] Carter, "Social Medicine and International Expert Networks."

The Decline of Social Medicine in the Early Cold War

The first wave of Latin American social medicine crested in the late 1940s and over subsequent decades the field and its integrative, holistic, and socially conscious philosophy were marginalized in favor of other, seemingly more "modern" models for improving population health. Examining this time of relative dormancy in social medicine during the 1950s and 1960s, rather than diverting us from the main story, is actually crucial for sharpening our understanding of social medicine, what it meant, and how it was changing.

Social medicine in Latin America faded in this period for many reasons, but two factors must be emphasized. First, the medical profession, on the whole, became more conservative and suspicious of state involvement in the health sector. By the 1960s, concerned over the threat of communism (which, after Cuba's revolution, no longer seemed abstract), doctors as an interest group began to push for greater autonomy from the state and sought distance from the often-chaotic realm of national politics. In Chile, the national medical union, the Colegio Médico, a descendant of the radical AMECH, increasingly acted as a bulwark against further centralization of health services under the SNS. In the early 1970s, the conservative Colegio Médico actively undermined the government of Allende – who had been the organization's first leader – and threw its support behind Pinochet's authoritarian regime.[25] In Argentina, the 1950s and 1960s witnessed doctors' strikes, fragmentation of health insurance and delivery into entities known as *obras sociales*, resistance to the politicization of medical education, and a search for international prestige in medical specialties, all of which prevented the establishment of a centralized health system.

Another important factor was the growth of a powerful international development apparatus that incorporated new social science approaches which, in turn, crowded out social medicine ideas and praxis. The apparatus of modern health planning that developed during this period drew the energy of public health personnel inward, into specialized, professionalized fields, and away from an engagement in the larger political realm to advocate progressive social policies. New "functional international organizations," such as the World Health Organization (WHO), Pan-American Health Organization (PAHO), UNESCO, and the Food and Agricultural Organization, along with international financial institutions (World Bank, IMF, and Inter-American Development Bank), provided career opportunities for health professionals and new ways of thinking about progress through research and planning. Specialized research centers, like the Comisión Económica para América Latina y el Caribe (United Nations

[25] Cueto and Palmer, *Medicine and Public Health*, 202–3.

Economic Commission for Latin America and the Caribbean, CEPAL) and Facultad Latinoamericana de Ciencias Sociales (Latin American School of Social Sciences, FLACSO), both headquartered in Santiago, trained a generation of social scientists to analyze the workings of national societies according to paradigms (positivism, functionalism, behavioralism) that were broadly acceptable internationally and shaped the mindset of mainstream international development institutions, which in turn affected health policy priorities across the region.[26] The idealism, passionate rhetoric, and radical proposals of social medicine were thus at odds with the increasingly technocratic procedures of national health planning in the postwar era.

For progress in health policy, the new social sciences were a double-edged sword: robust research paradigms, and investment in social science research programs, helped to refine and improve health policy but at the same time, the emphasis on rational planning of interventions according to the economic possibilities of each nation tended to sideline concerns over equity and marginalize ideas of the political left. A new generation of pragmatic international technocrats came to power, tailoring their words and actions to the dominant development discourse of the era.[27] The Cold War geopolitical priorities of the United States, as the hemispheric hegemon, promoted this shift in mentality. The Alliance for Progress of the 1960s, as a counter to the Cuban Revolution, intensified US backing of development projects in Latin America (Figure 3.2). And what some have labeled "medical McCarthyism" spread from the US to restrain leftist involvement in health politics across the region (see Fonseca, Chapter 8 in this volume).

It would be a mistake to think that the international health and development technocracy was merely an imposition from the outside; Latin American experts embraced this new "development apparatus," adapting to its norms and creating new possibilities within it. A collaboration between PAHO (Pan-American Health Organization, Organización Panamericana de la Salud, OPS), the CEPAL, and its affiliated economic research institution in Venezuela, the Centro de Estudios del Desarrollo (Center for Development Studies, CENDES), launched the influential OPS/CENDES health planning method, which trained over 5,000 health ministry bureaucrats from across the Latin America region.[28]

[26] On CEPAL's inner workings and international impact, see Margarita Fajardo, *The World That Latin America Created: The United Nations Economic Commission for Latin America in the Development Era* (Cambridge, MA: Harvard University Press, 2022).

[27] Arturo Escobar, *Encountering Development: The Making and Unmaking of the Third World* (Princeton, NJ: Princeton University Press, 1995), 86; Fernando A. Pires-Alves and Marcos Chor Maio, "Health at the Dawn of Development: The Thought of Abraham Horwitz," *História, Ciências, Saúde-Manguinhos* 22, no. 1 (2015): 69–93.

[28] Clara Fassler, "Transformación social y planificación de salud en América Latina," *Rev. Centroamericana de Ciencias de la Salud* 13 (1979): 151; author interview with Mario Testa, 2015.

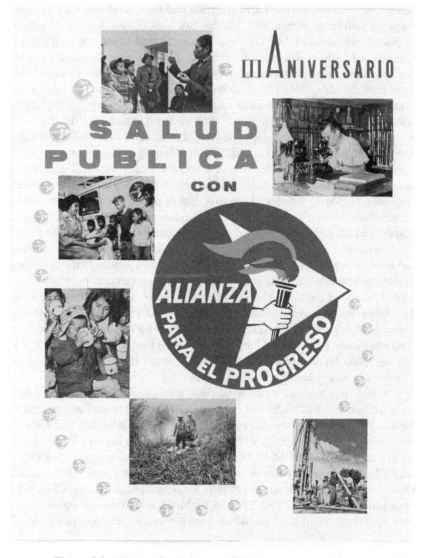

Figure 3.2 Alliance for Progress public health promotion poster. U.S. Information Agency. Bureau of Programs. Press and Publications Service. Publications Division. July 27, 1964. US National Archives, NAID 6949337.

Abraham Horwitz, a veteran of the Chilean SNS, who came to lead the PAHO from 1958 to 1974, embodied a pragmatic new approach, leveraging the resources of the new development apparatus (including funds from the Alliance for Progress) to create new professional opportunities for Latin American health workers, address persistent public health problems, and shield the health sector from the vicissitudes of national health politics. Benjamin Viel – like Horwitz, part of a nucleus of Chilean *salubristas* trained at Johns Hopkins' school of public health – found ways to use the flow of development money (for family planning projects in the 1960s, for example), to continue community-oriented, proto-PHC projects within the SNS.[29] Such projects were grounded in the model of "preventive medicine," which emphasized behavior modification to minimize health risks, while avoiding discussion of structural determinants of those risks.[30] Thanks to the influence of PAHO technical assistance, public health education in Argentina became increasingly professionalized and immersed in modernizationist theories of cultural change.[31]

Thus, social medicine was temporarily displaced in the discourses of medicine, public health, and health planning during the early Cold War period. Its holism, appeals to diverse philosophical influences, incoherence as a scholarly field, and lack of a research agenda all marginalized social medicine in the realm of medical education, increasingly under the hegemony of the ideas of Abraham Flexner and his reforms of medical education in the US, starting at Johns Hopkins.[32] Meanwhile, in response to geopolitical pressures and following the technocratic development logic of the Cold War, the WHO turned its back on rights-based, horizontal approaches that required comprehensive, critical analysis of social inequalities.[33]

As health system planners developed specialized expertise, they narrowed their scope of action and became more reductionist in their understanding of how to improve population health conditions. The growth of a postwar international development apparatus encouraged these habits of mind and ways of thinking; professional survival and advancement depended on incorporation

---

[29] Eric D. Carter, "Population Control, Public Health, and Development in Mid Twentieth Century Latin America," *Journal of Historical Geography* 62 (2018): 96–105; Jadwiga E. Pieper-Mooney, "From Cold War Pressures to State Policy to People's Health: Social Medicine and Socialized Medical Care in Chile," in Anne-Emanuelle Birn and Raúl Necochea López (eds.), *Peripheral Nerve: Health and Medicine in Cold War Latin America* (Durham, NC: Duke University Press, 2020), 187–210.

[30] Gustavo Molina Guzmán and Claudio Jimeno, "Teaching Social Science Concepts in a Clinical Setting in Preventive Medicine," *Milbank Memorial Fund Quarterly* 44, no. 2 (1966): 211–25; Porter, "How Did Social Medicine Evolve?," 1669.

[31] Federico Rayez, "La Organización Panamericana de la salud en Argentina. El caso de la Escuela de Salud Pública de la Universidad de Buenos Aires (1960–1976)," *Asclepio* 75, no. 2 (2023): e34; Carla Reyna, *Educación sanitaria y desarrollismo: Argentina, 1960–1970* (Buenos Aires: Biblos, 2023), 142–8.

[32] Porter, "Social Medicine and the New Society," 182.

[33] Marcos Cueto, Theodore M. Brown, and Elizabeth Fee, *World Health Organization: A History* (Cambridge: Cambridge University Press, 2019); Randall M. Packard, *A History of Global Health: Interventions into the Lives of Other Peoples* (Baltimore: Johns Hopkins University Press, 2016).

into techno-bureaucratic systems. The successful figures in Latin American health of this era – people like Horwitz, or Viel – "stayed in their lanes" not just for the sake of professional self-preservation but also because it promised the best chance for success, which they defined as measurable improvement in population health outcomes. Meanwhile, radical voices from early social medicine, like Josué de Castro of Brazil, found themselves increasingly out of step with the times. Though his famous book *The Geography of Hunger* featuring holistic, integrative, and politically charged analysis of the social causes of hunger, malnutrition, and child mortality was widely read for a while, he was increasingly alienated from the centers of power of the international development apparatus and exiled from Brazil soon after the military took over the government in 1964.[34]

Second Wave: A New Latin American Social Medicine

Disenchanted technocrats, not revolutionaries, would spark the second wave of Latin American social medicine in the 1970s. The political energy of the first wave of social medicine ebbed in the 1950s and 1960s, as international health institutions expanded and consolidated their power in a larger apparatus of modernization and development. As time went on, however, a small but influential faction of technical and administrative personnel in the international health and development apparatus grew disillusioned with ineffective bureaucratic routines and sterile, uncritical discourses about public health (including the field of "preventive medicine," which had become a politically neutered variant of social medicine). The harshly repressive dictatorships of the 1970s imposed severe constraints on the budding new wave of LASM, but such political pressures also fostered movement solidarity.

The new social medicine emerged during a period of broader intellectual ferment in Latin America. Overall, these intellectual influences can be described as leftist, anti-authoritarian, and skeptical of Western modernity. While not exactly part of the international "counterculture," the new generation of LASM was certainly stimulated by changing times, marked by decolonization, student protests, anti-war demonstrations, church reforms, new musical styles, and other signals of the disintegration of old orthodoxies and the crisis of modernity in the West. In the domain of development studies, dependency theory broke out of *cepalino* circles into the widely broadcast polemics of Andre Gunder Frank and Eduardo Galeano. Meanwhile, Paulo Freire, whose *Pedagogy of the Oppressed* was published in Brazil in 1968, explained how Western education tended to reproduce oppressive and hierarchical social structures. Che Guevara

---

[34] Carter, "Population Control, Public Health, and Development"; Federico Ferretti, "A Coffin for Malthusianism: Josué de Castro's Subaltern Geopolitics," *Geopolitics* (2019): 1–26.

was an indirect but potent influence on social medicine for his ideas of the communist "new man" and the "revolutionary doctor" but more importantly, as a model for turning ideology into decisive, radical action.[35] Older Marxist intellectuals, from Marx and Engels, to Gramsci and Mariátegui, were rediscovered, reread, and incorporated into the canon of university courses in politics and sociology in Latin America.[36] The political climate of the time, marked by the Cuban Revolution, student protests in Mexico in 1968, and the violent overthrow of Allende's government in 1973, added urgency to social medicine debates, and created the conditions for the formation of a core group of social medicine theorists in exile.

It was disaffected health technocrats who brought such social theory into conversations about medical education and health policy while also building the networks that would coalesce in the new wave of social medicine. In particular, the Argentinean Juan César García coordinated, sometimes covertly, the activity taking place in nodes of new social medicine thought. García skillfully leveraged his high-level position in PAHO's department of medical education to spread new ideas and, just as importantly, connect health workers across the hemisphere who were interested in critique of conventional health planning and more radical theories of social change. Mario Testa, a leader of the OPS/CENDES health planning program in the 1960s, became a fierce critic of such technocratic efforts. Health planning, he now argued, not only failed on its own terms, but also depoliticized the underlying problem of social inequality. For much the same reason, Sérgio Arouca took aim at conventional preventive medicine programs in Brazil.[37] Extending this critique, Francisco de Assis Machado, along with Arouca, Testa, and others, attempted to enact a new model of community-organized healthcare in the Montes Claros project, in the state of Minas Gerais.[38]

Social medicine's resurgence came amidst the brutality of dictatorship, and the experience of repression and exile forced the leftist-progressive group of Latin American doctors, health workers, and health social scientists to band together. From the mid-1960s until the mid-1980s, Argentina, Chile, and Brazil were under authoritarian governments for extended periods. Exiles from Argentina (such as Testa, José Carlos Escudero, and Hugo Mercer) and Chile (including numerous officials of the Ministry of Health or staff of the School of Public Health in Santiago during Allende's

---

[35] "Juan Carlos Concha, ex Ministro de Salud de Allende: 'Salud Integral e Igual para Todos.'" Red Digital, 22 October 2015, at: https://reddigital.cl/juan-carlos-concha-ex-ministro-de-salud-de-allende-salud-integral-e-igual-para-todos/

[36] Everardo Duarte Nunes, "Las ciencias sociales en salud en América Latina: Una historia singular," Espacio Abierto 6, no. 2 (1997): 228.

[37] Sérgio Arouca, O dilema preventivista (São Paulo: Unesp, [1975] 2003).

[38] Sonia Fleury Teixeira, Projeto Montes Claros: a utopia revisada (Rio de Janeiro: Abrasco, 1995).

ill-fated government, like Gustavo Molina Guzmán or Clara Fassler), found safe harbor in universities, hospitals, and health projects in other Latin American countries, the US, and Europe. Under more open political conditions, the ideas of the new social medicine might have been assimilated, as in the earlier period, into the structures of national welfare states and international health bureaucracies – tamed, so to speak. But in the 1970s, the group of leftist health workers in exile was too large and too unorthodox ideologically to be digested into the machinery of official international development. Instead, they formed a new identity as a cohesive outsider group through their far-flung networks.

The "second wave" of LASM was distinctive from what came before for many reasons, first among them a serious consideration of social theory. During social medicine's first wave, the social sciences as systematic disciplines were hardly known in Latin American universities. Thus, members of the early social medicine milieu were mostly medical doctors who employed eclectic conceptual frames that drew inspiration from natural sciences (positivism, eugenics, hygienism), along with Catholic social doctrine and medical humanism. By contrast, in the 1970s, new theoretical currents from the social sciences, including structural Marxism, feminism, post-structuralism, and post-colonialism, reinvigorated social medicine thought. The new generation in social medicine mobilized such theory to take on functionalism, positivism, behavioralism, and developmentalism (*desarrollismo*), which were the intellectual and ideological pillars of the international health and development apparatus. Though many in the second wave of social medicine were trained in medicine, scholars like Eduardo Menéndez, Susana Belmartino, and Maria Cecília Donnangelo were not health professionals but social scientists who trained their critical lenses on medicine as a socially powerful institution.[39]

The new wave of social medicine coincided with growing suspicion of Western medicine. In Brazil, living under a military regime sharpened the *saúde coletiva* group's critical portrayal of medicine as an institution of discipline, punishment, and social control. This perspective was informed by influences from abroad, such as the pioneering work of Michel Foucault (in books like *Discipline and Punish* or *The Birth of the Clinic*, which found a receptive audience in Brazilian academia – see de Camargo, Chapter 11 in this volume); the Italian mental health reform movement led by Franco Basaglia in the 1960s; and the critical humanism of Ivan Illich, the firebrand Catholic priest based in Cuernavaca, Mexico, whose book *Medical Nemesis* offered

---

[39] Vicente Navarro, based for much of his career at Johns Hopkins University, is Catalonian but closely tied to leftist solidarity networks in Latin American health; though known as a sociologist and political scientist, he was also trained in medicine.

a polemical takedown of the medical establishment.[40] Illich was also part of the Liberation Theology movement, which had an important, though sometimes latent, influence on the integration of a social justice vision into Latin American health systems. Most academics in social medicine avoided overt discussion of religion but coalition-building with ecclesiastical base communities (*comunidades eclesiais de base*) and Catholic charity groups was a crucial part of the long process of Brazilian health systems reform.

These new endeavors sought not only to improve population health, but also to change the prevailing *style of learning* that characterized international development work. This style of learning depended on the top-down transmission of models created by experts in specific domains, so that most health planners hardly understood their models and analytic procedures well enough to offer cogent critiques or adjust them to local circumstances. And yet, nearly all the institutions and projects central to the new social medicine – graduate programs in Mexico and Brazil, the Cuenca meetings, *Educación Médica y Salud*, the Montes Claros project – received funding and support from PAHO, USAID, or the US-based Kellogg Foundation. As a whole, the network placed more value on the open exchange of ideas and information, and the maintenance of protective friendships, than the enforcement of any one ideological party line. Thus, the many social medicine journals created in that decade – *Saúde em Debate, Salud Problema, International Journal of Health Services, Cuadernos Médicos Sociales* (of Rosario, Argentina) – aired theory from many different quarters, usually leftist but drawing from the many varieties of Marxist theory, post-structuralism, feminism, and phenomenology.[41] More broadly, we could say that LASM became a part of the international civil society milieu that developed starting in the late 1960s, from pro-democracy movements to human rights organizations like Amnesty International that put pressure on military dictatorships, international financial institutions, and multinational corporations. Eventually, soon after Juan Cesar García's untimely death in 1984, and coinciding with the slow return to democracy in the region, these networks coalesced in the formation of ALAMES, an international association of professionals in social medicine.

---

[40] Paula Gaudenzi and Francisco Ortega, "O estatuto da medicalização e as interpretações de Ivan Illich e Michel Foucault como ferramentas conceituais para o estudo da desmedicalização," *Interface-Comunicação, Saúde, Educação* 16 (2012): 21–34; Livia Penna Tabet, Valney Claudino Sampaio Martins, Ana Caroline Leoncio Romano, Natan Monsores de Sá, and Volnei Garrafa, "Ivan Illich: da expropriação à desmedicalização da saúde," *Saúde em Debate* 41 (2017): 1187–98; author interview with Fernando Pires and Carlos Henrique Paiva, July 26, 2017; author interview with Mario Rovere, 2015; John Foot, "Franco Basaglia and the Radical Psychiatry Movement in Italy, 1961–78," *Critical and Radical Social Work* 2, no. 2 (2014): 235.

[41] Spinelli, Librandi, and Zabala, "Los *Cuadernos Médico Sociales* de Rosario."

78   Eric D. Carter

Conclusions

Social medicine began as an offshoot of the hygiene movement, especially as public health policy concerns began to move away from infectious disease and sanitation, into more chronic population health issues, during the construction of Latin American welfare states. The first wave of social medicine, with its integrative, systemic, and holistic perspective, was helped along by support from international players like the League of Nations and ILO, although they were less important than networks of hygienists and health and social policy experts within Latin America. During the early Cold War period, social medicine faded internationally and in Latin America. A growing international health and development apparatus promoted narrow, specific projects and avoided contentious political questions. Social medicine seemed a relic alongside more scientific and supposedly apolitical approaches like health systems planning, preventive medicine, and disease eradication campaigns. But, disaffected technocrats within this larger apparatus proved to be the nucleus for the second wave of social medicine in Latin America in the early 1970s. The authoritarian regimes of the 1970s sent Chilean, Argentinean, and Brazilian health workers into exile, and they formed solidarity networks, programs of study in social medicine, new journals, and, eventually, international associations like ALAMES. The second wave of social medicine (in Brazil, collective health) led directly to major health systems reform in Brazil; offered imaginative ways of thinking about health, disease, and society; resisted the incursions of neoliberalism in the health sector; and shaped health policy of "Pink Tide" governments of the region, like Venezuela under Hugo Chavez, after the year 2000.[42]

From this analysis, I draw three major lessons, which might inform not only the historiography on health and medicine in Latin America, but also affect the way we understand social medicine's relationship to health systems in dynamic societies. First, we should be careful about linking LASM with European and North American intellectual and political movements. Certainly, there were influences on LASM from outside the region, but contrary to Virchow-centric histories, LASM was never in a state of ideological or intellectual dependency on European social medicine. Characteristically, LASM activist-academics have been engaged in deep analysis of national problems and connected in regional-scale (Latin American) expert networks. Such networks help to develop a geographical imaginary, a consciousness of Latin Americanism within (and against) the international economic and geopolitical order.[43] LASM has been fueled by homegrown or autochthonous

[42] Hartmann, "Postneoliberal Public Health Care Reforms"; Amy Cooper, *State of Health: Pleasure and Politics in Venezuelan Health Care under Chávez* (Berkeley: University of California Press, 2019).
[43] Fajardo, *The World That Latin America Created.*

social theories, whether dependency theory, liberation theology, or Freire's critical theories of education, or the *buen vivir* philosophy more recently. In this way, LASM is part of a larger trend of constructing an "alternative" and "decolonial" epistemology of health, from the Global South.[44] As part of this larger effort, argues Mexican anthropologist Paola Sesia, Latin American social medicine needs accurate and complete histories of its origins and development, to "counteract the epistemic injustice" of hegemonic, Eurocentric historical narratives of the field.[45]

Second, the history of LASM must be placed in the history of the social sciences in Latin America. In the early 1900s, the pioneers of LASM used eclectic analytical frames mixing social and natural sciences to analyze the roots of public health problems. As LASM matured, starting in the early 1970s, we see the development and influence of Marxist and poststructural theories that offered critical analytical tools to understand the role of health institutions in reproducing inequitable political-economic systems and cultural norms. Moreover, the professionalization and rising prestige of social scientists, especially sociologists, anthropologists, and historians, means that social medicine (and *saúde coletiva*), as an academic field, has considerable autonomy from the biomedical mainstream. While recent work like Margarita Fajardo's *The World That Latin America Created*, on the CEPAL and the complicated rise of dependency theory in development economics, represent tremendous progress, the historiography of the *social sciences* in the region is still in its infancy, as compared to the much deeper explorations of histories of natural sciences, medicine, and public health.[46]

Lastly, *social medicine's influence on health policy must be understood dialectically*. Social medicine promotes often radical transformation of the health sector. However, successful reforms produce technocratic institutions to implement and manage more equitable and far-reaching health policies (like primary healthcare). This institutionalization inevitably defuses the radical outsider spirit of social medicine. And while LASM has empowered the medical community, physicians' own professional and class interests often diverge, eventually, from a progressive health agenda. In this long-term dialectic process, militancy leads to policy achievements, which lead to institutionalization – a narrowing of focus and concentration of effort along technical lines. When the institutions are thrown into crisis, or fail to respond to the new demands of organized sectors, disillusionment and critique rise and may initiate new cycles

---

[44] Gonzalo Basile, "Hacia una salud desde el Sur: epistemología decolonial y de soberanía sanitaria," *Medicina Social* 15 (2022): 65–72; Hartmann, "Postneoliberal Public Health Care Reforms"; Jaime Breilh, *Critical Epidemiology and the People's Health* (Oxford: Oxford University Press, 2021).

[45] Sesia, "Global Voices for Global (Epistemic) Justice," 143.

[46] Fajardo, *The World That Latin America Created*.

of activism. When we think of social medicine dialectically – as a field of radical critique, interacting with the mainstream – we see that this relationship is laden with contradictions that keep social medicine from ever becoming the dominant principle or perspective in health politics.

From the 1920s to today, social medicine changes in response to dynamic political conditions and academic innovations. Like an organism that evolves in response to changes in the environment around it, social medicine has shed certain values, concepts, and associations (eugenics, medical paternalism, hygienicist moralizing) while gaining new ones (more sophisticated social theories, flattening hierarchies in the health field, stronger connections to other social movements, a commitment to participatory democracy). Despite its internal diversity and fluctuations in broader influence, social medicine nonetheless remains recognizable and consistent over the long run, with its critical perspectives on mainstream medicine, commitment to health equity, and advocacy for strong state involvement in the health sector.

4   Imperial Social Medicine in Southeast Asia

The Bandung Intergovernmental Conference on Rural Hygiene

Laurence Monnais and Hans Pols

In August 1937, more than 80 delegates from ten "Far Eastern" Asian colonized regions and three independent countries gathered in fashionable and cool Bandung, a new and modern city situated in a mountainous area immediately south of the slopes of the modestly active volcano Tangkuban Perahu ("upturned prau"), visible on the northern skyline on a clear day.[1] Bandung is a mere 160 kilometers southeast of Batavia (today's Jakarta), the capital of the Dutch East Indies, and can be reached by a scenic train ride. These delegates, joined by international health experts, assistants and observers including representatives from the Indian Research Fund Association, the League of Red Cross Societies, and the Rockefeller Foundation, long active in international health initiatives – nearly 200 individuals in all – attended the Intergovernmental Conference of Far-Eastern Countries on Rural Hygiene, organized by the League of Nations Health Organization (LNHO). The conference met at the main building of the recently established Technical School, which had a traditional Minangkabau appearance but was built with modern construction methods (Figure 4.1). It was accompanied by an impressive exhibition in the nearby trade fair building (Jaarbeurs).[2] The local hosts clearly hoped to impress the international visitors by presenting an event as lavish as the Depression era would allow. The postal service even set up a small post office close to the conference site where mail was stamped with "Rural Hygiene Conference" (Figure 4.2). Both Dutch and Malay Dutch East Indies newspapers reported extensively on the conference.

---

[1] The colonized areas represented were: Burma, French Indochina (Vietnam, Cambodia, and Laos), the Dutch East Indies (Indonesia), British India, Ceylon, British Malaya, British North Borneo, Fiji and the Western Pacific, Hong Kong, and the Philippines; independent countries represented included Japan, China, and Siam (Thailand). On the city of Bandung, see Farabi Fakih, "Colonial Domesticity and the Modern City: Bandung in the Early Twentieth-Century Netherlands Indies," *Journal of Urban History* 49, no. 3 (2023): 645–67.

[2] League of Nations Health Organization, *Guide Book for the Intergovernmental Conference of Far-Eastern Countries on Rural Hygiene* (Batavia: Kolff, 1937).

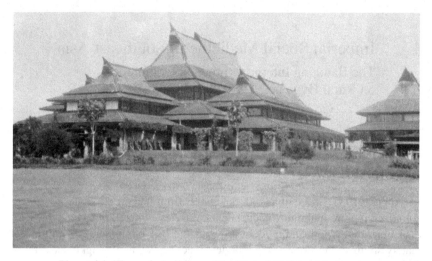

Figure 4.1 The main building of the Technical School in Bandung, erected in the style common among the Minangkabau of Western Sumatra. The meetings were held in this building. Image collection of the KITLV, housed at Leiden University Libraries, The Netherlands.

According to a Sundanese folktale, the Tangkuban Perahu volcano and the adjacent Bandung basin were created by a local deity who smashed the large prau he had just completed to assuage his anger and disappointment. As a child, he had been banished from the household of his mother, a princess who had been expelled from her parents' palace, after he had killed a large dog and gave its liver to his mother, who cooked and ate it. Unbeknownst to him, this dog was his own father. When mother and son reunited years later, they failed to recognize each other, fell in love, and planned to marry. Just before the marriage would take place, the princess recognized her son's birthmark and tried to avert their wedding by setting him an impossible task: to create, overnight, a lake (which later became the Bandung basin) and a large prau to traverse it.[3] Her plan was successful: her son was utterly disappointed, threw the prau away, and drained the lake. This Sundanese Oedipus had killed his father but did not get to marry his mother.

Several medical historians, global health experts, and international relations specialists have analyzed the legacy of the 1937 Bandung Conference in the areas of international health, social medicine, and primary healthcare.

---

[3] Oman Abdurahman and Denny Sukamto Kadarisman, "Geomythology as a Geotourism Attraction, Case Study: The Sangkuriang Legend in the Bandung Highland and Its Surrounding Areas Based on Geological to Hermeneutics Interpretation," *International Journal of Geotourism Science and Development* 2, no. 1 (2022): 34–40.

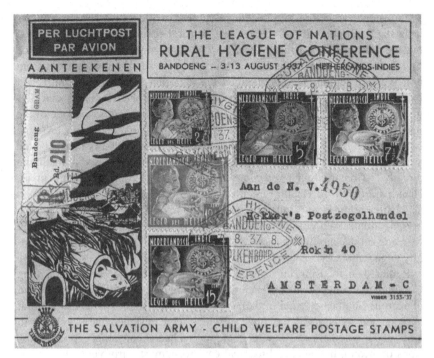

Figure 4.2 An envelope issued for the Bandung Conference with a special postage mark reading, "Rural Hygiene Conference, Bandoeng, Volkenbond [League of Nations]." A small post office was erected near the meeting hall to stamp all outgoing mail. The envelope displays a rat poking its head from a bamboo pole, which refers to the bubonic plague epidemic that had been ravaging Java over the previous twenty years. Note the stamps dedicated to the (Dutch) Salvation Army.

Most view it as a landmark event in the history of international health and a precursor to the 1978 Alma-Ata Declaration on Primary Health Care.[4] Theodore Brown and Elizabeth Fee, for example, characterize "Bandung" as

---

[4] Among these accounts are: Niels Brimnes, "Bandung Revisited: From Rural Hygiene to Primary Health Care," in Haakon A. Ikonomou and Karen Gram-Skjoldager (eds.), *The League of Nations: Perspectives from the Present* (Aarhus: Aarhus University Press, 2019), 172–81; Tomoko Akami, "Imperial Polities, Intercolonialism, and the Shaping of Global Governing Norms: Public Health Expert Networks in Asia and the League of Nations Health Organization, 1908–37," *Journal of Global History* 12, no. 1 (2017): 4–25; Randall Packard, *A History of Global Health: Interventions into the Lives of other Peoples* (Baltimore: Johns Hopkins University Press, 2016); Annick Guénel, "The 1937 Bandung Conference on Rural Hygiene: Toward a New Vision of Healthcare?," in Laurence Monnais and Harold J. Cook (eds.), *Global Movements, Local Concerns: Medicine and Health in Southeast Asia* (Singapore: National University of Singapore Press, 2012), 62–80; Iris Borowy, *Coming to Terms with*

a "milestone event" in health and development, while Randall Packard views it as the "culmination" of the interest in rural reconstruction and hygiene outside Europe.[5] According to Iris Borowy, the conference was one of the first major international public health meetings hosting representatives from non-Western regions who challenged the idea that there was one universal model for health.[6] The highly respected and outspoken Polish bacteriologist and LNHO medical director Dr. Ludwik Rajchman, who gave one of the opening addresses, was probably the first to revisit the meeting. In 1938, he extolled the "Bandung spirit" and argued that it "was probably the first time a governmental conference was able to face the problems of social medicine directly."[7] Constructing a genealogy to the Alma Ata conference on Primary Health Care, World Health Organization (WHO) General-Director Halfdan T. Mahler referred to "Bandung" to support his own agenda to replace the organization's then common techno-centrism and vertical interventions by focusing on decentralizing services, intersectoral collaboration, and community engagement.[8]

Rather than focusing on its legacy, this chapter focuses on the Bandung Conference's antecedents. We view "Bandung" as a synthetic formulation of various Southeast Asian initiatives, experiments, and experiences in rural hygiene and social medicine, most of which were designed and developed in areas under colonial rule. Experts in the region had already engaged in discussions on health, hygiene, and medical care for almost thirty years, for example at the biennial meetings of the Far Eastern Tropical Medicine Association (FEATM), which was founded in 1908.[9] Physicians, both European (colonial) and Southeast Asian (colonized), frequently traveled within the region to observe healthcare initiatives.[10] Through expert networks, meetings, and site visits, physicians and other experts collectively developed expertise in health relevant to Southeast Asia. At the time of the Bandung Conference, several

World Health: The League of Nations Health Organisation 1921–1946 (Frankfurt am Main: Peter Lang, 2014); Theodore M. Brown and Elizabeth Fee, "The Bandoeng Conference of 1937: A Milestone in Health and Development," *American Journal of Public Health* 98, no. 1 (2008): 40–3; Lion Murard, "Designs within Disorder: International Conferences on Rural Health Care and the Art of the Local, 1931–39," in Susan Gross Solomon, Lion Murard, and Patrick Zylberman (eds.), *Shifting Boundaries of Public Health: Europe in the Twentieth Century* (Rochester, NY: University of Rochester Press, 2008), 141–74; and Sunil S. Amrith, *Decolonizing International Health: India and Southeast Asia, 1930–1965* (Basingstoke: Palgrave Macmillan, 2006).

[5] Brown and Fee, "The Bandoeng Conference," 40–3; Packard, *History of Global Health*, 87.

[6] Borowy, *Coming to Terms*, 347–56.   [7] Guénel, "The 1937 Bandung Conference," 62.

[8] Halfdan Mahler, "Promotion of Primary Health Care in Member Countries of WHO," *Public Health Reports* 93, no. 2 (1978): 107–13.

[9] Akami, "Imperial Politics," 5–6.

[10] Claire Edington and Hans Pols, "Building Southeast Asian Psychiatric Expertise: Site Visits, Scientific Journeys, and Medical Exchanges between French Indochina and the Dutch East Indies, 1898–1937," *Comparative Studies in Society and History* 58, no. 3 (2016): 636–63.

colonial governments had implemented decentralization policies to deal with the economic consequences of the Great Depression. Their health departments followed suit but attempted to make a virtue out of necessity by claiming that health interventions were ideally designed to respond to local conditions and the health needs of rural communities.

The Great Depression hit the region hard, leading to increased poverty, malnutrition, and decreased expenditures on health and medical services. In the 1930s, malaria, famine, and colonial exploitation affected the already poor health of colonized populations, forcefully illustrating the social dimensions of health and well-being. The Depression also fueled political unrest in the region. Nationalist movements, in which indigenous health personnel played significant roles, became increasingly vocal, demanding improvements in healthcare provision for indigenous populations.[11] Politically, developing health solutions for the mostly rural Southeast Asian populations therefore became more urgent while the funds to implement these plans were scarcer than ever. During the 1930s, health departments aspired to do much more but had to do so with much less. Both factors, political unrest and a lack of meaningful financial resources, inspired the discussions at the Bandung Conference. In this chapter, we explore the meanings of social medicine and rural hygiene in Southeast Asian contexts, where health measures were tied to (colonial) economic objectives, health budgets were limited, and populations mostly rural. We primarily focus on French Indochina and the Dutch East Indies. With 21 delegates, French Indochina (9) and the Dutch East Indies (12), which hosted the event, clearly played a significant part in both organizing and running the conference.

Before "Bandung": Rural Hygiene and Social Medicine in Southeast Asia

After the First World War, international interest in medical care and public health intensified, initially focusing on preventing the global spread of epidemics. The various colonial empires became increasingly interested in improving the health of colonized populations. These interests motivated the establishment, in 1924, of the League of Nations Health Organization to collect and distribute information, organize international health projects, and advise the League of Nation's Council. Dr. Rajchman served as its medical director from its inception to 1939. Under his leadership, the LHNO promoted cooperation and exchange between countries through conferences and expert missions.

---

[11] Warwick Anderson and Hans Pols, "Scientific Patriotism: Medical Science and National Self-Fashioning in Southeast Asia," *Comparative Studies in Society and History* 54, no. 1 (2012): 93–113.

In 1915, the Rockefeller Foundation had established the International Health Board (IHB), directed by physician Victor Heiser, former Director of Health for the Philippines. The IHB funded most of the activities of the LHNO and various health initiatives worldwide. In 1925, the LNHO established an Eastern Bureau in Singapore to collect epidemiological intelligence; at the same time, the IHB started to promote intercolonial cooperation in Asia.[12] The Far Eastern Association for Tropical Medicine had been established in 1908 to provide physicians, public health, and other experts working in Southeast Asia with opportunities to exchange ideas, share discoveries and the results of local initiatives, and to present a voice to influence health-governing agendas.[13] These three organizations established and funded a dynamic intercolonial network of physicians working in Southeast Asia, who collectively developed a specifically Southeast Asian body of knowledge and expertise in health, hygiene, and medicine.

In the aftermath of the 1929 economic crisis, the LHNO encouraged further intercolonial cooperation. Colonial public health experts discussed how to improve the health of "rural masses," and the connections between poverty, malnutrition, and poor health, and came to emphasize the need for social and economic improvement through rural reconstruction.[14] According to Brimnes, rural hygiene connected health, nutrition, and agriculture to the principles of social medicine by promoting simple, broad, and affordable solutions to health problems such as general sanitation, better housing, improved nutrition, and expanded educational facilities.[15] Because health was related to several social and economic variables, health experts became increasingly convinced that these variables needed to be addressed as well.

In 1930, the LNHO organized a conference on rural health centers – clinics offering basic medical services – in Budapest.[16] In July 1931, it held it first rural hygiene conference in Geneva, focusing on Europe, followed by two Pan-African conferences. The first one, held in 1932, called for an integrative approach to curative and preventive interventions and services, and for cooperation among different fields of expertise and departments – agriculture, veterinary services, and education. The second one, held in 1935, recommended that local healthcare infrastructure were staffed with local personnel and emphasized the importance of economic growth for health. In Asia, the League of Nations organized several meetings on "social questions," including opium control (Bangkok, 1931) and the trafficking of women and children

---

[12] Amrith, *Decolonizing International Health*, 25. One of its first meetings was the International Sanitary Convention, which was held in Melbourne, Australia. See Anne Sealey, "Globalizing the 1926 International Sanitary Convention," *Journal of Global History* 6, no. 3 (2011): 431–55.

[13] Akami, "Imperial Polities," 5–6, 10.   [14] Murard, "Designs within Disorder," 141–74.

[15] Brimnes, "Bandung Revisited," 172–81.   [16] Borowy, *Coming to Terms*, 330–3.

(Bandung, 1937). In the meantime, Heiser, as head of the IHB, started participating in debates taking place in the region and insisted on developing closer ties between the LNHO and FEATM.[17] At successive meetings of the FEATM, ecological approaches to malaria eradication, nutrition and deficiency diseases such as beriberi, and "social diseases" (i.e., pathologies that were related to living conditions and social behavior such as sexually transmitted diseases, leprosy, cancer, or addictions) were discussed. These health issues and social medicine were already at the core of colonial healthcare policies in the region.

In both French Indochina and the Dutch East Indies, various initiatives in social medicine and rural hygiene had been discussed for some time and some initiatives already been undertaken at the time of the Bandung Conference. The health services of both colonies had hired an increasing number of indigenous physicians to staff rural services. In both regions, there was also some discussion about the potential role of traditional medicine and traditional practitioners while nationalist movements were becoming increasingly active.

Health in the Colonies and the Indigenization of Colonial Medical Services

To address health and disease among indigenous populations in the French Empire, the Assistance Médicale Indigène (Native Medical Assistance, AMI) was founded in Madagascar in 1899 as part of France's *mission civilisatrice*, inducing colonized populations to accept Western civilization through medicine. AMI was established in French Indochina in 1905 and focused primarily, with the help of a medical (mostly military at the time) corps, on public health – sanitation and the prevention and control of epidemic diseases – rather than medical care. It organized (smallpox) mass immunization programs and various vertical initiatives targeting one pathogen at a time. From the outset, it faced the challenge of managing pathological environments characterized by a volatile combination of high morbidity and mortality rates, especially in infants and children. Despite the civilizing rhetoric and the insistence on free care, colonial medical initiatives in Indochina remained minimal and focused on the large urban centers, where sanitation was improving and a network of medical facilities had been established. In rural areas, a modest number of medical outposts, first-aid posts, infirmaries, and maternity clinics had been established but their numbers were grossly insufficient and chronically understaffed. Life-threatening epidemic and endemic diseases continued to be omnipresent. Although the challenges were enormous, the AMI received a modest and inconsistent budget from the French Government-general in Hanoi. It was

[17] Akami, "Imperial Polities," 15.

impossible to combat malaria with strictly biomedical measures, as complex local environmental variables, economic exploitation, the plantation economy, forest clearing, and increased human mobility all played a role. Effective measures, such as general sanitation, better housing, and improved nutrition were, unfortunately, expensive. From the very beginning, AMI officials were facing tremendous challenges which they were supposed to attack while they were supported with minimal and ever dwindling resources.

After the First World War, AMI resources increased in the context of the French *mise en valeur* ("colonial development" or "improvement") policy,[18] and more Vietnamese personnel – auxiliary doctors and nurses were cheaper than European physicians and considered closer to the indigenous population – were hired. New investments in maternal and child health led to the creation of maternity wards, specialized consultation services, and milk stations and the training of midwives. Attention to rural needs was growing among Vietnamese auxiliary doctors trained at the Indochina Medical College (since 1902) who were generally sent to the countryside. In 1926, one of them, Henri Marcel, strongly criticized the growing gap in health services between Tonkin (Northern Vietnam) provinces, the major urban centers, and "the rest."[19] The French local director of health in Cochinchina (Southern Vietnam), Dr. A. Lecomte, admitted that rural hygiene had thus far been neglected and announced several new initiatives, such as the creation of a body of "hygiene agents" who, after a brief education, would be able to detect cases of contagious diseases, and of mobile teams of health professionals who would assist bringing clean drinking water everywhere, and ensure the cleanliness of public places, schools, and homes. This "applied hygiene" would require legislative tools and be under the control of "local hygiene committees" (made of French civil servants: medical doctors, public works engineers, policemen). Rural hygiene, according to the director, was vertical in nature and costly; it would not take local specificities, needs, or social practices into consideration.[20]

As maternal and child health was nevertheless improving (neonatal tetanus, for instance, vanished from the hospital statistics in the 1920s[21]), in 1927, the AMI launched a "program of rural assistance" (Programme d'Assistance Rurale), providing basic medications to rural populations and disseminating small outposts staffed primarily by indigenous physicians, nurses, and

[18] Martin Thomas, "Albert Sarraut, French Colonial Development, and the Communist Threat, 1919–1930," *Journal of Modern History* 77, No. 4 (December 2005): 917–55.
[19] Henri Marcel, "L'hygiène Publique dans une Province du Tonkin (Hadong)," *BSMI* 4, no. 2 (1926): 40–57.
[20] A. Lecomte et al., "Sur l'hygiène rurale en Cochinchine," FEATM Conference Proceedings, Tokyo (1925), 961–78.
[21] Laurence Monnais-Rousselot, *Médecine et Colonisation: L'Aventure Indochinoise, 1860–1939* (Paris: CNRS Editions, 1999), 181–2.

midwives. It emphasized close cooperation between administrative services – departments of public works, education, agriculture, and, of course, health – but remained biomedical, vertical, and centralized. One of its most interesting initiatives was the "re-education" of traditional birth attendants (*Ba mu*). The two Western-style midwifery training schools that had opened in the 1900s had never attracted many students. Now, traditional birth attendants received a six-month training at the maternity hospital closest to their village of origin after which they were sent back to their community, which was expected to pay their salaries, at least in part. Their role in childbirth was initially strictly codified: they were only meant to attend normal deliveries and refer risky pregnancies and deliveries to the nearest doctor and hospital. Nevertheless, their duties quickly expanded "on the ground" to include a variety of maternal and childcare services, such as vaccinations, eye care, emergency first aid, and even monitoring daycare facilities.[22]

In 1901, the Dutch Queen announced the Ethical Policy, a new approach to its colonies. Instead of viewing them as a source of financial gain for the Dutch Treasury or private initiative, the Dutch government now accepted the ethical responsibility to guide the further development of indigenous populations to higher levels of welfare.[23] The Ethical Policy inspired new initiatives in public health and medical care, which started including the Indonesian population. Various new medical initiatives were announced but insufficiently funded. Previously, the colonial administration had maintained a military health service; the health and medical care of the indigenous fell outside its remit, except in the prevention and management of epidemics. The extensive smallpox inoculation campaigns, initiated in the 1830s, probably constitute one of the few health initiatives that reduced mortality among Indonesians.[24]

Medical care and public health initiatives for Indonesians were primarily provided through private initiative – plantations, sugar factories, and mines – or through various Protestant (*Zending*) and Catholic (*Missie*) missionary initiatives. After the turn of the twentieth century, the immensely profitable tobacco plantations in the Deli area surrounding Medan (North Sumatra) pioneered public health initiatives to increase labor vitality and longevity,

[22] Laurence Monnais, "Les Premiers Pas Inédits d'une Professionnelle de Santé Insolite: La Sage-femme Vietnamienne dans les Années 1900–40," in Gisèle Bousquet and Nora Taylor (eds.), *Le Vietnam au Féminin/Viêtnam: Women's Realities* (Paris: Les Indes Savantes, 2005), 67–106.

[23] Robert Cribb, "Development Policy in the Early 20th Century," in Jan-Paul Dirkse, Frans Hüsken, and Mario Rutten (eds.), *Development and Social Welfare: Indonesia's Experiences under the New Order* (Leiden: KITLV Press, 1993), 225–45; Suzanne Moon, *Technology and Technical Idealism: A History of Development in the Netherlands East Indies* (Leiden: CNWS, 2007).

[24] Peter Boomgaard, "Smallpox, Vaccination, and the Pax Neerlandica, Indonesia, 1550–1930," *Bijdragen tot de Taal-, Land- en Volkenkunde* 159, no. 4 (2003): 590–617.

supported by several hospitals and a medical laboratory.[25] An evaluation of these initiatives in 1909 indicated that mortality rates had dropped markedly – from 60 to 0.95 per 1,000 per year.[26] While the colonies had been "off limits" for missionary activity so as not to antagonize the mostly Muslim population, they started to become active in healthcare at the same time, after colonial officials realized that they were willing to establish much needed schools and hospitals (thereby fulfilling the Ethical Policy "on the cheap"). Protestant and Catholic organizations soon built hospitals, clinics, and other health facilities, which became their modus operandi as the population preferred them over preaching and attempts at conversion. The first missionary hospital was established in Mojowarno (near Surabaya) in 1894 and had a stellar reputation. The extensive Petronella Hospital in Yogyakarta, operated by the Gereformeerde Church (Calvinist) and headed by Dr. J. Offringa, was often cited as an example of the benefits of denominational initiatives in the Dutch East Indies.

The Civil Medical Service, established in 1911, operated a limited number of medical services. It preferred to subsidize the health initiatives undertaken by private initiative and missionary groups, either by offering the services of Indies physicians (graduates of the Batavia Medical College (founded in 1851) and the Surabaya Medical College (founded in 1913), providing medical equipment, or through grants. It also offered salary supplements to physicians practicing in rural areas, which required them to provide medical services to the indigenous population for free. The obligations these physicians had half-heartedly accepted to supplement their meager income grew exponentially with the aim of providing more medical services, leading to much unhappiness among them. Semarang's city physician, W. T. de Vogel, campaigned to transform the colonial medical service into a colonial public health service, which would relinquish physicians of providing ever more medical services.[27] As city physician in Semarang, he had successfully implemented malaria prevention programs, the provision of fresh drinking water, a sewage system, and kampung (indigenous neighborhood) improvement programs. According to

[25] Hans Pols, "Quarantine in the Dutch East Indies," in Alison Bashford (eds.), *Quarantine: Local and Global Histories* (Basingstoke: Palgrave Macmillan, 2016), 85–102; Budi Agustono, Junaidi, and Kiki Maulana Affandi, "Pathology Laboratory: An Institution of Tropical Diseases in Medan, East Sumatra, 1906–1942," *Cogent Arts & Humanities* 8, no. 1 (2021), doi.org/10.1 080/23311983.2021.1905261. See also Jan Peter Verhave, *The Moses of Malaria: Nicolaas H. Swellengrebel (1885–1970) Abroad and at Home* (Rotterdam: Erasmus Publishing, 2011).

[26] W. Schüffner, and W. A. Kuenen, "Die Gesundheitlichen Verhältnisse des Arbeiterstandes der Senembah-Gesellschaft auf Sumatra während der Jahre 1897 bis 1907: Ein Beitrag zu dem Problem der Assanierung Großer Kulturunternehmungen in den Tropen," *Zeitschrift für Hygiene und Infektionskrankheiten* 64 (1909): 167–257.

[27] W. T. de Vogel, "Memorie Betreffende den Burgelijken Geneeskundigen Dienst," *Bulletin van den Bond van Geneesheeren in N.-I.*, no. 14 (Augustus 1906): 17–44.

him, the Civil Medical Service should focus its efforts on public health, leaving medical care to private initiative. De Vogel was promptly appointed as head of the Civil Medical Service; initially, he tasked with addressing Java's plague epidemic. He initiated a widespread (and expensive) program of housing improvement, as the rats that spread the plague were fond of living in the bamboo poles which Indonesians used to build their houses.[28] In 1925, the Civil Medical Service was transformed into the Public Health Service. Offringa – even though he was a "hospital man" and knew little about public health – became its head.

The Great Depression and Rural Hygiene in Southeast Asia

The Great Depression hit colonial economies hard. According to some studies, 12.8 percent of the peasantry in the Red River Delta, Northern Vietnam (8 million people) suffered from severe malnutrition in the mid-1930s; despite efforts at double cropping, food often ran out only two months after harvest,[29] while the price of rice dropped rapidly. The colony's allocation to health and sanitation dropped as well, from 10,034,000 piasters in 1931 to 6,935,000 in 1935.[30] Poverty, overpopulation, and famine fostered the radicalization of nationalist and anti-colonial sentiment – the Indochinese Communist Party, established in 1930, became very popular among peasants. More than ever, providing basic medical care in the countryside became politically imperative.

Budgetary and personnel challenges became unusually pressing, especially in Annam (Central Vietnam), the most rural area of Vietnam and the cradle of the opposition to French rule in the late nineteenth century. Annam's facilities consisted of small medical posts and dispensaries lined up along the coast and a few hospitals concentrated in the cities. Medical officers often complained about the lack of resources and personnel in the region, which made it virtually impossible to send nurses on tours or maintain daily consultation services. In 1932, Dr. Pierre Chesneau, who had been a military physician before joining the AMI and had worked extensively in Annam from the early 1920s, estimated that the average medical facility in Annam only served an "attraction perimeter" of maximum 10 kilometers, unless it was located close to a

---

[28] Maurits Bastiaan Meerwijk, *A History of Plague in Java, 1911–1942* (Cornell, NY: Cornell University Press, 2022).

[29] Thuy Linh Nguyen, "Overpopulation, Racial Degeneracy and Birth Control in French Colonial Vietnam," *Journal of Colonialism and Colonial History* 19, no. 3 (2018), doi.org/10.1353/cch.2018.0024.

[30] Health comprised less than 1 percent of the general budget for Indochina and only 10–15 percent of local budgets during the first half of the 1930s (Monnais-Rousselot, *Médecine et Colonisation*, 80–2).

market or in areas where malaria was prevalent.[31] He recommended that rural infirmaries be strategically located and that medical tours not only distribute basic medications but also educated locals about available services. He emphasized that malaria was still the prime cause of child mortality in the region, particularly when associated with overcrowding, malnutrition, and comorbidities. Posted in the province of Thanh Hoa for a couple of years, he reported on fertility issues in women and strongly advocated for "rural midwives" and regular screening for trachoma, a prevalent social disease often leading to blindness, in local schools.[32]

In 1937, a rural assistance program specifically designed for Annam was launched. Chesneau's "rural assistance" and "social medicine" work in Thanh Hoa had already received praise for increasing the local population's trust in what the AMI, biomedicine, and French physicians had to offer.[33] The program divided Annam into twenty-two "sectors," which were further divided into "health itineraries" (*itinéraires sanitaires*) by grouping ten to fifteen villages together, established after consultation with local authorities. Both decentralization and mobility were key. Re-educated *Ba mu* were to be trained and hired locally; villages were to be regularly visited by rural nurses who would screen for diseases, provide emergency care and hygiene advice, and draw a health sheet (*fiche sanitaire*) for each village.[34] The sheets were to be transmitted to sectors' doctors who would check on the sick monthly, send the most serious cases to the provincial hospital (conditions were identified by index cards to facilitate triage), and educate audiences in "basic hygiene principles" (Figure 4.3). This approach was still top-down and biomedical in nature; health promotion initiatives were limited. Although food hygiene and fresh drinking water were considered important, scarce resources continued to limit attention to the "most devastating (epidemic) diseases" for which education and vaccinations to prevent them were prioritized.[35]

[31] Pierre Chesneau, "Le Rayonnement des Infirmeries d'une Province du Sud Annam," *Annales de Médecine et de Pharmacie Coloniales* 31 (1933): 638–42.

[32] Pierre Chesneau and Nguyen Huy Soan, "L'inspection médicale des écoles d'une province du nord-Annam," *Annales de Médecine et de Pharmacie Coloniales* 34 (1933): 995–1015; Archives Nationales du Viêt nam (ANVN), Centre no. 2 (Saigon), Fonds de la Résidence Supérieure d'Annam (RSA)/HC, dossier 37903, "Rapport du Dr. Chesneau sur la cécité dans la province de Thanh Hoa, 1937."

[33] René Lays, "En Annam: Un Apôtre de l'Assistance Rurale: M. le Dr. Chesneau," *Le Nouvelliste d'Indochine*, September 12, 1937.

[34] A manual (the *Rural Nurse Handbook*), written by Chesneau and translated into *quoc ngu* (romanized Vietnamese) accompanied every nurse (ANVN, Saigon, RSA, dossier 3362, "Organisation de l'assistance rurale en Annam, 1935–1937"). Chesneau also published a magazine twice a month, *Le Journal de l'Infirmier de Thanh Hoa*, which was distributed to all nurses.

[35] ANVN, Saigon, RSA, dossier 3362, "Programme de développement de l'Assistance rurale en Annam, 1937."

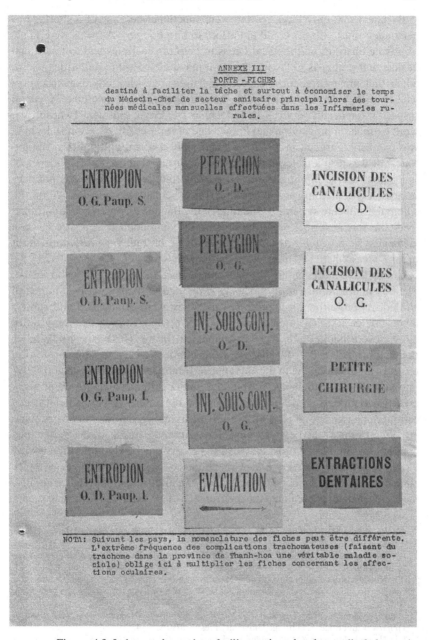

ANNEXE III
PORTE - FICHES
destiné à faciliter la tâche et surtout à économiser le temps
du Médecin-Chef de secteur sanitaire principal, lors des tour-
nées médicales mensuelles effectuées dans les Infirmeries ru-
rales.

ENTROPION O. G. Paup. S.

PTERYGION O. D.

INCISION DES CANALICULES O. D.

ENTROPION O. D. Paup. S.

PTERYGION O. G.

INCISION DES CANALICULES O. G.

INJ. SOUS CONJ. O. D.

ENTROPION O. G. Paup. I.

INJ. SOUS CONJ. O. G.

PETITE CHIRURGIE

ENTROPION O. D. Paup. I.

EVACUATION

EXTRACTIONS DENTAIRES

NOTA: Suivant les pays, la nomenclature des fiches peut être différente.
L'extrême fréquence des complications trachomateuses (faisant du
trachome dans la province de Thanh-hoa une véritable maladie sociale) oblige ici à multiplier les fiches concernant les affec-
tions oculaires.

Figure 4.3 Index cards used to facilitate triage by the medical doctor in charge of a health sector, Thanh Hoa Province (Annam), 1937. The cards show the local prevalence of eye infections. League of Nations Archives (LofNA), R6197-8D17773-341.

By late 1938, only three sectors were functional because of a shortage of personnel; most villages could not afford to hire *Ba mu*.[36] Appeals were made to private charities and the Red Cross to help run facilities and to traditional healers and druggists to "reach the rural masses."[37] Health authorities had to admit that money remained exceedingly tight, requiring pragmatism everywhere, beyond Annam. In addition, "tolerating traditional medicine," General Inspector for health services in Indochina Dr. Pierre Hermant (whose own work on malaria prevention and knowledge of rural health issues in Indochina was extensive) argued in 1937, "was not only a moral and political obligation ... it was also a material imperative" to ensure that the 25,000 villages of Indochina receive minimal care.[38] Involving traditional healers was not necessarily a first step toward integrating Sino-Vietnamese medicine within the colonial healthcare system. At the time of the Bandung Conference, traditional medicine was nevertheless in the process of being defined as a second-class medical system, *complementary* to biomedicine or, rather, an *alternative* to it in rural areas where resources were particularly scarce.[39]

Until 1925, the economy of the Dutch East Indies was in good shape. The colonial administration modestly supported various initiatives in health and education, although it preferred that they were established and run by others. After 1925, colonial profits and tax revenue started declining; after 1929, severe budget cuts were implemented. In the 1920s, the Rockefeller Foundation had sent J. L. Hydrick to the Indies to establish demonstration projects in rural hygiene in the Banyumas (Central Java) area. Instead of relying on technology-intensive hospitals in major urban centers, these projects established modest clinics in rural areas and ran extensive public health education campaigns (Figure 4.4).[40] Their overarching motive was to provide effective forms of medical care that were within the means of the indigenous population – in other words, they had to be very cheap. Hydrick often waxed lyrical about how villagers under his guidance made toothbrushes and other cleaning utensils from coconut hulls, twigs, and different materials. Initially, the Dutch had not appreciated the interference of an American in their hygienic

---

[36] ANVN, Saigon, RSA, dossier 37911, "Organisation et fonctionnement de la médecine rurale en Annam, 1938."

[37] ANVN, Saigon, RSA, dossier 3362, "Lettre de Terrisse au Ministre de l'économie rurale, Hué, 22 juillet 1935."

[38] [French] Archives Nationales d'Outre-Mer, Aix-en-Provence, Fonds de la Commission Guernut Bc, "Programme d'organisation des services d'Assistance et d'hygiène en Indochine, 1937."

[39] Laurence Monnais, *The Colonial Life of Pharmaceuticals: Medicines and Modernity in Vietnam* (Cambridge: Cambridge University Press, 2019), 242–4.

[40] J. L. Hydrick, *Intensive Rural Hygiene Work and Public Health Education of the Public Health Service of Netherlands India* (Batavia: Author, 1937); Eric Andrew Stein, "Colonial Theatres of Proof: Representation and Laughter in 1930s Rockefeller Foundation Hygiene Cinema in Java," *Health and History* 8, no. 2 (2006): 14–44.

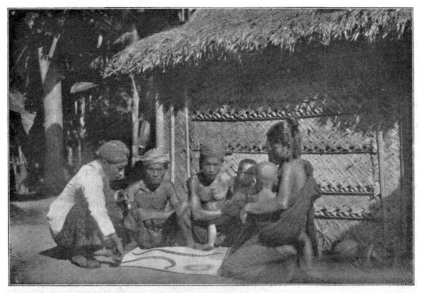

9. HUIS- OF FAMILIE-DEMONSTRATIE GEHOUDEN DOOR EEN DER MANTRI'S VOOR KAMPONG-HYGIËNE.

Figure 4.4 A *mantri* (health worker) educates a family about the intricacies of hygiene (in this case hookworm) at their home. Instructions for home visits stipulated the hygiene *mantris* would squat at the same level as the families they visited, indicating equality. Image originally distributed by the Dutch East Indies Public Health Service in 1937, most likely for use at the exhibition at the Bandung Conference.

affairs; the Public Health Services either ignored Hydrick's work or were obstructive.[41] After the economic situation darkened, however, it warmed to his ideas as they indicated how health could be purchased at bargain-basement prices. Offringa, the head of the Public Health Service, now saw Hydrick's program – a combination of public health education, public health measures, and local health centers – as key to the decentralization of health services and reducing health expenditures. Indonesian physicians had embraced Hydrick's work with great enthusiasm from the outset. Abdul Rasyid, a physician, politician, member of the colonial parliament, and, after 1938, president of the Indonesian Association of Physicians, viewed it as an example of how health and medicine could be organized to meet the needs of average Indonesian and

[41] Terence H. Hull, "Conflict and Collaboration in Public Health: The Rockefeller Foundation and the Dutch Colonial Government in Indonesia," in Milton Lewis and Kerrie L. MacPherson (eds.), *Public Health in Asia and the Pacific: Historical and Comparative Perspectives* (New York, NY: Routledge, 2007), 139–52.

modeled his ideas on medical nationalism on Hydrick's work. For the same reason, he embraced traditional herbal medicine as Indonesia's own medicine: it was cheap, its ingredients were available everywhere, and it was one of Indonesia's own products.[42]

Another expert in economizing health expenditures was psychiatrist W. F. Theunissen, a prominent psychiatrist not known for his research but for his organizational skills in managing large mental hospitals at minimal cost.[43] In 1917, he published a programmatic article on the current state and future development of healthcare provisions for the (indigenous) insane.[44] As demand would always expected to exceed supply, Theunissen argued that more much needed beds could become available when expenses per bed were reduced, which could be achieved by building and running institutions as cheaply as possible and by increasing revenue. Unlike the first and very expensive modern mental hospital in the Indies, located near Buitenzorg (Bogor), pavilions at the Magelang and Lawang mental hospitals, where only Indonesian patients were institutionalized, were not built with bricks and mortar but with much cheaper bamboo. Theunissen argued that these pavilions were much more comfortable for Indonesian patients because they resembled the housing of the indigenous population. He also advocated occupational therapy because it enabled patients to learn skills that would enable to earn their living upon discharge as well for its potential to reduce the cost of running asylums. Housing patients with their families living near mental hospitals also promised to reduce expenses. Similar initiatives had been undertaken with leprosy patients.

Once economic problems increased in the colonies, Theunissen expanded occupational therapy in the large agricultural colonies surrounding mental hospitals by introducing several new crops, fishponds, and orchards. After purchasing machinery to process rice, the hospital sold the surplus. Cattle, chicken, and duck farms were established, in addition to large vegetable gardens and small plots for the cultivation of tobacco and sugar cane. Kapok trees, which produce material to fill mattresses and pillows, were planted. Theunissen also introduced cotton plants. In 1935, the Lawang asylum was able to sell large quantities of surplus food. Patients also made and repaired furniture and buildings. Female patients worked in batik workshops and products were either sold or used by patients. Patients made mats from coconut fiber to sleep on. Almost everything used and consumed at the asylum,

---

[42] Hans Pols, *Nurturing Indonesia: Medicine and Decolonisation in the Dutch East Indies* (Cambridge: Cambridge University Press, 2018), 148–53.

[43] Hans Pols, "The Psychiatrist as Administrator: The Career of W.F. Theunissen in the Dutch East Indies," *Health and History* 14, no. 1 (2012): 143–64.

[44] W. T. Theunisse [sic], "Het Krankzinnigenwezen in Nederlandsch-Indië," *Koloniale Studiën* 2, I (1917): 434–78.

a journalist noted, had been grown, produced, or manufactured there.[45] Occupational therapy motivated patients to work to improve their own condition and had a salubrious healing effect. It also reduced expenses significantly. Theunissen also introduced new residences for psychiatric patients who could no longer benefit from treatment; they were housed more cheaply elsewhere. These patients were placed in simple housing, built by patients themselves, on the slopes of Bromo volcano and tended crops with minimal supervision. Even though these initiatives are not strictly speaking social medicine, they reduced expenditures by transforming care provided in large institutions into initiatives resembling village care. His accomplishments – activating patients to contribute to their own care – did not go unnoticed and became central in later health initiatives.

In 1935, Theunissen was appointed acting head of the Public Health Service and became head in 1938. While holding the first position, he was tasked with preparing the Bandung Conference as the head of the Dutch delegation. He and other medical experts from the Dutch East Indies and French Indochina actively participated at the 1937 conference, preparing and attending it because of their experience with rural health initiatives that had become more pressing after the onset of the Great Depression.

Preparing and Attending the Bandung Conference

To prepare for the conference, the LHNO proposed to establish a small preparatory committee to make site visits all over South and Southeast Asia to consult with local health officials, visit medical institutions, and observe initiatives in public health and social medicine. Coordination problems and chronic medical staff shortages in all participating countries made it difficult to appoint expert rapporteurs who could dedicate their time to prepare the meeting, which was consequently postponed.[46] While the preparatory work was enormous, it was done carefully. The LNHO appointed A. S. Haynes, former colonial secretary of the Federated Malay States; Professor C. D. de Langen, former dean of the Batavia Medical School; and Dr. E. J. Pampana, Secretary of the Malaria Commission of the Health section of the League of Nations secretariat to the preparatory committee. These three men toured South and Southeast Asia (bypassing China and Japan) from April to August 1936. They met colonial health administrators and officers of the Rockefeller Foundation IHB and consulted local public health staff. Based on these surveys, the final conference program had five main topics: health and medical services; rural

---

[45] "Een Bezoek aan Soember Porrong: Genezing door Arbeid," *Indische Courant*, March 10, 1934, part IV, p. 1.
[46] LofNA, R6197-8D17773-341, "Eastern Bureau of Singapore: Annual Report, 1934."

reconstruction and collaboration of the population; sanitation and sanitary engineering; nutrition; and measures for combatting specific diseases in rural districts. Preparatory reports on each of these topics were prepared by physicians appointed by the organizing committee. The report of the preparatory committee was made available before the start of the conference.[47] In addition, every participating country was asked to name delegates and to submit a national report addressing these five issues. Reports included surveys, elaborate descriptions, and photos of local rural hygiene initiatives.[48] Most of the delegates to the Bandung Conference had spent long periods in Asian colonies and were intimately familiar with health and medical conditions there. They had extensive experience in matters related to rural health.

Most delegates from French Indochina (six out of nine) were health professionals and had been associated with the AMI for years. Dr. Pierre-Marie Dorolle, the delegation's vice president, had accompanied the preparatory mission during their visit to Indochina in June 1936 and co-wrote the preparatory report on Health and Medical Services. Starting in 1925, he had built a career in Vietnam and became involved in the LNHO and the Eastern Bureau by participating in several international missions. He was first active in malaria prevention and was concerned with accessibility issues – he had observed that the high price of quinine restricted its impact.[49] In 1933, he specialized in psychiatry and was put in charge of the most important local asylum, the Bien Hoa asylum. He had visited the Dutch East Indies to explore more affordable options for housing psychiatric patients.[50] Dorolle was accompanied by Dr. Chesneau, who had co-authored the preparatory report on rural reconstruction, Dr. Henry G. S. Morin, a famous malaria expert interested in the prevention, treatment, and ecology of malaria in rural Southeast Asia,[51] Professor Henri Galliard from the Faculty of medicine in Hanoi, and Tran Van Thin, an AMI physician. They were joined by Marcel Autret, a military pharmacist who specialized in potable water in rural centers; he was also interested in nutritional deficiencies as well as quinine fraud and traditional herbal remedies.[52]

---

[47] LNHO, *Intergovernmental Conference of Far-Eastern Countries on Rural Hygiene: Report of the Preparatory Committee* (Geneva: LNHO, 1937).

[48] LofNA, R6096-8A26763-8855, "Rural Hygiene: Far East Conference – Government Reports."

[49] Pierre Dorolle, "Le Paludisme à Ha Giang (Tonkin)," *Bulletin de la Société de Pathologie Exotique* 20 (1927): 921.

[50] Edington and Pols, "Building Psychiatric Expertise."

[51] In several of his publications, Morin had analyzed the influence of the climate and socioeconomic factors on the prevalence of this disease in particular.

[52] The delegation president, A. F. X. Vinay, was a civil servant, G. Kaleski, a public work engineer, and G. J. Oudot, an agricultural engineer. Interestingly, the delegation originally proposed by the Governor-general was larger and counted more Vietnamese members ("L'Hygiène Rurale en Extrême-Orient," *Les Annales Coloniales*, July 23, 1937).

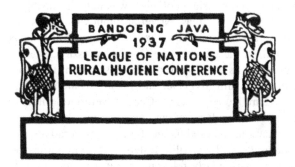

Figure 4.5 Name badge for the delegates to the Bandung Conference. From: League of Nations Health Organization, *Guidebook for the Intergovernmental Conference of Far-Eastern Countries on Rural Hygiene* (Batavia: Kolff, 1937), 20.

The delegation from the Dutch East Indies was headed by Theunissen. The Dutch East Indies were eager to show off their psychiatric services, the most extensive in Asia, at the conference.[53] He was joined by Professor J. E. Dinger, director of Batavia's Institute of Hygiene and Bacteriology and member of the preparatory committee on Nutrition; Professor W. F. Donath of the Batavia Medical School, a specialist on diet and nutrition; Dr. J. G. Overbeek, director of the malaria control services, and M. S. W. de Wolff, head of the West Java Health Service. Hydrick (who chaired the Health and Medical Services preparatory committee) was joined by his associate Arifin *gelar* Sutan Saidi Maharaja, an aristocrat from Sumatra's Minangkabau area and Head of the Division of Medical and Hygiene propaganda of the Public Health Service, and, for several years, member of the *Volksraad*, the colonial parliament.[54] Hydrick also was a member of the preparatory commission on rural reconstruction.

Dr. Offringa, the head of the Dutch Indies Public Health Service, presided over the Bandung Conference while the leaders of each delegation served as vice presidents (Figure 4.5). The purpose of the meeting was to propose measures that could improve the health of indigenous populations in Asia, over 90 percent of whom lived in rural areas which could be implemented with severely limited funds. Building hospitals and clinics, as was commonly

---

[53] Hans Pols and Sasanto Wibisono, "Psychiatry and Mental Health Care in Indonesia from Colonial to Modern Times," in Harry Minas and Milton Lewis (eds.), *Mental Health in Asia and the Pacific: Historical and Comparative Perspectives* (New York, NY: Springer, 2017), 205–21.

[54] Hydrick's book on his program, *Intensive Rural Hygiene Work*, was given to all conference attendees.

done in the urban centers in Asia's colonies, was neither feasible not useful in Southeast Asia's vast rural areas. Novel and innovative approaches were needed; fortunately, several promising experiments had already been conducted in the region. In the midst of the Great Depression, health interventions had to be effective as well as affordable. Discussions therefore focused on prevention, public health, hygiene, and health promotion – rather than individualized and curative approaches. Central were mosquitos, sanitation, water supply, sewers, waste disposal, and vaccinations, but also agricultural improvements, education, and establishing farming cooperatives. Social medicine was heralded as the "only possible system in these countries that are still poor," and hence not particularly relevant in Europe and North America.[55] To improve the health of rural populations, delegates argued that more than medicine was needed: improvements in agriculture, credit provision, and education were needed, as well as cooperatives and representative bodies, all of which were placed under the heading "rural reconstruction." To realize change, intersectoral collaboration was necessary, as well as an intensive focus on specific and local health conditions.

From its inception, it was obvious that the Bandung Conference was a conference on colonial public health and social medicine. Virtually all conference attendees originated from Europe and North America and had spent a considerable time of their careers in Asia working within the colonial health services; many of them had developed expertise on social diseases broadly defined (from malaria and trachoma to mental health issues) and experience with rural health issues (accessibility to medical personnel, facilities, essential medicines). Even though there were a small number of Asian participants, they hardly played a meaningful role. All public health initiatives discussed at the meeting were organized and implemented by colonial physicians, at times with the assistance of their local colleagues working under their guidance and direction. Only a few colonized and Asian people present at the meeting were participants, most Indonesians were there as spectacle.[56] The most striking absence at the conference were physicians and experts from the Philippines: the

---

[55] LNHO, *Report of the Preparatory Committee*, 21.
[56] The local exclusively European club, the Concordia, for example, arranged a *wayang wong* ballet performance for the delegates. Other Indonesians inhabited the model housing in a local *kampong* (indigenous neighborhood) erected by the city of Bandung, which apparently greatly impressed the international delegates ("Excursie door Gemeentelijke Kampongs: Vijftig Conferentie-Deelnemers Bezichtigden den Kleinwoningbouw en Kampongverbeteringen," *Algemeen Indisch Dagblad: De Preangerbode*, August 7, 1937, Section IV, 1). A rural school had been transplanted to the exhibition area for the duration of the conference as well. Delegates could observe a home visit of the propaganda *mantri* (health assistant), his conversation with the family and how school hygiene was taught in order for local children to be trained to "develop good habits from an early age" ("Hygiënsiche Tentoonstelling te Bandoeng," *Soerabajasch Handelsblad* 1937, Section II, 1).

American colony only sent one representative. In 1935, the Philippines had been granted Commonwealth status by the United States with the expectation that it would gain full independence in ten years. Its health services were already almost exclusively staffed by locals and many initiatives in rural health developed there were exemplary. Medical professionals from the Philippines might not have been interested in attending a meeting where the white man abounded on the health needs specific to the region.

The most interesting part of the conference dealt with rural reconstruction. Delegates assumed that the health problems among indigenous populations in the region had worsened as an effect of the Depression. Health experts therefore had to pay attention to social and economic factors affecting these populations beyond a fixed list of social diseases and how they could be addressed. Improvements in health, they agreed, would be the outcome of rural reconstruction, which included the introduction of innovative agricultural practices, the establishment of farming cooperatives and representative bodies, education, and cooperation. Yet the most difficult obstacle in realizing this was the difficulty in motivating the indigenous population to improve its own fate along indicated lines. Rural health in Southeast Asia was about implementing community health initiatives but the roles the members of the community itself could play were reduced to a minimum.

Traditional medicines were mentioned at the conference but did not attract much attention. Involving re-educated birth attendants, traditional healers, indigenous pharmacists, and local remedies was merely instrumental to reduce expenses and, probably, to create the appearance of doing something. The need for accessible and affordable medical care was clear at a time of growing anti-colonial sentiment in Southeast Asia. In the 1930s, several Western-trained Vietnamese and Indonesian physicians were discussing the "right to health," claiming that indigenous populations needed accessible and cheap medications. Several came to advocate pluralistic therapeutic practices and even self-medication.[57]

The "native" did not understand what we colonial health experts were up to and was passive and inert, Offringa, the president of the conference, opined in his opening address (Figure 4.6). He heralded the "Victory March of Western Medicine" and bemoaned the lack of understanding of indigenous populations of hygienic measures for their own benefit. Too often, he stated, prejudice and ignorance, stemming from a different psychological orientation among local populations, resulted in most health initiatives remaining fruitless.[58] As the final conference report states:

---

[57] Monnais, *The Colonial Life*, 237–41; Pols, *Nurturing Indonesia*, 156–9.
[58] "Streven naar Bevordering Volkshygiëne: Moelijkheden Verbonden aan Opbouw," *De Koerier*, August 3, 1937, Part III, 1.

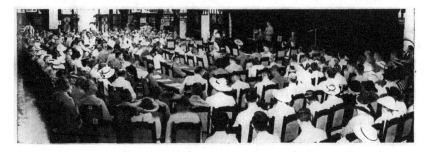

Figure 4.6 The opening ceremony of the Bandung Conference on August 3, 1937. Photo published in the *Java Bode* (August 4, 1937), part IV, p. 13. From: Newspaper Collection, The Hague, Royal Library of the Netherlands.

no remedy or plan of work however well conceived or well intentioned can effect the desired changes and improvements for the well-being and happiness of the rural population unless there is genuine desire on the part of the people in the rural areas to accept them and voluntarily work for them. No legislation, no efforts can help those who are not determined to help themselves. *The problem becomes thus fundamentally psychological.*[59]

When the delegates pondered "enrolling the local people themselves to co-operate in the task of their own improvement," the locals could have been suspicious and interpreted this as an attempt to reduce services and cut spending by transferring them from the colonial state to colonial subjects.[60] The proposed interventions, although intersectoral and holistic, were still fundamentally vertical, biomedical, and colonial in nature, as state-driven intervention toward a "civil society" that had local needs into account.

Needless to say, when indigenous populations were characterized by apathy, ignorance, and lack of initiative, the realization of the high ambitions of the conference necessarily remained unattainable. If the problem was both "psychological" and intractable, all possible health interventions would come to nothing. Fortunately, the attendees were much more comfortable discussing the last topic of the conference: specific diseases – malaria, plague, ancylostomiasis, and tuberculosis. They were, as it were, on "home" ground. The emphasis on individual diseases and their prevention (BCG vaccinations were

---

[59] LNHO, *Report of the Intergovernmental Conference on Far-Eastern Countries on Rural Medicine, Held at Bandoeng (Java)* (Geneva: League of Nations, 1937), 40. Emphasis added.

[60] LNHO, *Report on Rural Medicine*, 42. Even though there were three psychiatrists present, no proposals were ventured to address this psychological problem, despite several Dutch psychiatrists working in the Dutch East Indies having proposed a "psychological colonial policy" for quite some time. See Hans Pols, "Psychological Knowledge in a Colonial Context: Theories on the Nature of the 'Native' Mind in the Former Dutch East Indies," *History of Psychology* 10, no. 2 (2007): 111–31.

discussed at length in the French Indochina preparatory report) resembled earlier vertical approaches and interests in infectious disease, despite the holistic emphasis of the conference.

Conclusions

In Southeast Asia, interest in social medicine and rural hygiene become pronounced in the 1930s as it promised to deliver substantial health improvements at a fraction of the price of curative medical initiatives. Rural hygiene included the provision of basic medical care for the masses, and cheap creative solutions for ever-increasing health problems. (It appears that the health of city-dwelling indigenous populations was not considered similarly pressing, as most participants agreed that urban centers had ample medical institutions, making innovative approaches such as those proposed for rural areas appear unnecessary.) The delegates to the Bandung Conference, in particular those from French Indochina and the Dutch East indies, had been familiar with debates on rural hygiene and had been involved in implementing such initiatives for at least two decades. The conference allowed them to showcase their initiatives and formulate a synthetic statement based on their experiences.

We have situated "Bandung" in the context of imperial medicine and the Great Depression to provide a genealogy of its proposals in social medicine as the combination of political pressure to do something about the health of the rural masses with an exceedingly small budget. This complicates other assessments that have heralded it as a precursor for later initiatives in primary healthcare. We assume that, in general, large international events accompanied with ample press which are presented as ultimate "landmarks" or point of departure for global health transformation are best analyzed based on what happened before (their genealogy) rather than what happened after (their legacy).

The delegates at the conference proposed highly idealistic programs that could not possibly be realized. Consequently, all lofty plans turned into a mirage that symbolically absolved colonial administrations from their responsibility to safeguard their subject's health. This somewhat negative conclusion contrasts with the more positive appraisals the Bandung Conference has received from historians and health professionals previously. Iris Borowy, for example, has asserted that the Bandung Conference "may have been one of the first, if not indeed the first, major international event in public health in which Asian voices were heard" and that it "helped challenge the idea of a universal Western model for world health."[61] Borowy is correct that the delegates at the conference continuously emphasized the local and the specific and that health measures needed to be tailor-made for specific contexts. They

---

[61] Borowy, *Coming to Terms*, 355.

consequently argued that solutions that appeared feasible in Europe could not simply be transplanted to the "Far East." The colonial health experts gathered at the conference continuously emphasized specific local factors related to climate, agricultural conditions, and socioeconomic factors. Conservative views that had been common among colonial physicians, emphasizing the primitive and backward nature of the "natives," had mostly disappeared – the specificity of the "East" lay in socioeconomic factors, not in racial ones. Yet the "Asian voices" she refers to were almost all the voices of Western health experts working in Southeast Asia, as indigenous voices were mostly either silent or absent. The indigenous-looking building where the meeting took place – erected with the most advanced Western engineering techniques and sporting the appearance of a Minangkabau dwelling, an ethnic group residing 2,000 kilometers westward on the island of Sumatra, best symbolizes the Asian involvement at the conference – its appearance was local but its essence Western.

The proposals for public health measures and medical services ventured at the conference were primarily motivated by economic and political pressures. Colonial physicians remained in charge of designing and implementing programs. Delegates viewed increasing the number of indigenous auxiliary health personnel as fundamental, while the re-education of traditional birth attendants and research in traditional medicine were pragmatic propositions – and most probably added some exotic flourishes to the discussions. The proposals discussed at the meeting went beyond earlier vertical approaches, which had viewed natives as primitive, undeveloped, and apathetic, indicating that change had to be brought about by force and compulsion. Instead, indigenous populations were invited to participate in health initiatives led by indigenous physicians while designing these programs remained in the hands of biomedically trained colonial physicians. According to Packard, the Bandung Conference reflected the continued entanglement of international health organizations, colonial medicine, and rural hygiene was mainly an issue of colonial governance.[62] We agree with this assessment: social medicine at Bandung was a tool for colonial governmentality at a time when colonial empires were contested and weakened.

Progressive voices had discussed a type of colonialism that disdained compulsion and the use of force and, instead, recognized individual or community agency when it came to health. The colonialism on display at the Bandung Conference was empathic and reasonable, suffused with a moralistic and paternalistic feelings. It was an example of empire by persuasion, education, and argument, of necessity guided by the best interests of its subject population and ample attention to its specific and crucial needs at a time of global economic turmoil. Unfortunately, despite the best of intentions, health professionals often reported that their attempts were thwarted by indigenous

[62] Packard, *History Global Health*, 89.

misunderstanding, irrational prejudice, and obstruction. The conference's high ideals soon became an upturned boat as it caught in the floods of the Great Depression and Japan's military expansion – the lack of indigenous appreciation for colonial health initiatives had little to do with it. The somewhat Oedipal motives inspiring it – the caring and morally infused feelings cherished by Western physicians for indigenous populations – could not hide that they were projecting their own image on those silenced Others. After independence, however, Southeast Asian physicians continued to be inspired by these programs and were successful in implementing them as they viewed rural hygiene initiatives as essential components in nation-building.

5   Social and Socialist
Ideas of Health, Medicine, and Society
across the Iron Curtain

Dora Vargha

Socialist medicine, its priorities, healthcare organization, and underpinning ideology was an important aspect of the Cold War world, through which East and West set themselves apart. Following Western medical tourists who studied the new Soviet system in the first half of the twentieth century – among them Henry Sigerist – the geopolitical divisions of the post-First World War era accentuated the marked differences in approaches to health, even as overlaps remained in basic concepts. Through an Eastern European lens, this chapter explores the definition of socialist medicine in tandem with that of social medicine to ask if the difference between social and socialist that became more and more stark in the Cold War, was in name only, or if it represented different historical pathways.

Social medicine and its relation to socialist medicine occupies a particularly useful analytical terrain on the boundaries of the political and professional and the medical and social. Taking together the social and socialist, we can situate health and medicine in (state) socialist contexts into broader conversations around definitions of health, responsibilities for and methods of maintaining it, and on guiding concepts behind healthcare structures. Integrating socialist health into the history of social medicine challenges conventional Cold War divisions in separate "Western" and "Eastern" narratives in the politics of health, broadening an understanding not only of how we approach social medicine and its meanings, but also of what the Cold War itself meant in terms of health and its politics.

The intertwined ideas of social and socialist medicine lead us to further reconsiderations of how we can understand socialist medicine as a phenomenon and, more broadly, where we place the role of ideology within it. Historian Mat Savelli, in his analysis of Yugoslav psychiatry, differentiates between "socialist by design" and "socialist by default."[1] The former refers to practices

---

[1] Mat Savelli, "Beyond Ideological Platitudes: Socialism and Psychiatry in Eastern Europe," *Palgrave Communications* 4, no. 1 (2018), doi.org/10.1057/s41599-018-0100-1.

and concepts that were ideologically infused, engaging some way with socialist ideas and aims – these did not necessarily need to be in socialist countries.
Socialist by default, in turn, refers to medicine and health in state socialist
contexts that do not necessarily have anything to do with ideology or particular political and social infrastructure – they just happen to be in state socialist
countries. What we can see in the overlaps of, and interactions between, social
and socialist medicine is the combination of the two: continuities in social
medicine that are then framed and molded in a particularly socialist, ideology-
infused manner.

Social Medicine before State Socialism

Social medicine has always been an explicitly political project. In Eastern
Europe, the interwar era became a high point in the expansion of social medicine, as new states and regimes struggled with redefining nation and health
on the ruins of empires. Eastern European pioneers of social medicine were
in continuous exchange and conversation with their Western counterparts and
had a significant global impact through international organizations. As Patrick
Zylberman points out, social medicine in the East and the West were not very
far apart but it was more incendiary in the East, as it quickly gained an overall aim of modernization (economy, society, the nation on the whole) instead
of its Western, more modest aims of reforming medicine as a field.[2] At its
conception and development, however, Eastern ideas about social medicine
and social hygiene and Western concepts and practices were fundamentally
connected.

   Building on ongoing reform in hygiene reaching back to the nineteenth century, social hygiene became a distinct field in the Soviet Union shortly after the
Russian Revolution of 1917, with dedicated departments in medical schools
starting to appear in 1922. Soviet social hygienists were proponents of the
well-being of the whole population, positioning themselves between a sociological and a biological approach. They focused on the description of social
factors that contributed to ill health and proposed social measures as disease
prevention. The field as such was heavily supported by the revolutionary government, which eventually put social hygienists in an uncomfortable position:
they were, in essence, paid by the state to point to its shortcomings and call out
the lack of promised social reforms.[3]

   Soviet social hygienists did not work in isolation. They followed closely,
adapted ideas from, and were in conversation with key figures in German

---

[2] Patrick Zylberman, "Fewer Parallels than Antitheses: René Sand and Andrija Stampar on Social
   Medicine, 1919–1955," *Social History of Medicine* 17, no. 1 (2004): 77–92.
[3] Susan Gross Solomon, "The Limits of Government Patronage of Sciences: Social Hygiene and
   the Soviet State, 1920–1930," *Social History of Medicine* 3, no. 3 (1990): 405–35.

social medicine via medical journals and personal correspondence and translated many influential works into Russian.[4] Historian Susan Solomon argues, however, that Soviet social hygienists saw their work as differing from that of the Germans as it was animated by a "social thrust", and they also set themselves apart from previous Russian efforts as the units of analysis were class-based, rather than territorial.[5] At the same time, soviet hygienists were, at least in the early Soviet Union, working in a very international environment.[6] Soviet healthcare became an object of intense international attention, its underpinning ideas and system held up as exemplary by many who visited there in the 1920s and 1930s, publishing their praises of social and socialized medicine in the Soviet Union. The most well-known among them are Arthur Newsholme's *Red Medicine* and Henry Sigerist's *Socialized Medicine in the Soviet Union.*[7]

Experiments in social hygiene and medicine were rife elsewhere in Eastern Europe in the interwar era as well, although not all social hygiene experiments were successful. In Czechoslovakia, for instance, a pilot project in Prague to coordinate social and health work failed in a combination of the ageing of the main protagonists driving the project, the loss of the Rockefeller Foundation's support, and the rapidly changing national and geopolitical circumstances.[8] Still, Eastern European social medicine and social hygiene models created a significant impact and the region became an international leader in social hygiene, rural health, and healthcare reform.

Contrary to usual historical representations of the region as isolated, participation in international medical networks in Eastern Europe was very much part of forming nationhood. Katharina Kreuder-Sonnen applies Geert Somsen's term "Olympic Internationalism" to describe this interwar transnational medical mobility through the case of Poland.[9] Social hygiene became central to international health, specifically the League of Nations Health Organization

[4] For more on interwar Russian–German connections in medicine, see Susan Gross Solomon, *Doing Medicine Together: Germany and Russia between the Wars* (Toronto; Buffalo: University of Toronto Press, 2006).

[5] Solomon, "The Limits of Government Patronage of Sciences," pp. 414–15.

[6] See Susan Grant, *Russian and Soviet Health Care from an International Perspective: Comparing Professions, Practice and Gender, 1880–1960* (New York, NY: Springer International Pub. AG, 2017).

[7] Arthur Newsholme and John Adams Kingsbury, *Red Medicine: Socialized Health in Soviet Russia* (Garden City, NY: Doubleday, Doran & company, Inc., 1933); Henry E. Sigerist, *Socialized Medicine in the Soviet Union* (New York, NY: W. W. Norton & Company, 1937).

[8] Hana Masova, "Social Hygiene and Social Medicine in Interwar Czechoslovakia with the 13th District of the City of Prague As Its Laboratory," *Hykiea Internationalis* 6, no. 2 (2007): 53–68.

[9] Katharina Kreuder-Sonnen, "From Transnationalism to Olympic Internationalism: Polish Medical Experts and International Scientific Exchange, 1885–1939," *Contemporary European History* 25, no. 2 (2016): 207–31; Geert J. Somsen, "A History of Universalism: Conceptions of the Internationality of Science from the Enlightenment to the Cold War," *Minerva* 46, no. 3 (2008): 361–79.

and later informed basic tenets or the World Health Organization through key Eastern European actors: the Polish Ludwik Rajchman and the Yugoslav Andrija Štampar.[10]

Intertwining of the socialist, social, and socialized emerged in the interwar era with various configurations. Sara Silverstein points out that Andrija Štampar was, already in the 1930s, a critic of the American private health system and saw that social and socialized went hand in hand. Štampar argued that applied sociology in health would lead to "an understanding of society that would form the basis for establishing egalitarian access to health services."[11] The centrality of socioeconomic development and equality in accessing health coupled in convenient and logical ways, whether as part of a nation-building, democratic project in Yugoslavia or as part of flagship projects of new and groundbreaking ideas in healthcare in the Soviet Union.

Socialist Medicine

The stark distinction between social and socialist medicine is partly the product of Cold War politics. After the Second World War, newly established communist governments and officials consistently narrated their policies and the reconfiguration of the state which was set up against both the interwar period and the West. Furthermore, the self-distancing from social medicine could serve as a way to skirt around social hygiene's uncomfortable history with eugenics.[12] On the Western side, the thought that very similar ideas in Eastern European authoritarian regimes might underpin health movements that have been constituted as "progressive" in the West could have been troubling enough to reinforce the distinction between the two political contexts. Before turning to the question of overlaps and differences between social and socialist medicine, we need to take a look at how health and medicine was imagined in socialist contexts, what ideas guided healthcare organization, and what frameworks set priorities in building new health infrastructures.

---

[10] Theodore Brown and Elizabeth Fee have written extensively on this early history of international social medicine, including Štampar, Rajchman, and Sigerist. See, for example, Theodore M. Brown and Elizabeth Fee, "Andrija Štampar," *American Journal of Public Health* 96, no. 8 (2006): 1383; Marcos Cueto, Theodore M. Brown, and Elizabeth Fee, *The World Health Organization: A History* (Cambridge: Cambridge University Press, 2019); Elizabeth Fee, "Henry E. Sigerist: From the Social Production of Disease to Medical Management and Scientific Socialism," *Milbank Quarterly* 67 (1989): 127–50.

[11] Sara Silverstein, "The Periphery Is the Centre: Some Macedonian Origins of Social Medicine and Internationalism," *Contemporary European History* 28, no. 2 (2019): 220–33.

[12] Christian Promitzer, Sevvasti Trubeta, and Marius Turda (eds.), *Health, Hygiene, and Eugenics in Southeastern Europe to 1945* (Budapest and New York, NY: Central European University Press, 2011). For global context, see Alison Bashford, "Sex: Public Health, Social Hygiene and Eugenics," in Bashford, *Imperial Hygiene: A Critical History of Colonialism, Nationalism and Public Health* (London: Palgrave Macmillan UK, 2004), 164–85.

Socialist health and medicine in Eastern Europe – and beyond – was far
from uniform in practice and concepts, just as approaches to and practices of
socialism varied widely across the world. Moreover, socialist state structures,
ideologies, and socialist networks shifted and changed over time, with their
timelines peppered with revolutions, retributions, freezes, and thaws, or with
intermittent socialisms appearing and disappearing as organizing forces (either
in state or health care) beyond the Soviet Bloc, for instance in Ghana, Chile,
or even in England, where the Socialist Medical Association played an important role in what became the National Health Service but had been side-lined
in the process.[13]

As fragmented as the socialist world may seem, ideologically, geographically, and temporally, we can identify certain fundamental approaches that
connected the various healthcare structures. Some of these concepts stem from
core ideas underpinning a wide range of ideologies on the left, which aim to
further the well-being of the masses – workers and peasants, whether formulated by Engels or Mao. Furthermore, the movement and exchanges of people,
materials, ideas, and practices continued throughout the Cold War era. A Cuban
mission toured Eastern Europe to search for applicable models in the development of the new revolutionary healthcare system and Eastern European physicians and nurses helped the Cuban government in providing rural healthcare
in the early 1960s, while Soviet and Czechoslovak researchers participated in
setting up polio-vaccination efforts that became a calling card of early Cuban
health policy.[14] From the first dispatch of Chinese medical experts to Algeria
in 1963, Chinese medical assistance expanded to twenty-two African countries by the 1970s.[15] In the immediate post-war era, Eastern European countries, together with China, collaborated and provided medical aid in the form
of pharmaceuticals, medical care, and hospital-building in North Korea and
later, in Vietnam.[16] From the 1950s onward, socialist states' health ministers,

[13] Hilary Modell and Howard Waitzkin, "Medicine and Socialism in Chile," *Berkeley Journal of Sociology* 19 (1974): 1–35; Constantin Katsakioris, "Nkrumah's Elite: Ghanaian Students in the Soviet Union in the Cold War," *Paedagogica Historica* 57, no. 3 (2021): 260–76; John Stewart, *'The Battle for Health': A Political History of the Socialist Medical Association, 1930–51* (London: Routledge, 1999).

[14] E. Beldarraín, "Poliomyelitis and Its Elimination in Cuba: An Historical Overview," *MEDICC Rev.* 15, no. 2 (2013): 30–6; Dora Vargha, "The Socialist World in Global Polio Eradication," *Revue d'etudes comparatives Est-Ouest* 1, no. 1 (2018): 71–94.

[15] Xiangcheng Wang and Tao Sun, "China's Engagement in Global Health Governance: A Critical Analysis of China's Assistance to the Health Sector of Africa," *Journal of Global Health* 4, no. 1 (2014): 010301; Anshan Li, *Chinese Medical Cooperation in Africa, with Special Emphasis on the Medical Teams and Anti-malaria Campaign*, Discussion Paper 52 (Uppsala: Nordiska Afrikainstitutet, 2011).

[16] Young-Sun Hong, *Cold War Germany, the Third World, and the Global Humanitarian Regime* (New York, NY: Cambridge University Press, 2015); Bogdan C. Iacob, "Paradoxes of Socialist Solidarity: Romanian and Czechoslovak Medical Teams in North Korea and Vietnam (1951–1962)," *Monde(s)* 20, no. 2 (2021): 117–40; Dora Vargha, "Technical Assistance and Socialist

including those of Mongolia, Cuba, Vietnam, and Eastern European countries, met annually to align healthcare policies and international health strategies and develop exchanges in training, technical assistance, and medical technology.[17] Thus, common threads among the very diverse set of actors were partly due to common ideological underpinnings but were also shaped by various collaborations among members of socialist networks.

Three common themes emerge more strongly than others in approaches to health in socialist contexts. First, all health was seen as public. While in practical terms, public health as a term officially retained its focus of engaging with living and working conditions and epidemiology, it was clear that there was no distinction between private and public health – all aspects of health became a public concern in a socialist society, which the state was responsible for, therefore achieving the true meaning of public health.[18] Second, socialist medicine placed a strong emphasis on prevention and its integration with therapy. Third, socialist medicine was statist medicine, in other words, socialized. The aim was to provide equal healthcare access to all members of society without cost, in a system where all health institutions are organized, managed, and financed by the state and in which medical professionals are all state employees.

Historian Bradley Moore argues that Czechoslovak hygienists saw Western medicine as reductionist, which "biologised" the social and environmental determinants of health.[19] Socialist medicine presented itself as an alternative. Emphasis lay on the integration of health and medicine in the workplace, the home, in education, and to address factors external to the body, placing special focus on prevention. Since health was a social and political project, this approach was seen as inseparable from what the West termed as socialized medicine, that is free and universal access to healthcare for everyone. Health thus became an integral part of the revolutionary process. As society's ailments were caused primarily by social ills (hunger, poverty, dire working conditions, environmental factors, etc.), society itself needed to transform along with healthcare structures and priorities.

In an article providing an overview of the history of healthcare organization in the Soviet Union published in the main Hungarian medical journal *Orvosi Hetilap*, the essence of health was laid out: "First, we have to mention the healthcare's state characteristic, the organic and inseparable connection of

International Health: Hungary, the WHO and the Korean War," *History and Technology* 36, no. 3–4 (2020): 400–17.

[17] Bogdan C. Iacob, "Health," in James Mark and Paul Betts (eds.), *Socialism Goes Global: The Soviet Union and Eastern Europe in the Age of Decolonisation*, new ed. (New York, NY: Oxford University Press, 2022), 255–89.

[18] István Simonovits, *Társadalomegészségtan és egészségügyi szervezéstudomány* (Budapest: Medicina Könyvkiadó, 1966), 85.

[19] Bradley Matthys Moore, "For the People's Health: Ideology, Medical Authority and Hygienic Science in Communist Czechoslovakia," *Social History of Medicine* 27, no. 1 (2014): 122–43.

health to the building of socialism [építőmunka]. The prophylactic direction of medicine and health – the other most important conceptual trait – is the consequence of soviet healthcare's stateist characteristic, it originates from the socialist state's nature."[20] The heavy (or nearly exclusive) involvement of the state and the focus on prevention were intertwined with the ideology that underpinned the system.

The article also emphasized that therapy and hygiene must be connected. Here, Boris Dmitrievich Petrov, a Soviet historian of medicine who had widely published on the history of Soviet public health, pit Virchow against Pavlov. Virchow, in his understanding, has furthered the specialization of medical knowledge and its separation based on the locality of the body (organs, tissues, cells), thus did not allow for the unity of therapy and hygiene and disregarded the importance of the environment in health. Pavlov, on the other hand, placed emphasis on prevention, as illness forms in the body of the patient before they would encounter medical examination. Therefore, the main goal of medicine was to address the factors that caused illness and disease in the first place.

The concept of a legal right to health was just as fundamental to the socialist state and society and a key aspect of the role of socialist health in the revolutionary project. The new Polish constitution of 1952 stated that the state will ensure the continuous improvement of the standard of health protection and culture and stipulates that this health protection is a legal right of citizens and must be achieved through preventative measures.[21] In a similar vein, the 1949 Hungarian constitution declared the protection of citizens' health to be an obligation of the state through the organization of healthcare and wide social security.[22] This concept was very much verbalized in early interactions between Eastern European countries and international organizations as the right to health, coupled with the right to relief in a postwar environment,[23] and framed expectations from, and frustrations with, international organizations such as the World Health Organization (WHO).[24]

---

[20] B. D. Petrov, "A szovjet egészségügy megalapozása," *Orvosi Hetilap* 45, (November 11, 1967): 2146.

[21] B. Kozusznik, "Az egészségügy fejlődésének 15 éve a Lengyel Népköztársaságban," *Orvosi Hetilap* 11 (1962): 2162.

[22] "A Magyar Népköztársaság Alkotmánya. VIII. Fejezet. Az állampolgárok jogai és kötelessé- gei," in *1949. évi XX. törvény* (Budapest, 1949). For commentary and context on legal and orga- nizational frameworks, see Jenő Lukács et al., "Die Entwicklung des Gesundheitswesens in der Ungarischen Volksrepublik," in Kurt Winter et al. (eds.), *Sozialismus und Gesundheitswesen. Probleme der Gesundheit und der physischen Entwicklung des Menschen* (Jena: VEB Gustav Fischer Verlag, 1979).

[23] Jessica Reinisch, "Internationalism and Relief: The Birth (and Death) of UNRRA," *Past and Present* 210, 6 (2011): 258–89.

[24] Vargha, "Technical Assistance."

Eastern European and state socialist healthcare systems always clearly presented the intertwining of medicine and politics in the foreground, not merely as priorities and policies that are underpinned by politically informed views of society, but as direct and explicit political projects that are instrumentalized by the state, party, or political models of the Cold War East.

Social and Socialist

Even as social hygiene was central to socialist medicine and Western engagement and influence on it was openly discussed already in the interwar era, it also set itself apart from Western social medicine in various ways. One central element to this difference was the relationship between biomedical and social, which in many understandings of social medicine are oppositional. In the socialist mindset, they were inseparable parts of medicine and health, in postwar Eastern European contexts and across the wider socialist world, as Sean Brotherton demonstrates in the case of Cuba in this volume. The explanation for the socialist intertwining of the biomedical and the social is situated in the particular political understanding of health on the one hand and the immediate effects of war, destruction, and economic hardship, on the other.

While there was a new and pronounced distancing from Western approaches to medicine with the emergence of the Cold War, continuities with interwar social hygiene projects remained influential. Moore in his work on Czechoslovak social hygienists puts forth that rather than a product of Sovietization and the enforcement of Soviet or socialist models on a profession externally, social hygienists in Czechoslovakia took advantage of the new political emphasis on concerns with environmental and social factors in medicine and of the new state support to realize goals they had been unable to achieve before the war.[25] It was not the result of a clear-cut or even hazy case of Sovietization, but the realization of longer standing goals of social hygienists taking on board the ideological and organizational framework of state socialism, which fit well with their existing intentions.

Continuities in concepts and, indeed, people involved in social medicine and social hygiene were not particular to the Czechoslovak case. In 1966, István Simonovits, a key member of the Ministry of Health between 1945–63 and later head of the Health Organization Institute at Semmelweis University, published a medical textbook titled *Social Hygiene and Health Organization Studies*. In its historical overview, Simonovits clearly connected Virchow's attention to social contexts in health and Grotjahn's social hygiene with "nervismus" (Pavlov's theories) and functionalist approaches that privilege the focus on

---

[25] Moore, "For the People's Health."

environment (mentioning Edwin Chadwick) and with hygienists such as Max Joseph von Pettenkofer.

In theory, Simonovits extrapolates, social hygiene and health organization studies are distinct. Social hygiene or social medicine (treated as synonyms in Hungarian) is on the boundary of social sciences and medicine and sees beyond the biological unit of the human body to look to the social unit: in other words, it investigates the interaction between people's social status, living and working conditions, and their health. "Health organization studies emerges to the scene with socialism, in the active phase of establishing socialist health, as a further development of social hygiene," Simonovits argues. Its goal is to provide scientific base for the effective and economic development and operation of healthcare. This is only achievable by keeping in mind the social conditions, therefore, naturally, it is permeated by social hygiene.[26] The two, then, are actually connected and complementary and combine a top-down, biomedical organization that integrates the ground-level social, rather than the Western bottom-up, approach of social medicine.

Continuities between social and socialist, with the latter encompassing the biomedical and hierarchical, was widespread in Eastern Europe and at least partly utilitarian. Gabriele Moser, in her analysis of social hygiene and public health in the Weimar Republic and early German Democratic Republic points to continuities between the two, following an older generation of social hygienists' role in establishing new healthcare structures. Moser argues that ideas of social hygiene from the 1920s had resurfaced in the immediate postwar era, although these were somewhat stifled by the "crisis medicine" to address the immediate challenges of wartime destruction and epidemic outbreaks and which favored the microbiological approach over a focus on social aspects.[27] Historian Donna Harsch sees this strong presence of the biomedical as a deviation from social medicine: a "medicalized social hygiene," a blend of medical treatment instead of preventative social interventions, and social hygienic concerns instead of a focus on individual rights.[28]

First, "crisis medicine" and its necessary foregrounding of biomedical approaches cannot be understated and is valid across Eastern Europe. The Second World War had left the region devastated and much of health infrastructure was destroyed or had to be repurposed. For instance, according to a report from 1948, in Pest-Solt-Kiskun county in Hungary, hospital beds were

[26] Simonovits, *Társadalomegészségtan és egészségügyi szervezéstudomány*, 10–18.
[27] Gabriele Moser, *"Im Interesse der Volksgesundheit …" Sozialhygiene und öffentliches Gesundheitwesen in der Weimarer Republik und der frühen SBZ/DDR. Ein Betrag zur sozialgeschichte des deutschen Gesundheitswesens im 20. Jahrhundert* (Frankfurt: Vas, 2002), 174–201.
[28] Donna Harsch, "Medcalized Social Hygiene? Tuberculosis Policy in the German Democratic Republic," *Bulletin of the History of Medicine* 86, no. 3 (2012): 394–423.

down by 28 percent compared to before the war and nearly three times as many beds were needed in the region to reach the national, prewar average. Many hospitals were damaged, while 45 villages were left without any access to healthcare.[29]

Addressing immediate and urgent needs had to be combined with a revolutionary project that aimed to solve those same needs in the longer term. In a 1986 article, Patricia Kullerberg argued that in the Hungarian case, several reasons led to the process in which scientific medicine was uncontested in the transition in which social and socialist ideas merged in the postwar era. She cited the inefficiency of political indoctrination in vulgar Marxist courses at medical schools; the utility of a narrower concept of disease for economic development and political control of the state; the enforcement of scientific medicine as an avenue to retain physicians' control and power; and the indestructible avenue for private medical care that was (and has been ever since) an unofficial part of the healthcare system.[30] The conclusion, then, is that biomedicine as a remainder from the interwar era persisted due to economic concerns and the continuity of capitalist structures in the medical profession.

The inseparability of the social and biomedical was not merely a pragmatic issue, however. Instead of seeing it as a deviation, the strong biomedical and state organization of health and medical training in Eastern Europe and the Soviet Union may be considered as a particular direction in which social medicine developed. Vilém Škovránek, Chief Officer of Public Hygiene in Czechoslovakia, outlined the importance of the integration of the social and biomedical, making a case that hygiene needs to be seen as a field that brings together specialized scientific branches, such as epidemiology and microbiology, communal hygiene, hygiene of work, children and adolescents, and nutritional hygiene as organized around the same objective, "working out scientific and medically justified precepts for the active guidance of all strata of the population, especially economic and technical experts, as well as ordinary citizens, toward the creation of the most favourable conditions necessary for the consolidation, protection and development of the physical and mental health of people living and working in a certain environment." This work, according to Škovránek, needed to be harmonized within the medical service and outside it, as public hygiene needed to be "an integral connection with the basic aim and mission of the entire community in the public health welfare."[31]

---

[29] Közegészségügy, 1948, XIX-C-2-s, Simonovits István iratai, 16. doboz, Magyar Nemzeti Levéltár, Budapest.

[30] Patricia Kullberg, "Social Visions and Social Control: The Evolution of Medical Thought in Postwar Hungary," *International Journal of Health Services* 16, no. 3 (1986): 391–408.

[31] Vilém Škovránek (ed.), *Public Hygiene Service and Infectious Disease Control in Czechoslovakia*, The Collection of Foreign-Language Publications of the Ministry of Health (Prague: Press Department of the Ministry of Health in Czechoslovak Medical Press, 1967), 12–13.

The biomedical and social were entangled in the Soviet Union as well and the Soviet view of the Alma-Ata Conference in 1978 can be instructive to understand this convergence. Based on Soviet archives, historians Anne-Emanuelle Birn and Nikolai Krementsov argue that Soviet health officials like Deputy Health Minister Dimitri Venediktov had very different ideas about primary healthcare to those of Western colleagues at the WHO, such as its director-general, Halfdan Mahler. While the latter conceptualized community-based medicine as primary healthcare, for the Soviet Union, the point of pride was the ability to provide medical care very much based on biomedical practice in an established healthcare infrastructure that reached the whole population, including rural areas.[32] While community-based healthcare was a way to overcome and meager resources and lack of access, the socialist aim was to provide the resources to the whole of society instead.

This was a major departure from the way primary and community healthcare was understood in Western non-socialist or other socialist contexts outside of Eastern Europe. In fact, while drawing on drastically different political contexts, socialist models significantly informed the renewed approach to primary healthcare that led to the Alma Ata declaration. One often heralded successful approach was Indian rural medicine in Kerala, where the Communist Party had been in power since 1957 and its primary healthcare system and achievements attracted widespread international attention.[33] Another notable approach to improving health in the so-called developing countries was the Chinese model of barefoot doctors, even as China itself did not participate in the Alma-Ata Conference due to growing tensions with the Soviet Union following the Sino-Soviet split that began in 1956.[34] Chinese healthcare organization and priorities in healthcare delivery shifted in the early 1960s, in the aftermath of the famine recovery process of agricultural production. As Xun Zhou points out, there was a marked shift from the top-down organization of disease eradication to prevention and the provision of basic care, in part to address the dire scarcity of medical provisions and hygienic infrastructure and in part as an opposition to what Mao saw as flawed in the Soviet system: too many specialized doctors, who were, in Mao's eyes, bourgeois and not needed in great numbers. Instead, public health work was prioritized, particularly in rural areas, which, in the combination of severe shortages of medical staff and the basic tenet of community involvement, eventually led to the development of the barefoot-doctor

---

[32] Anne-Emanuelle Birn and Nikolai Krementsov, "'Socialising' Primary Care? The Soviet Union, WHO and the 1978 Alma-Ata Conference," *BMJ Global Health* 3, 3 (2018): e000992.

[33] V. Raman Kutty, "Historical Analysis of the Development of Health Care Facilities in Kerala State, India," *Health and Policy Planning* 15, no. 1 (2000): 103–9; Vicente Navarro, "Has Socialism Failed? An Analysis of Health Indicators under Capitalism and Socialism," *Science & Society* 57, no. 1 (1993): 583–601.

[34] Cueto, Brown, and Fee, *The World Health Organization*, 171, 176.

scheme, integrating the use of Western and Traditional Chinese Medicine.[35] Thus, the Chinese pursuit of communist utopia in healthcare was at least partly set up against not only Western, but the Soviet socialist model, which they saw as too biomedical. The connecting socialist tissues that remained were a continued focus on prevention as a priority, the view that health is as much a medical as a social and environmental question, and the concept that health and healthcare are integral parts of the revolutionary and political project, even in their nuance.

Rural healthcare, which also became a central feature of the revolutionary overhaul of health organization and priorities in Cuba, remained to be an important feature of socialist medicine in Eastern Europe. However, like in the Soviet Union, the organization of healthcare in rural contexts was not based on community, rather on a network of epidemiological and hygiene stations, healthcare organized in workplaces, and schools and was based on local districts and on centralized control of hygienic practices in agriculture. In the 1967 informational volume on public hygiene in Czechoslovakia, Karel Symon from the Public Hygiene Institute of Prague did not even mention community participation in the discussion on rural hygiene. The focus instead was on the improved living conditions of farmers with the establishment of large-scale agricultural production and on the perils of the environmental impact and challenges in pollution that had resulted in the shift to collectives.[36]

In Hungary, Simonovits connected peasants' improved access to healthcare with the transformation of the agricultural structure and the establishment of cooperatives (which were done mainly through forced collectivization, beginning in the early 1950s) and saw room for improvement in integrating the local and factory healthcare units with the hospital system, while promoting the unity and decentralization of healthcare provision, involving community action and self-care. This latter was to be achieved through education of the population and propaganda, with the active involvement of the Hungarian Red Cross.[37] Thus, Hungarian healthcare organization saw social hygienic aims to be achieved through a horizontal biomedical infrastructure that is coordinated vertically, along with the organization of local community action in the form of committees and through workers' unions and schools. However, on the ground, access to healthcare remained a challenge. A 1964 article in the

---

[35] Xun Zhou, *The People's Health: Health Intervention and Delivery in Mao's China, 1949–1983* (Montreal, Kingston, London, and Chicago, IL: McGill-Queen's University Press, 2020), 178–216. For more on the barefoot doctors, see Xiaoping Fang, *Barefoot Doctors and Western Medicine in China* (Rochester, NY: University of Rochester Press, 2012). Miriam Gross, "Between Party, People, and Profession: The Many Faces of the 'Doctor' during the Cultural Revolution," *Medical History* 62, no. 3 (2018): 333–59.

[36] Karel Symon, "Rural Hygiene," in Škovránek (ed.), *Public Hygiene Service*, 69–73.

[37] Simonovits, *Társadalomegészségtan és egészségügyi szervezéstudomány*, 73–5.

national daily *Népszabadság* highlighted the development of rural healthcare as a pressing priority, with a lack of doctors in rural areas and calling on aspiring medical students to work in villages and outside of urban areas.[38]

Divergence and Convergence

While we can see definite distinctions among various framings of medicine and health between East and West, engagement with social and socialist medicine did not cease on either side. The Iron Curtain was not impermeable throughout the Cold War era, particularly regarding medicine and biomedical sciences.[39] Eastern Europeans continued to engage with Western social medicine, while Western experts had a continued interest in socialist medicine.

A clear interest in Western social medicine and its compatibility with socialism is illustrated by an article published in 1964 in, *Valóság*, the journal of the Hungarian Society for Dissemination of Scientific Knowledge. Titled, "The Sociology of Medicine and Healthcare," the social psychologist, Béla Buda, provided a lengthy discussion on the importance of integrating a sociological viewpoint into medical theory and practice, relying heavily on American literature.[40] In the closing pages, Buda turned his attention to the particular Hungarian case and lamented the point that research in medical sociology has mainly been conducted in capitalist health contexts, within the methodological and theoretical atmosphere of bourgeois sociology (as opposed to Marxist, materialist sociology).

This has obscured the most important correlations, Buda argued:

Among the analysis of various classes and social groups' lifestyles based on extensive data, their illnesses and the particularities of health organization, the broader context that provides a comprehensive interpretation was lost: the significance of the social system. They did not notice the huge role the essence of the social system – in this case, capitalism – the distribution of wealth, the prominent interests and values play both in the distribution of disease and the functioning of healthcare. There is scarce Western research that focuses on e.g., questions of coverage and accessibility of healthcare services for various social groups, and the importance of state investment and action in the quality of public health.[41]

---

[38] Ferenc Lovászi, "Akik végeztek és akik most indulnak," *Népszabadság* (Budapest), June 7, 1964.

[39] Nisonen-Trnka Riikka, "Soft Contacts through the Iron Curtain," in Sari Autio-Sarasmo and Katalin Miklóssy (eds.), *Reassessing Cold War Europe* (London: Routledge, 2010), 100–18. Dora Vargha, "Between East and West: Polio Vaccination Across the Iron Curtain in Cold War Hungary," *Bulletin of the History of Medicine* 88, no. 2 (2014): 319–43.

[40] Béla Buda, "Az orvostudomány és az egészségügy szociológiája," *Valóság* 7, no. 10 (1964): 52–64.

[41] Buda, "Az orvostudomány és az egészségügy szociológiája." p. 61.

Conversely, Hungarian medical professionals have not paid enough attention to the thorough investigation of social factors with the help of sociological methods and theories. This, Buda continues, could be particularly interesting, given the enormous and fundamental changes in social structures within a relatively short time and was especially important, due to cultural differences, the social factors and causal mechanisms of the same diseases based on Western research could not be applicable in places like Hungary.

In this scientific treatise then, Buda formulated critique for both sides and argued for the combination of perspectives among Western social medicine and the socialist view of health. In his understanding, the value of sociology in medicine was undisputed. Furthermore, he acknowledged the leading role particularly American researchers were taking in this discipline and saw the lack of such a strong field in Hungary as a weakness. However, without fundamental political engagement, the Western analysis has been incomplete and this is what socialist medicine brings to the table: it is not possible to improve human health, no matter if there is attention to detail for social factors, if the overarching political structures that frame social ones, among them access to healthcare and distribution of resources, are unaddressed.

On the other side, the most comprehensive source through which Western experts could learn about the healthcare structure and priorities of Eastern European countries was Richard Weinerman's book *Social Medicine in Eastern Europe: The Organization of Health Services and the Education of Medical Personnel in Czechoslovakia, Hungary and Poland*, written in collaboration with his wife, Shirley Weinerman, and published in 1969. The Weinermans, advocates of social medicine and Richard being Professor of Public Health and Medicine at Yale University at the time,[42] compiled this book as a follow-up to their earlier one, *Social Medicine in Western Europe*, published in 1951.[43] They spent a month in each country in 1967, sponsored by the respective Ministries of Health, and visited national research institutes, schools of medicine, postgraduate-training institution, regional and district health departments, hospitals, local healthcare offices, industrial medical units, and sanitation and epidemiological stations.

The Weinermans' visit was, of course, carefully curated. While they were quick to note that they were not hindered in their movements during the visits in any way, the trips were organized by the ministries, complete with chauffeurs

---

[42] The Weinermans died a year after the book was published when a bomb was detonated in a plane he was on, traveling from Geneva to Tel Aviv. Herbert K. Abrams et al., "E. Richard Weinerman, M.D.," *American Journal of Public Health and the Nations Health* 60, no. 5 (1970): 797–95.

[43] E. Richard Weinerman, *Social Medicine in Western Europe: Report of a World Health Organization Traveling Fellowship, Summer 1950* (Berkeley: University of California School of Public Health, 1951).

and translators, and held in a select number of institutions. Still, the analysis and observations of the volume provide a relatively thorough analysis of the guiding principles that served as a framework for Eastern European organization of healthcare, highlighting historical roots, local specifications – even if the reality on the ground might have been quite different.

In its general observations, the book identified formulations that characterized all three countries' guiding principles, among them were emphases on prevention, raising the standard of living through public health, and centrally organized planning with decentralized responsibility.[44] What becomes immediately clear is that the list was written for an American audience, from an American perspective, and four of the seven points – public responsibility for health, free and accessible healthcare, public education and research, and universal social insurance – addressed socialized medicine. An understanding of Eastern European healthcare structures and priorities and the interpretation of what the Weinermans had seen in the three countries therefore needs to be situated in the American context as well: the intense debates in the 1960s about Medicare and Medicaid, resulting in the 1965 legislation.[45] From the early Cold War onward, socialized medicine had increasingly become a symbol of the socialist world and had become vilified in the 1960s, with heavy involvement by the American Medical Association. As one of the first inroads to the world of politics, the young Ronald Reagan recorded a speech in 1961 titled, "Ronald Raegan Speaks Out against Socialized Medicine," which was available for listening at home, getting the message into households about the dangers of such an approach.[46] As Greene, Podolsky, and Jones point out Chapter 7 in this volume, the blurring of the boundary between social and socialized served the purpose of undermining social medicine in the United States by invoking the Red Scare. However, this was not particular to American distinctions because the blurry boundaries became inconvenient for the same reason elsewhere in the West, too, and the coupling was explicitly pushed back against by proponents of social medicine such as Rene Sand, who proclaimed after the Second World War, setting himself apart from Eastern European counterparts: "Social medicine does not mean socialist or socialized."[47]

---

[44] E. Richard Weinerman, *Social Medicine in Eastern Europe: The Organization of Health Services and the Education of Medical Personnel in Czechoslovakia, Hungary and Poland* (Cambridge, MA: Harvard University Press, 1969), 16.

[45] Edward Berkowitz, "Medicare and Medicaid: The Past as Prologue," *Health Care Financing Review* 27, no. 2 (2005): 11–23.

[46] Jeffre St. Onge, "Operation Coffeecup: Ronald Reagan, Rugged Individualism and the Debate over 'Socialized Medicine,'" *Rhetoric and Public Affairs* 20, no. 2 (2017): 223–51.

[47] Quoted in Zylberman, "Fewer Parallels than Antitheses," 90.

Conclusion

Through the lens of Eastern Europe and beyond, we can see defined lines of differentiation along political ideologies but also an ebb and flow of ideas and practices across divisions, which characterized both social and socialist medicine. Looking at the establishment of healthcare systems and medical thought in Eastern Europe and the socialist world in the Cold War era, we can broaden how we understand social medicine itself. Social and socialist were intertwined in their concepts and aims and as historians, we need not necessarily follow Cold War politics in keeping them wholly separate. Rather, instead of a terminology based on mainly Western sources and practitioners and instead of dismissing Eastern European socialist medicine as irrelevant or a deviation, we might include them as a particular direction in which social medicine developed. This can then enable us to move beyond dichotomies set up in a Western understanding. Socialist approaches point to the integration of the biomedical and social in a way that shows them inseparable and as parts of the same political project, rather than opposing sides of medicine. They work with practices that entwine vertical and horizontal interventions in public health and combine a top-down and bottom-up organization of healthcare.

Integrating the particularities of socialist medicine in Eastern Europe, its continuities with and iterations of social hygiene, and health organization studies into a Western history invites us to reconsider what social medicine is on the whole. Along with rural health and the primary healthcare movement, Chinese barefoot doctors and Cuban medical internationalists, the inclusion of Eastern European socialist medicine is important.

Of course, more research is needed to see the changes over time in the approach of socialist medicine and the role and conceptualization of social medicine within, and to investigate, furthermore, how socialist medicine was represented by Eastern Europeans to the so-called Third World and how competing ideas of social medicine were negotiated and integrated into these interactions. This, hopefully, can eventually connect missing pieces that can provide us with a more comprehensive view of social and socialist medicine.

6   Social Medicine in Social Democracy

Anne Kveim Lie and Per Haave[*]

The concept of social medicine, pioneered by activists and leftist medical professionals in Denmark, Norway, and Sweden during the 1930s, played a significant role in reshaping the Scandinavian societies. Initially characterized by its political radicalism, social medicine's principles were integrated after the war into the prevailing social democratic ideology. Many of its early proponents assumed influential positions within the state medical apparatus, thus wielding considerable influence in crafting national health policies during the "golden age" of the Scandinavian welfare states (1940s–1970s), as well as playing important roles on the international scene.

This chapter explores the emergence and evolution of social medicine within the context of the Scandinavian welfare states, tracing its transition from being a catalyst for revolutionary change to a discipline instrumental in bolstering the foundations of the burgeoning welfare state. What happened to social medicine's ambitions to disrupt the current power balances in society when the persons proposing them were themselves in hegemonic positions? The chapter examines the trajectory of social medicine in late twentieth-century health policy, research, and clinical practice, while shedding light on some of its inherent limitations and subsequent demise.

Although the historiography of social medicine has been predominantly Eurocentric, it has been Eurocentric in a particularly narrow way. As Timmermann relates in Chapter 1 in this book, it is the narrative of social medicine that George Rosen found it appropriate to tell that has formed the history of social medicine that we know. Hence the history we have told our colleagues and students has started with Virchow in Germany and discussed

[*] The authors are grateful to fruitful comments from the delegates at the workshop on the Global Histories of Social Medicine in Rosendal, Norway, in 2022, and to Sunniva Engh, Niels Brimnes, Oivind Larsen, and Gunnar Mæland for helpful comments on an earlier draft. Anne Kveim Lie also thanks Jeremy Greene and Warwick Anderson for important conversations during this process. The research which this chapter is based on was funded by the Norwegian Research Council for the project Biomedicalization from the Inside Out, where both authors were members. Sadly, Per Haave passed away before the completion of the final manuscript but acceptance for publishing has been secured from his next of kin.

some of the UK histories. However, his narrative not only fails to adequately acknowledge the broader global context, as the contributions to this volume show to the full extent, it also omits large parts of what happened within non-anglophone parts of Europe. The history of social medicine in Scandinavia is in many ways different from what we are told by Rosen and later authors.[1] It is more sharply grounded in social theory, at least in the 1930s (in contrast to Latin America, where social theory becomes important in the 1970s, as we learn in Chapters 3, 8, and 11), it becomes a proper medical specialty and is tightly involved in the welfare state, both as theory and field of practice. It also offers an important counterpoint to traditional chronologies, for instance by revealing how social medicine, evolving within the framework of social democracy, achieved its greatest impact in the 1950s and 1960s, at a time when social medicine was struggling in the Americas.

Social Medicine in the Interwar Years

Concerns about the social dimensions of health and disease had been raised and approaches discussed during the nineteenth and early twentieth centuries in Scandinavia. People's living conditions, like housing and nutrition, were increasingly becoming an object of medical interest.[2] Different professional and voluntary organizations made efforts to improve the overall health and well-being of the population, termed "folkhälsan" or "folkehelse" (there is no real equivalent to public health in the Scandinavian languages).[3] The emergence of social medicine as a pivotal concept in the region first occurred in 1923. Then, the Swedish Medical Association replaced the term "state medicine" with "social medicine." The subsequent year, in 1924, marked the release of the inaugural issue of the *Journal of Social Medicine* in Sweden, enabling a dedicated scholarly platform for the exploration of social medicine.

During the early decades of the twentieth century, the first women physicians across Scandinavia pioneered new and socially pertinent realms of medicine. They championed initiatives such as assistance for unmarried women, support for vulnerable children, sexual education, and guidance on contraception.

---

[1] See, for example, Dorothy Porter, *Health Citizenship: Essays in Social Medicine and Biomedical Politics* (San Francisco: University of California Health Humanities Press, 2011).

[2] Aina Schiøtz, Maren Skaset, and Una Thoresen Dimola, *Folkets helse – landets styrke 1850–2003*, vol. B. 2 (Oslo: Universitetsforl, 2003), 38 ff.

[3] On the term "the health of the people," see Annika Berg and Teemu Ryymin, "The Peoples' Health, the Nations' Health, the World's Health: Folkhälsa and Folkehelse in the Writings of Axel Höjer and Karl Evang," in Sophy Bergenheim, Johannes Kananen, and Merle Wesse (eds.), *Conceptualising Public Health: Historical and Contemporary Struggles over Key Concepts* (London and New York, NY: Routledge, 2018), 76–100. See also Motzi Eklöf, *Läkarens Ethos: Studier i den svenska läkarkårens identiteter, intressen och ideal 1890–1960* (Malmköping: Exempla, 2018), 33.

Moreover, they actively engaged in political endeavors aimed at reshaping the societal structures contributing to poor health outcomes.[4] Ideologically, most of these physicians aligned themselves in the tradition of social hygiene and social medicine.[5] One notable figure was the Norwegian pediatrician Kirsten Utheim Toverud. She utilized her research on child nutrition and her leadership position within the Norwegian pediatric association to advocate for the establishment of guidance stations tailored to pregnant women and single mothers.[6] Through her multifaceted approach, Toverud not only addressed immediate medical needs but also sought to address systemic issues underlying public health challenges.

Socialist Physicians and Social Medicine

In the context of economic and social crisis of the 1920s and 1930s, young leftist physicians across Scandinavia started arguing for social medicine as an approach grounded in social theory based on readings of Marx and Freud. For them, social medicine by necessity implied not only describing and mapping inequity but also working for societal change. They took a critical stance on what they described as the technical and reductionist character of medicine (including hygiene, which they described a "bourgeois ideology"), which neglected the social and economic influences on health. In a decade characterized by unemployment, poverty, and social unrest, the socialist doctors set themselves the goal of developing a kind of medicine that included the economic and social aspects of sickness, prevention, and treatment, anchored in a socialist ideology of social reform.[7] They wanted to disrupt the system of power balances and transform the capitalist society into a socialist society.

Many of them became active members of the International Federation of Socialist Physicians, which inspired the creation of socialist medical associations in all three countries.[8] Together, these Scandinavian socialist medical

[4] Cecilie Arentz-Hansen, *"Kvinder med begavelse for lægevirksomhed": Norges første kvinnelige leger, og tiden de virket i* (Oslo: Cappelen Damm, 2018): 105–214.
[5] Aina Schiøtz, "'Gjør deres plikt- Men la all ting skje i stillhet': kvinner i folkehelsearbeidets tjeneste," *Michael* 11, no. 1 (2014): 28–44.
[6] Aina Schiøtz, "'Gjør deres plikt- Men la all ting skje i stillhet'," 37–8.
[7] Axel Strøm, "En sosialmediciner ser tilbake," *Tidsskrift for den Norske Lægeforening* 91, no. 31 (1971): 2239–44; Siv Frøydis Berg, *Den unge Karl Evang og utvidelsen av helsebegrepet: en idéhistorisk fortelling om sosialmedisinens fremvekst i norsk mellomkrigstid* (Oslo: Solum, 2002), 33–83; Trond Nordby, *Karl Evang: en biografi* (Oslo: Aschehoug, 1989), 38–42 and 54–9; Niels Brimnes, "Mahler before India," unpublished manuscript, 2024; Annika Berg, *Den gränslösa hälsan: Signe och Axel Höjer, folkhälsan och expertisen* (Uppsala: Uppsala University, 2009).
[8] The International Federation was founded in Karlovy Vary (Karlsbad) in Czechoslovakia in 1931, on the initiative of the Verein sozialistischer Ärzte (Federation of Socialist Physicians). Jonathan Høegh Leunbach from Denmark and Karl Evang from Norway were elected to the new federation's international bureau. "Karlsbader Tagungen der sozialistischen Ärzte," *Der Sozialistische Arzt. Monatszeitschrift des Vereins Sozialistischer Ärzte* 7, no. 7 (1931): 197.

associations engaged in the "culture wars" against fascism and Nazism, partly by building on a common platform. The journal of the Norwegian Socialist Medical Association, *Socialistisk Medisinsk Tidsskrift* (1932–9) soon developed into a journal for the Scandinavian section of the International Federation of Socialist Physicians.[9] By joining the international federation, the organized left-wing doctors in Scandinavia affiliated to a global movement for a social medicine that professed "socialism and class struggle."[10]

To the young Norwegian physician Karl Evang and his progressive Scandinavian colleagues, social medicine was a crucial advance forward in the development of academic medicine. "The wildest confusion" prevailed, Evang argued, regarding the concept "social."[11] First of all, social medicine was not the same as socialized medicine. Social medicine was destined to study the conditions of health under a capitalist world order (as an object of critique). Social medicine, he continued, did not mean a health system financed by the state, nor was it merely a term for the health of a population. Finally, although social medicine took a special interest in conditions caused by society, such as alcoholism, poverty, or criminality, this was only a part of the field. Rather, social medicine was dedicated to (a) understanding the socioeconomic causes of ill health, (b) criticize and change the individualistic and reductionistic modern healthcare, and (c) change how society organized healthcare.

Paraphrasing the first German professor in social hygiene Alfred Grotjahn, whose book *Social Hygiene* he read when imprisoned for conscientious objection in 1930, Evang contended that the organization of society played a crucial role in determining how external factors which can be detrimental to health, affect individuals.[12] Illness was not a random occurrence; rather, it was heavily influenced by the socioeconomic factors humans were exposed to. Acting for change was a crucial part of social medicine and social medicine as a field could provide the tools for doing so.

In Denmark, Mogens Fog, the first chairman of the Danish socialist medical association, commented that doctors "often encounter conditions, which lies beyond our narrow field, but nevertheless touches on our profession. We encounter housing conditions, states of nutrition and environments, which make our prescriptions illusory." In conclusion, he asked: "Can we simply close our door and wash our hands?"[13]

---

[9] "Aus der sozialistischen Ärztebewegung," in *Internationales Ärztliches Bulletin. Zentralorgan der Internationalen Vereinigung Sozialistischer Ärzte* 1 (January 1934): 20.

[10] "Karlsbader Tagungen der sozialistischen Ärzte."

[11] Karl Evang, "Av en innledning til en studiecirkel i sosialmedicin," *Æskulap* 12 (1931): 2–8.

[12] Karl Evang, "Socialmedisinske fremtidsperspektiver," in S. Kjølstad (ed.), *Socialhygiene og folkehelse* (Oslo: Stenersen, 1938), 69–71.

[13] Quoted from Brimnes, "Mahler before India," 8–9.

Sex Education and Reproductive Rights

Freud's ideas greatly influenced young socialist physicians across Scandinavia.[14] They actively advocated for sexual education and the decriminalization of abortion, aligning themselves with the radical women's movements and collaborating with reproductive rights activists.[15] Notable examples include Elise Ottesen-Jensen in Sweden and Katti Anker Møller in Norway, who left indelible marks on the sociomedical landscape of Scandinavia.

Ottesen-Jensen, along with Gunnar Inghe (who in the 1960s became professor of social medicine) founded the Swedish Association for Sexuality Education (RFSU), an organization that continues to advocate for sexual health and LGBT rights.[16] Similarly, Møller advocated for single mothers and campaigned for the legalization of abortion. She also established Norway's first women's health center, laying the foundation for the establishment of similar centers across the country, and influenced the social medical physicians with her thinking.[17] In Denmark, Jonathan Leunbach was a co-founder of the World Liga for Sexual Reform and fought for the right to induced abortion.[18]

Building on their work, proponents of social medicine published a *Popular Journal for Sex Education* in the three Scandinavian countries from 1932 to 1935, reaching diverse audiences. Its content ranged from advocating for women's unfettered access to abortion services to promoting sexual pleasure, while emphasizing the importance of using contraceptive methods such as condoms and pessaries to alleviate women's concerns about unwanted pregnancies. According to Evang, the Norwegian edition alone sold an impressive 120 000 copies of one of its first issues and the editorial team were inundated with 3,000 letters within a two-year span, underscoring its profound impact on public discourse and awareness.[19]

Eugenics and Sterilization in Scandinavia

In the 1990s, a major public upheaval was caused by the fact that the Scandinavian welfare states, which were supposed to protect the marginalized, had engaged in eugenics from the interwar years. In Scandinavia, laws permitting sterilization for eugenic and social reasons were introduced in Denmark,

---

[14] Nordby, *Karl Evang: en biografi*, 35–53.
[15] Kari Tove Elvbakken, *Abortspørsmålets politiske historie: 1900–2020* (Oslo: Universitetsforlaget, 2021): 78–9.
[16] Lena Lennerhed, "Sex Reform in the 1930s and 1940s: RFSU, the Swedish Association for Sex Education," in Lars-Göran Tedebrand (ed.), *Sex, State and Society: Comparative Perspectives on the History of Sexuality* (Umeå: Nyheternas tryckeri KB, 2000): 403–7. The organization had 33,000 members in 1933 and 65,000 members in 1940.
[17] Schiøtz, "Gjør deres plikt- Men la all ting skje i stillhet."
[18] Elvbakken, *Abortspørsmålets politiske historie*, 38.
[19] Karl Evang, *Fred er å skape.* (Oslo: Pax, 1964): 68. Kari Hernæs Nordberg, "Ansvarlig seksualitet: Seksualundervisning i Norge 1933–1935," PhD, University of Oslo, 2013.

Norway, and Sweden between 1929 and 1941. Sterilizations for eugenic and/ or social reasons,[20] mainly of women, peaked from the 1930s to the 1950s. By the mid 1950s, a shift occurred toward voluntary sterilization for contraceptive purposes, moving away from coercive measures.

The development of eugenics in Scandinavia is an example of the well-established links between eugenics and progressive social thought.[21] How did social medicine in Scandinavia relate to these practices? Alfred Grotjahn was a major source of inspiration in Scandinavian social medicine. He had introduced eugenics as one way to solve what he called "social pathologies" and the members of the International Federation of Socialist Physicians did not distance themselves from eugenics.[22] Scandinavian advocates of social medicine, particularly those with radical socialist leanings, however, vehemently opposed the interpretation of eugenics propagated by the radical right and the Nazis as well as its endorsement by "bourgeois scientists." They criticized the unscientific, "race-chauvinistic," and "reactionary" literature associated with eugenics.[23] However, they did not outright reject eugenics itself. Axel Höjer, the Swedish General Director of Health, and prominent public figures Alva and Gunnar Myrdal in Sweden supported the Swedish sterilization laws. The Norwegian Karl Evang viewed the concept of eugenics as – in principle – fundamentally rational. Since the primary cause of intergenerational suffering in his view lay in socioeconomic inequality, however, eugenics would only be justifiable in a society devoid of class distinctions, where socioeconomic disparities had been eradicated.[24] Upon assuming the position of General Director of Health in 1938, Evang, alongside his Swedish counterpart Axel

[20] See Gunnar Broberg and Nils Roll-Hansen, *Eugenics and the Welfare State: Sterilization Policy in Denmark, Sweden, Norway and Finland*, 2nd ed. (East Lansing, MI: Michigan State University Press, 2005), 265. Mattias Tydén, *Från politik till praktik: de svenska steriliseringslagarna 1935–1975* (Stockholm: Almqvist & Wiksell International, 2002); Lene Koch, "The Meaning of Eugenics: Reflections on the Government of Genetic Knowledge in the Past and the Present," *Science in Context* 17, no. 3 (2004), at: doi.org/10.1017/S0269889704000158; Lene Koch, *Racehygiene i Danmark 1920–56* (Copenhagen: Gyldendal, 1996); Lene Koch, *Tvangssterilisation i Danmark 1929–67* (København: Gyldendal, 2000); Per Haave, *Sterilisering av tatere 1934–1977: en historisk undersøkelse av lov og praksis* (Oslo: Norges forskningsråd, 2000).
[21] Paul Weindling, "International Eugenics: Swedish Sterilization in Context," *Scandinavian Journal of History* 24, no. 2 (1999), doi.org/10.1080/03468759950115791; Paul Weindling, *Health, Race, and German Politics between National Unification and Nazism, 1870–1945* (Cambridge; New York: Cambridge University Press, 1989).
[22] See Michael Schwartz, *Sozialistische Eugenik. Eugenische Sozialtechnologien in Debatten und Politik der deutschen Sozialdemokratie 1890–1933* (Bonn: Dietz, 1995).
[23] Karl Evang and Ebbe Linde, *Raslära, raspolitik, reaktion* (Stockholm: Clartés förlag, 1935): e.g., 17, 47, 88.
[24] Karl Evang, "Rassenhygiene und Sozialismus," in *Internationales Ärztliches Bulletin. Zentralorgan der Internationalen Vereinigung Sozialistischer Ärzte* 1, no. 9 (1934): 130–5. Evang and Linde, *Raslära, raspolitik, reaktion*; Karl Evang, *Rasepolitikk og reaksjon* (Oslo: Fram forlag, 1934).

Höjer, nevertheless found themselves intricately involved in the implementation of sterilization laws. This involvement was unavoidable given their roles as directors of their respective countries' national public health services, regardless of their personal endorsements.[25]

Nonetheless, in the broader context of social reform, eugenics and sterilization remained relatively minor issues within Scandinavian social medicine. The primary focus remained on the prevention of unjust disparities in morbidity and mortality through socioeconomic and political measures.[26]

Social Medicine and the Post-war Welfare State: The Expanded Concept of Health

During the interwar years, leading intellectuals like Alva and Gunnar Myrdal in Sweden, along with radical physicians across Scandinavia, saw medicine as having a political role in reshaping industrial society. They pushed for the welfare state's construction through science, with social medicine as a key tool.[27]

After the Second World War, social medicine proponents from the 1930s rose to influential positions in Scandinavian welfare states.[28] For instance, Karl Evang became Norway's General Director of Health from 1938 until 1972, interrupted by wartime exile. In Denmark, Johannes Frandsen led the national board of health from 1928 to 1961, and Axel Höjer served as Sweden's General Director of Health from 1935 to 1952. All of them anchored their social medicine in socialist ideology of social reform.[29]

One crucial component of social medicine as a normative and practical field was the expanded concept of health, which was clearly rooted in the politically radical social medicine that the Scandinavian social medicine advocates had championed since the 1930s,[30] rejecting what they deemed a reductionist and "primitive" view in contemporary medicine. While in exile during the war, Karl Evang built a broad network of social medicine allies in the US and Europe, who shared this vision. He participated in the technical preparatory committee for the International Health Conference in Paris in 1946, working on the draft with the preamble for the new World Health Organization (WHO), which contained the definition of the expanded concept of health. When the conference took place in New York in June, he was appointed chair

---

[25] Tydén, "Från politik till praktik."   [26] Berg, *Den gränslösa hälsan*, 269.
[27] Alva Myrdal and Gunnar Myrdal, *Kris i befolkningsfrågan* (Stockholm: Albert Bonniers Förlag, 1934).
[28] Berg, *Den unge Karl Evang og utvidelsen av helsebegrepet*; Berg, *Den gränslösa hälsan*.
[29] Berg and Ryymin, "The Peoples' Health"; Haave Per, "The Winding Road of the Norwegian 'Welfare State,'" in Nils Edling (ed.), *The Changing Meanings of the Welfare State: Histories of a Key Concept in the Nordic Countries* (New York, NY: Berghahn Books, 2019), 179–224.
[30] Berg, *Den unge Karl Evang og utvidelsen av helsebegrepet*.

of the subcommittee tasked with finishing the constitution for the WHO.[31] Throughout his tenure as General Director of Health and at the WHO, Evang viewed the expanded concept of health not as empty rhetoric but as a catalyst for health policy action, advocating for its implementation beyond hospitals.

Evang remained committed to the expanded concept of health that throughout his life, both in his role as General Director of Health and in that at the WHO. He did not regard it as an empty concept but as a powerful source of health policy action,[32] and wanted the health service outside of hospitals to be organized and filled with content that involved a realization of the extended concept of health.[33]

The sociomedical thinking expressed in the expanded concept of health fitted the intention of the ruling Labour Party in the three countries to secure lives from the cradle to the grave. In varying degrees drawing on the Beveridge Report,[34] the healthcare systems in Scandinavia rose within a welfare model, which would later become known as the Scandinavian or Nordic welfare model.[35] Social medicine helped to form the theoretical basis for health and social policy and the public administration of health was reorganized to construct all those procedures, techniques, institutions, and knowledges that together could empower the application of social medicine.[36]

While rooted in socialist ideology, proponents of social medicine transitioned from revolutionary figures to empowered experts advocating for social integration and justice within the state apparatus. Figures like Karl Evang shifted their focus to using the state to ensure public health rather than viewing it as a repressive entity.[37] The former revolutionary doctors had become nation-builders; a medical expertise in the making of "the good society," and the capital invested to "safeguard the health of the people" was not unproductive, rather "in the truest sense productive capital."[38]

---

[31] Nordby, *Karl Evang*, 138.

[32] Kari Martinsen, *Omsorg, sykepleie og medisin: historisk-filosofiske essays* (Oslo: TANO, 1989), 239.

[33] Seip, *Veiene til velferdsstaten*, 351.

[34] Aina Schiøtz and Maren Skaset, *Folkets helse – landets styrke 1850–2003* (Oslo: Universitetsforlaget, 2003), 314–15; Nordby, *Karl Evang*, 118; Brimnes, "Mahler before India."

[35] P. Kettunen and Klaus Petersen, "Images of the Nordic Welfare Model: Historical Layers and Ambiguities," in Haldor Byrkjeflot, Lars Mjøset, Mads Mordhorst, and Klaus Petersen (eds.), *The Making and Circulation of Nordic Models, Ideas and Images* (London: Routledge, 2021), 13–33.

[36] Aina Schiøtz and Maren Skaset, *Folkets helse – landets styrke 1850–2003* (Oslo: Universitetsforlaget, 2003), 344–7; Anne-Lise Seip, *Veiene til velferdsstaten: norsk sosialpolitikk 1920–75* (Oslo: Gyldendal, 1994), 313–56.

[37] Engh, "The complexities of postcolonial international health," 28.

[38] K. Evang, "Det norske forslag til folketrygd," public speech, 194, Ra/Pa-386/J/L0082; Anne Lise Ellingsæter, Aksel Hatland, Per Haave, and Aksel Hatland (eds.), *Den nye velferdsstatens historie: ekspansjon og omdanning etter 1966* (Oslo: Gyldendal, 2020), 79.

The advocates of social democracy wanted to create systems aiming to "make life worth living for us all," with healthcare as a crucial element.[39] All citizens, regardless of social class or geographical location, were supposed to get the same chances of being included as citizens in the welfare state.[40] The provision of equal access to health services was a crucial policy goal from the immediate afterwar years.[41] An important aspect was that people should not be humble applicants of social and health services but have their rights defined – in terms of services in kind and of financial support. The welfare state rested on a redistribution of money by direct and indirect taxation and improving the people's health was an integral part of social democratic policy to play down social differences.[42] Universalism was the underlying principle – in theory at least, all citizens of the welfare state should have the same rights and the state was given the responsibility to ensure their well-being.[43]

The work of social medicine proponents within the frames of the expansive social and work policy of the Scandinavian welfare states implied that these goals to a certain extent were reached: social medicine actors were important both for the normative reform work and its practical implementation in the Scandinavian welfare states from the end of the war to the 1970s. As Ida Rosenstam has argued, the postwar years were the golden age of social medicine, when the influence of social medicine on the sociopolitical debate and practice was considerable.[44]

Building a Health System: The Example of Norway

The plan for the restructuring of the health system after the war was built on the Norwegian Public Health Act of 1860, which had located the responsibility for the health of the people to Health Councils in the municipalities. These councils consisted of lay people and politicians and was headed by the respective district health officer, appointed by the state. The health officer and a locally appointed community nurse, constituted the core of primary healthcare in the municipality.[45] The attractiveness of this system was

[39] Nordby, *Karl Evang*, 156, 71–72; Rune Slagstad, *De nasjonale strateger* (Oslo: Pax, 2001), 209–12, 308–11.
[40] Teemu Ryymin and Astri Andresen, "Effecting Equality: Norwegian Health Policy in Finnmark, 1945–1970s," *Acta Borealia* 26, no. 1 (2009), doi.org/10.1080/08003830902951565. Seip, *Veiene til velferdsstaten*, 357–9; Slagstad, *De nasjonale strateger*, 210–11, 310–11.
[41] Schiøtz and Skaset, *Folkets helse*, 313–14.
[42] Karl Evang, *Gjenreisning av folkehelsa i Norge* (Oslo: Fabritius, 1947); Nordby, *Karl Evang*; Slagstad, *De nasjonale strateger*, 210–11, 310–11.
[43] Nordby, *Karl Evang*, 171–2; Slagstad, *De nasjonale strateger*, 209–10.
[44] Ida Ohlsson Al Fakir, *Nya rum för socialt medborgarskap: Om vetenskap och politik i "Zigenarundersökningen" – en socialmedicinsk studie av svenska romer 1962–1965* (Växjö: Linnaeus University Press, 2015), 97–8.
[45] Schiøtz and Skaset, *Folkets helse*, 332.

that it ensured decentralized and democratic control in matters of health but also a strong position for the central health administration in social matters. Explicitly drawing on inspiration from Andrija Štampar, Evang advocated participatory democracy at the district level, an idea rooted in the nineteenth-century educational tradition typical of the Scandinavian countries, which, in turn, had inspired Štampar's ideas of social pedagogy in the 1920s.[46]

When it came to primary healthcare within the municipalities, Norwegian health authorities considered publicly funded interdisciplinary health centers to be the best way to achieve an approach anchored in the expanded concept of health.[47] They were inspired by the *basic health services* approach in the WHO. Ideally, the health centers should have a fourfold task: carry out preventive work and curative activities, organize home-nursing care, be responsible for social provision in the municipalities, and be responsible for most of the public provision of health and social care.

However, in a system based on a considerable local political autonomy, this idea was never more than partially realized. Neither in the 1950s nor the 1960s did the health center idea gain traction with the county and municipal health authorities. The development of hospitals was given political priority, demanding the bulk of financial resources. Primary healthcare remained a functional periphery during the development of the welfare state in the post-war period.[48] The Hospital Act of 1969 reinforced the functional "distribution crisis" between the health service inside and outside the institution. In fact, during the post-war period, the Scandinavian healthcare system became more hospital-centered than healthcare systems in other Western countries.[49] In addition, both the Norwegian medical association as well as the municipalities preferred a system of mainly private family doctors to the system of health centers with publicly funded staff.

Although some interdisciplinary health centers emerged across the country over the next decade, shifting policy priorities gradually overshadowed their prominence, particularly the focus on curbing hospital expansion. In the health service reorganization planned in the latter part of the 1970s, the interdisciplinary health center lost its status as a pivotal institution. Simultaneously, the social medical vision integral to these centers faded

---

[46] Patrick Zylberman, "Fewer Parallels than Antitheses: René Sand and Andrija Štampar on Social Medicine, 1919–1955," *Social History of Medicine* 17, no. 1 (2004), doi.org/10.1093/shm/17.1.77.

[47] Martinsen, *Omsorg, sykepleie og medisin*, 240–1.

[48] Finn Henry Hansen, "Helsesektoren i velferdsstaten: kjempevekst og fordelingskrise," *Tidsskrift for samfunnsforskning* 20 (1979): 219–40.

[49] Per Haave, "The Hospital Sector: A Four-Country Comparison of Organisational and Political Development," in Niels Finn Christiansen, Klaus Petersen, Nils Edling, and Per Haave. (eds.), *The Nordic Model of Welfare. A Historical Reappraisal* (Charlottenlund: Museum Tusculanums Forlag, 2006), 215–42.

from health policy,[50] signaling a departure from the dominant social medical orientation of health policy since 1945.[51] Subsequently, in the 1990s, many of the health centers established in the 1970s and 1980s underwent privatization.[52]

Notwithstanding, Evang was content with the fact that they had managed to secure access to free healthcare to all. In 1964, he was taken on a tour of a hypermodern hospital at the University of California, Los Angeles, together with the sociologist, Milton Roemer. The director of the hospital, who was showing them around, halted in front of an advanced X-ray machine and asked Evang whether Norway had something similar. Evang praised the technology but added: "the advantage with our system is that we only need to take one image. Here you have to take two – one of the patient, and one of his wallet."[53]

Social medicine did not penetrate the medical system in a way that the socio-medically oriented health reformers across Scandinavia had wanted. The great paradox of Evang's career was that when he retired in 1972, close to 80 percent of health expenditures in Norway went to hospitals, even though he had been advancing prevention, rehabilitation, and primary care throughout his more than thirty years in office. Looking back, Evang argued that the majority of physicians were still practicing within an old and "outdated" reductionist biomedical mindset.[54] Throughout Scandinavia, in spite of the efforts of the leaders of the central health administration, social medicine became marginalized in a health service characterized by the growth of specialized hospitals, which developed into resource magnets – monopolizing investments, personnel, technology, and patients at the expense of primary healthcare.

Exploring the Margins of the Welfare State: Social Medicine As Academic Field

In 1967, the book, *The Unfinished Welfare* (*Den ofärdiga välfärden*), garnered widespread public attention in Sweden, to the dismay of the Minister of Social Welfare, who criticized it for undermining the welfare state. The authors argued that society tended to overlook silent suffering, which contradicted the welfare state's self-image. Utilizing statistics, they demonstrated how class disparities affected access to medical care, higher education, mental health, and mortality rates. Additionally, the book featured field descriptions and interviews with homeless individuals. The book was authored by Swedish

---

[50] Martinsen, *Omsorg, sykepleie og medisin*, 249; Seip, *Veiene til velferdsstaten*, 353.
[51] Seip, *Veiene til velferdsstaten*, 355.   [52] Schiøtz and Skaset, *Folkets helse*, 357–8.
[53] Nordby, *Karl Evang*, 55.
[54] Karl Evang, *Helse og samfunn. Sosialmedisinsk almenkunnskap* (Oslo: Gyldendal, 1974).

Professor of Social Medicine at Karolinska Institutet in Stockholm Gunnar Inghe and his wife, social worker Maj-Britt Inghe. It drew partly on Gunnar Inghe's groundbreaking PhD thesis of 1958,[55] published in Swedish in 1960 under the title, *Poor in the People's Home* (*Fattiga i folkhemmet*). The book sought to understand and address the root causes of poverty, illness, and marginalization within the welfare society.[56] Whereas sociomedical professionals in the health administration contributed to the building of the welfare state and assumed hegemonic positions, professionals within the academic sociomedical field sought to illuminate the shadows of the welfare state and expose the ill health and lack of access to the welfare state among people in marginalized positions.

Social medicine research had been performed by left-wing doctors in the 1930s, drawing inspiration from international social medicine research activities to explore nutrition and housing related to poverty in Scandinavia, and on the health conditions of people from disadvantaged backgrounds.[57] After the Second World War, social medicine gained recognition as a separate subject within the medical curriculum, complete with its own professorship. This first occurred in Norway in 1952, followed by Sweden in 1958, and Denmark in 1969. Across all three countries, this establishment involved the separation of social medicine from hygiene within the medical field.

The professors in social medicine, like Gunnar Inghe in Sweden, Poul Bonnevie in Denmark, and Axel Strøm in Norway, formed a generation of sociomedical professionals with their teaching and textbooks in social medicine. They were also people with significant influence in their own societies. For example, Strøm had served as President of the Norwegian Medical Association (1948–51) when he accepted his professorship. Following his tenure, he assumed the role of Dean of the Medical Faculty at the University of Oslo for seven years, from 1956 to 1964.

In Sweden, a committee appointed by the government recommended in 1953 that social medicine should be based on research related to the social context of clinical practice and on heredity, environment, and social determinants of health and disease, based in interdisciplinary research centers.[58] The first two professorships in social medicine with attached sociomedical clinics were established in 1958 in Gothenburg and Lund, followed by

---

[55] G. Inghe, "Mental and Physical Illness among Paupers in Stockholm," *Acta Psychiatrica Neurol Scandinavica* 33, Suppl 121 (1958): 1–316.

[56] Ohlsson Al Fakir, *Nya rum för socialt medborgarskap: Om vetenskap och politik i "Zigenarundersökningen" – en socialmedicinsk studie av svenska romer 1962–1965*.

[57] Karl Evang and Otto Galtung Hansen, *Norsk kosthold i små hjem : virkelighet og fremtidsmål* (Oslo: Tiden, 1937), 7.

[58] *Swedish Government Official Reports* (*SOU*), 1953: 7 Läkarutbildningen (on Medical Education) (Stockholm: Ministry of Education, 1953), 253–4.

professorships in three other universities by 1963, and ultimately in Linköping in 1969.[59] One of the early Swedish professors in social medicine was before mentioned Gunnar Inghe, who like the first professor in social medicine in Norway, Axel Strøm, had been one of the pioneers of the radical social medicine movement in the 1930s and then above all, for the more social-political line of social medicine.[60] In Denmark, Paul Bonnevie was the driving force in separating hygiene and social medicine. He was Professor in Hygiene at the University of Copenhagen from 1948. He rapidly expanded the subject to also include social medicine, which he called "the ecology of human beings,"[61] taking the post as the first Professor in Social Medicine in 1969.[62] In Norway, Per Sundby researched somatic health problems among patients with alcohol dependence, whereas Berthold Grunfeld continued the tradition of sexual health and reproductive rights in social medicine from the 1930s. His doctoral thesis from 1973 focused on women and abortion in Norway,[63] and had significant implications for the breakthrough of the new Norwegian legislation on voluntary abortion, which came into effect when the "abortion law" of 1975 was amended in 1978.

Social medical research in Scandinavia centered mainly on underprivileged groups in society – for example, on access to abortion services, alcoholism, substance use problems, venereal diseases, and national minorities.[64] A defining feature of the research in this period was its interdisciplinary nature, incorporating both natural and social sciences. It employed biomedical approaches alongside methods derived from the social sciences, encompassing clinical practice, research directed at policy and clinical practice, and investigations conducted at both individual and population levels. Moreover, funding for this research came from governmental authorities, public institutions, and universities alike. Thus, it was the transboundary character of social medicine that enabled the expansion of social medicine as an academic field.

[59] Urban Janlert, Socialmedicinens väg till specialitet, Socialmedicinsk tidskrift 5 (2009): 402–9. Umeå, Uppsala and Stockholm and Linköping.

[60] Jan Halldin, "Gunnar Inghe – de fattigas advokat Sveriges förste sociålläkare inspirerande lärofader," Läkartidningen 96 (1999): 2895–7. Other politically minded social medicine proponents were Gustav Jonsson and John Takman, whereas Ragnar Berfenstam, who was a professor in Uppsala argued for a more "descriptive" social medicine without normative dimensions.

[61] Steen Brock, Folkesundhed. Perspektiver på dansk samfundsmedicin (Aarhus: Philosophia), at: https://samples.pubhub.dk/9788793041189.pdf.

[62] Povl Riis, "Poul Bonnevie," in Den Store Danske lex.dk, at: https://denstoredanske.lex.dk/Poul_Bonnevie.

[63] Berthold Grünfeld, Legal abort i Norge: legalt svangerskapsavbrudd i Norge i tidsrommet 1965–1971: en sosialmedisinsk og sosialpsykiatrisk undersøkelse (Oslo: Universitetsforlaget, 1973).

[64] Ida Ohlsson Al Fakir, Nya rum för socialt medborgarskap: Om vetenskap och politik i "Zigenarundersökningen" – en socialmedicinsk studie av svenska romer 1962–1965 (Växjö: Linnaeus University Press, 2015), 96.

Social Medicine As a Medical Specialty

Social medicine as a clinical practice in Scandinavia during the postwar years was directed toward the multifaceted origins of diseases and disabilities, the importance of interdisciplinary collaboration, and advocacy for social reforms and collective care across various sectors such as education, healthcare, and social insurance. In all three countries, specialties in social medicine were created but took different forms.

One significant common feature was the development of social medicine as an important field in the disability benefit policy. This led to a new and broader client group, including the elderly, children, and other persons outside the labor market. From now on, experts in social medicine dominated the growing field of disability benefit policy. The new laws on disability pensions stressed the need to exhaust all available measures before granting pensions, a concept hailed by the General Director of Health in Norway as a "truly revolutionary sociomedical breakthrough."[65] Sociomedical advocates asserted that social medicine should play a pivotal role in a holistic and socially conscious rehabilitation, distinct from the biomedical approach.[66] Clinics were established in certain state and regional hospitals and primarily catered to a select group of complex patients while also serving as training facilities. In Sweden, Professor Gunnar Inghe held the position of clinic head at the Karolinska Hospital, whereas Strøm was the clinic head at the social medicine clinic at Rikshospitalet.[67]

In 1959, Norway was the first country in Scandinavia to establish a specialty in social medicine.[68] However, the proposed sociomedical departments that were supposed to give these new specialists a job and secure their specialization failed to materialize adequately due to low prioritization by regional authorities and societal stigma surrounding the specialty and its patients.[69] Instead, more biomedically oriented rehabilitation services began to dominate the hospital landscape. Additionally, primary healthcare, predominantly composed of general practitioners in private solo practices, was tasked with the responsibility of sociomedical rehabilitation, effectively diminishing the necessity for dedicated departments of social medicine. In 1986, social medicine ceased to exist as a medical specialty. A new specialty of physical medicine and rehabilitation was supposed to continue "the individual aspect" of

---

[65] Evang, *Helse og samfunn: sosialmedisinsk almenkunnskap.*
[66] Marte Feiring, "Fra revalidering til rehabilitering – en dansk begrebshistorie," *Tidsskrift for Professionsstudier* 13, no. 24 (2017): 86–97.
[67] Evang, *Helse og samfunn: sosialmedisinsk almenkunnskap.*
[68] Per Haave, *I medisinens sentrum. Den norske legeforening og spesialistregimet gjennom hundre år* (Oslo: Unipub, 2011), 92. See also the proposition:
[69] Anders Chr Gogstad, "Klinisk sosialmedisin: lavstatusposisjon i helsevesenet?," *Tidsskrift for Den norske lægeforening* 102, no. 31 (1982): 1619–21.

social medicine. Another new specialty, community medicine, was supposed to harbor the "population aspect" of social medicine, in addition to public health work in the municipalities.[70] In contrast to what Anderson, Dunk, and Musolino show in Chapter 12 in this volume, the authorities considered these new tasks to be "too important" to be left to "economists, experts on health administration, statisticians, lawyers or health educators" and wanted doctors in top positions in the local health administration.[71] Social medicine was supposed to be one of several disciplines contained within community medicine but it remained marginal in the new specialty.

In Denmark, social medicine, while similar to Norway, was important for rehabilitation in the early postwar years and defined as a proper clinical practice, a specialty devoted to social medicine alone never developed. However, in 1989, a specialty in community medicine (established in 1987) was expanded to include social medicine as a proper subspecialty (health administration is the other subspecialty). The specialty has, in contrast to Norway, maintained the combination of individual and population level focus so characteristic of social medicine in Scandinavia in the early days. The subspecialty in social medicine mainly focuses on sociomedical problems in individual patients, drawing on theory and methods from public health, sociology, epidemiology, law, and clinical medicine.

In Sweden, social medicine was suggested as a specialty by the highly influential scholars Gunnar and Alva Myrdal already in 1934,[72] but although it was defined as a clinical area in the 1950s, the specialty was only formed 1974. Until the 1990s, social medicine in Sweden had a clinical basis which was mainly concerned with work and rehabilitation toward full employment and many of the specialists worked as social physicians in interdisciplinary teams at regional level. However, as a consequence of the restructuring of the health system and finances, social physicians could no longer be employed at a district level and the specialty stopped being anchored in a clinical field. From then on, the Swedish specialty social medicine has been predominantly oriented toward population-oriented health policy and management, health promotion, prevention, and social epidemiology. The specialty still exists,

---

[70] One reason for the establishment was that the more than 120-year history of the centrally appointed District Medical Officer came to an end as a result of the new Act and was replaced by a physician appointed by the local government who was given the responsibility for the provision of healthcare in the community.

[71] Per Haave, *I medisinens sentrum: Den norske legeforening og spesialistregimet gjennom hundre år* (Oslo: Unipub, 2011), 271–3.

[72] Alva Myrdal and Gunnar Myrdal, *Kris i befolkningsfrågan* (Stockholm: Albert Bonniers Förlag, 1934); James M. Nyce and Toomas Timpka, "The reformist triad and Institutional Forgetting of Culture: A Field Study into Twentieth-Century Swedish Social Medicine" *International Journal of Health Services* 42, no. 1 (2012): 95–107.

although it is struggling due to a lack of places for the young specializing physicians to practice,[73] and its existence has been threatened.

Scandinavian Social Medicine Actors on a Global Scene

Social medicine protagonists in Scandinavia sought inspiration among likeminded colleagues abroad, first and foremost in the activities at the WHO. For small countries such as the Scandinavian, global engagements offered means to reassert themselves in an era of emerging powers and geopolitical crises. By collaborating with each other on a common social democratic agenda and with the non-aligned countries on political reform in the 1970s, the Scandinavian countries were able to maintain their status as important international actors, despite their small size.

As Sunniva Engh has shown, Norwegian Karl Evang played a more important role in the early process of the creation of the WHO than has been acknowledged in the anglophone literature on the WHO.[74] According to Szeming Sze, Evang was a driving force behind the proposal of the formation of a world health organization.[75] He continued to be an active member of the WHO and chaired all Norwegian delegations to the yearly assemblies until his retirement in 1972. Furthermore, he served as president and vice president at the second and fourth World Health Assemblies in 1949 and 1951, respectively, and as chairman of the Executive Board in two sessions.[76] In 1966, he received the Léon Bernard Foundation Prize for outstanding contribution to social medicine.[77]

While chairing the Panel on Public Health Administration, Evang, together with Andrija Štampar and others, formulated the Basic Health services idea in 1951. Carrying forward ideas from the Bandung Conference of 1937, they attempted to launch a new primary healthcare offensive, at a local level, with involvement of the local population and collaboration with different sectors of society.[78]

The most controversial field, however, was family planning and women's health. Partly relying on previous experiences with sex education and domestic

---

[73] Urban Janlert, Socialmedicinens väg till specialitet, *Socialmedicinsk tidskrift* 5 (2009): 402–9.
[74] Szeming Sze, "The Birth of WHO: Interview [with] Szeming Sze," *World Health*, May 1989. See also Sunniva Engh, "The Complexities of Postcolonial International Health: Karl Evang in India 1953," *Medical History* 67, no. 1 (2023): 29.
[75] Sunniva Engh and Niels Brimnes, "Scandinavian Entry Points to Social Medicine and Postcolonial Health: Karl Evang and Halfdan Mahler in India," *Medical History* 67, no. 1 (2023): 1–4.
[76] In the 36th and 37th session.
[77] https://apps.who.int/gb/awards/pdf_files/Bernard/Winners_en.pdf.
[78] Martin Gorsky and Christopher Sirrs, "From 'Planning' to 'Systems Analysis': Health Services Strengthening at the World Health Organization, 1952–1975," *Dynamis (Granada, Spain)* 39, no. 1 (2019), doi.org/10.30827/dynamis.v39i1.8672.

concern over child poverty and depopulation from the interwar period and forward, Norway and Sweden pushed an early maternal- and child-oriented agenda. In 1952, Evang suggested that an expert committee should investigate and deliver a report on the health aspect of birth control and family planning.[79] He received support from representatives from both Ceylon and India but had to withdraw the suggestion after heated debate.[80] In 1958, Sweden responded to a request from Ceylon and later Pakistan to provide development assistance for family planning.[81]

Both Höjer and Evang were impressed and inspired by the work of the Indian delegation during the first years of the WHO, an impression that also led both of them to develop projects with Indian collaborators. It was Sir Arcot Lakshmanaswami Mudaliar, a key figure both within the WHO and Indian health and education policy-making,[82] who convinced Axel Höjer to leave his post as General Director of Health in Sweden and instead help develop medical education in Kerala, India.[83]

As Niels Brimnes has recently shown, WHO Director General Halfdan Mahler's views on healthcare were formed by his experience of social medicine in India between 1951 and 1961, where he was inspired by indigenous traditions, community orientation, and a broad approach to health,[84] described by Baru in Chapter 11 in this volume. The election of Halfdan Mahler as Director-General of the WHO (1973–88) also led the push for a more radical international health agenda, based on equity and social justice and the emergence of a new health for all paradigm in the Alma-Ata Declaration of 1978.

[79] World Health Organisation (WHO). 1952. Fifth World Health Assembly, 8, 237–8, https://iris .who.int/bitstream/handle/10665/85641/Official_record42_eng.pdf

[80] According to Milton Roemer, this event was the reason why Evang had lost his chances of becoming the next Director-General of WHO: "He [Karl Evang] is, in my opinion, the best public health administrator in the world and would undoubtedly have been the next Director-General of W.H.O., had he not brought the Catholics down on him by being outspoken on birth control" (Letter from Roemer to Sigerist, Regina, January 29, 1955, at: www.img.unibe.ch/ e40437/e40444/e153944/section154575/files154580/CorrespondenceHenryE.Sigerist-MiltonI. Roemer_ger.pdf). Vicente Navarro held Evang to be one of the most important persons he had met: "my professional life in the health area was most influenced at that time by Evang and Brotherston. It was they who, with Štampar from Yugoslavia, wrote the famous definition of health in the 1948 World Health Organization Constitution" (Vicente Navarro, "A Historical Review (1965–1997) of Studies on Class, Health and Quality of Life: A Personal Account," *International Journal of Health Services* 28, no. 3 (1998): 389–406).

[81] Sunniva Engh, "The Rockefeller Foundation, Scandinavian Aid Agencies and the 'Population Explosion,'" in Klaus Petersen, John Stewart, and Michael Kuur Sørensen (eds.), *American Foundations and the European Welfare States* (Odense: Syddansk Universitetsforlag, 2013), 181–202.

[82] Roger Jeffery, *The Politics of Health in India & London* (Berkeley: University of California Press, 1988).

[83] Berg, *Den gränslösa hälsan.*

[84] Niels Brimnes, "Negotiating Social Medicine in a Postcolonial Context: Halfdan Mahler in India 1951–61," *Medical History* 67, no. 1 (2023), doi.org/10.1017/mdh.2023.11.

More than fifty years after Karl Evang had taken part in the first general
health assembly in the WHO, the Norwegian physician and politician Gro
Harlem Brundtland became Director General of the WHO. "There is a very
close connection between being a doctor and being a politician," Brundtland
said in an interview with *Time* magazine in 2001. "The doctor first tries to prevent illness, then tries to treat it if it comes. It's exactly the same as what you
try to do as a politician, but with regard to society."[85]

When the young and politically relatively inexperienced physician Gro
Harlem Brundtland was called to be Minister of Environment in 1974, she felt
competent because she compared environmental politics to health promotion.
She had a Public Health degree from Harvard and had worked in the Social
Medicine Department, first at the Norwegian Directorate of Health, then at the
Oslo City Health Council (on the subject of school health). At the time when
she got the call from the prime minister, she had started a PhD on the social
determinants of health and had initiated her public life as an abortion activist,
applying her medical experience to bring about political change. Her outspoken pro-choice lobbying brought her into the public eye in the early 1970s and
to the attention of the power circles in the Labour Party.[86] After having served
five successful years as a minister of the environment, she was prime minister
first in 1981, then in 1986–9 and 1990–6. In 1984, she was asked by the United
Nations Secretary General Perez de Cuellar to preside over the newly created
World Commission on Environment and Development.

With more of a willingness to compromise on humanitarian idealism than
Karl Evang, she brought what Simon Reid-Henry has called "a distinctly
Nordic brand of humanitarian internationalism" to the emergent environmental
politics of the time.[87] The commission's landmark report *Our Common Future*,
also known as the Brundtland report, published in 1987, coined the value-
based concept of sustainable development, defined as "development that meets
the needs of the present without compromising the ability of future generations
to meet their own needs."[88] In the report, social, economic, and environmental
concerns were inextricably linked and the policy solutions they suggested integrated social equity, economic growth, and environmental problems.

Although both the commission's extensive community engagement in the
form of hearings and the report's call for "vigorous redistributive policies" in

[85] N. Gibbs, "Norway's Radical Daughter," *Time*, June 24, 2001.
[86] Steinar Hansson, *Makt og mannefall: historien om Gro Harlem Brundtland*, ed. Ingolf Håkon
Teigene (Oslo: Cappelen, 1992).
[87] Simon Reid-Henry, "The Pragmatarian Style: Environmental Change, Global Health, and Gro
Harlem Brundtland's Nordic Internationalism," in Antoine de Bengy Puyvallée and Kristian
Bjørkdahl (eds.), *Do-Gooders at the End of Aid: Scandinavian Humanitarianism in the Twenty-
First Century* (Cambridge: Cambridge University Press, 2021), 194–221.
[88] World Commission on Environment and Development, *Our Common Future* (Oxford: Oxford
University Press, 1987), 43.

economic growth,[89] were completely in balance with Brundtland's own egalitarian and social democratic ideas as Iris Borowy has shown,[90] it opened up a path for addressing structural problems via market logics and instruments. Therefore, although it initially had quite a radical agenda, it has been criticized for having made change dependent not upon solidarity but on self-interest.[91] However, it is hard to overestimate the impact the value-based concept of sustainable development has had and there is certainly important social medicine elements in the Commission's early work on popular engagement.

After returning to Norway to serve as prime minister once more – first from 1986 to 1989 and again from 1990 to 1996 – Brundtland later reemerged on the global stage when she was elected as the new Director-General of the WHO in 1998, a post she had until she resigned when term ended in 2003. When taking office, one of her two announced priorities was tobacco control and, in 2003, the World Health Assembly adopted the WHO Framework Convention on Tobacco Control. This landmark agreement introduced regulations governing tobacco production, sale, distribution, advertisement, and taxation, marking a watershed moment for international public health.[92]

During her leadership, WHO projects moved away from the health systems approach of Mahler. She was determined to reposition WHO as an important global player and strengthen the organizations position in an era with a growing dominance of neoliberal globalization and the entry of a whole series of new actors on the global arena, in the fragmented and complex landscape characterizing this transition from international health to global health.[93] Building on her extensive political experience, she contributed to a more political approach to health within the WHO. She also sought to strengthen the difficult financial situation of the WHO by opening it up for private–public partnership, thereby increasing the number of actors within global health, but also address the lack of governance.

Social Medicine: Still in Search of a Lost Discipline?

In the first decades of the post-war society, what had been radical left-wing social medicine became close to self-evident policies and the 1930s pioneer

[89] World Commission on Environment and Development, *Our Common Future*, 50.

[90] Iris Borowy, *Defining Sustainable Development for Our Common Future: A History of the World Commission on Environment and Development (Brundtland Commission)* (London: Routledge, 2014).

[91] Reid-Henry, "The Pragmatarian Style."

[92] R. Roemer, A. Taylor, and J. Lariviere, "Origins of the WHO Framework Convention on Tobacco Control," *American Journal of Public Health* 95, no. 6 (June 2005), doi.org/10.2105/ajph.2003.025908.

[93] Theodore Brown, Marcos Cueto, and Elizabeth Fee, "The World Health Organization and the Transition from 'International' to 'Global' Public Health," *American Journal of Public Health* 96, no. 1 (2006): 62–72, doi: 10.2105/AJPH.2004.050831.

generation saw many of their central ambitions fulfilled and important tasks solved, both in academia (professorships in social medicine) and in bedside medicine (social medicine clinics), in a growing welfare state that built on the expanded notion of health. The political radicalism of social medicine receded to the background and practitioners of social medicine as well as academics focused increasingly on vulnerable groups and their precarious position within the health and welfare services and most of its practitioners left its revolutionary ambitions.

During the 1980s and 1990s, social medicine experienced a notable decline, which was particularly evident in Norway. This period saw the closure of social medicine departments in regional hospitals and the discontinuation of the medical specialty in social medicine in 1986. Instead of being housed in hospital departments, academic social medicine became based in university departments, without any real connection to clinical practice. Reflecting the shift from the hospital sector to primary healthcare within community medicine, professors of social medicine during the 1990s were recruited mostly from academic general practice, rather than from psychiatry.[94]

For example, Per Fugelli assumed the position of professor in Social Medicine at the University of Oslo in 1992, after having established an academic department of general practice in Bergen. In Oslo, he embarked on a lengthy career as a public intellectual, addressing topics such as medicalization, social justice, and death and dying.

To a lesser extent, he focused on cultivating a new generation of researchers and did not succeed in building an academic field in the same way as he had done for general practice a decade earlier.[95] However, during the 1990s, he established an interest group for medical students called "The Patient Earth," which attracted many students who would later play significant roles in the Norwegian medical community. This group aligned with his passion for ecology and the environment at the time. In 1993, before the concept of planetary health emerged, he wrote an article about "the patient Earth," urging doctors to diagnose the diseases of the planet and recommend treatment.[96] Fugelli's influence extended to a broad public audience, as evidenced by the front-page coverage of his death in 2017 by all major newspapers.

In Sweden and Norway, the reorganization of academic departments in the latter part of the twentieth century ultimately diminished the status of social medicine as an independent discipline. It was consolidated with other fields

---

[94] K. Haug, P. Fugelli, G. Høyer, and S. Westin, "Sosialmedisin – på sporet av det tapte fag," *Tidsskrift for Den norske lægeforening* 120 (2000): 3057–61.

[95] K. Malterud and S. Hunskår, "Per Fugelli – en allmennmedisinsk biografi. I: S. Hunskår (red.)," *Akademisk allmennmedsin i Bergen 50 år: 1972–2022, Michael* 19, suppl 29 (2022): S61–8.

[96] Per Fugelli, "In Search of a Global Social Medicine," *Forum for Development Studies* 20, no. 1 (1993/01/01 1993), https://doi.org/10.1080/08039410.1993.9665937, https://doi.org/10.1080/08039410.1993.9665937.

into larger units, where various subjects were merged under a single umbrella, both in research and teaching.[97] In 1999, the *Nordic Journal of Social Medicine* was rebranded as the *Scandinavian Journal of Public Health*, reflecting the fading prominence of the term "social medicine." According to the editors, it had been concluded that "despite the strong sentiments attached to the historical, ideological and professional connotations of 'social medicine', ... the broader term 'public health' would better convey the Journal's scientific orientation and sphere of interest."[98]

In the 2000s, research on social inequality in health surged, partly influenced by the Marmot Report. However, this research, mainly register-based and population studies, focused on the overall gradient of inequality in the population rather than addressing the sociomedical concerns of marginalized groups and the pathology of poverty. Furthermore, new dynamic research groups in international health, medical anthropology, and general practice, often adopting a social medicine perspective, opted against associating themselves with the label. The decline of the academic core environments for social medicine was partly due to the emergence of these new, vibrant research groups but also to a clear shift of research toward epidemiology and population-wide studies, where methodological challenges often took precedence and statistically trained researchers took the lead.

Today, the presence of academic chairs in social medicine has dwindled notably across Scandinavia, with Denmark showing a slightly more favorable situation compared to the other two countries. The calls for social medicine that became evident during the Covid-19 pandemic in other parts of the world remained almost silent in Scandinavia, despite its once prominent role as a core element of the welfare state. Consequently, social medicine, rooted in principles of social justice and the social determinants of health, has receded to the background.

---

[97] John Gunnar Mæland, "Samfunnsmedisin og folkehelsearbeid," *Michael* 13 (2016); John Gunnar Mæland, "Den norske akademiske sosialmedisins fall 1990–2024," unpublished manuscript, 2024.

[98] "From *Scandinavian Journal of Social Medicine* to *Scandinavian Journal of Public Health*: A Change of Name but Not of Vision," *Scandinavian Journal of Public Health* 27, no. 1 (1999): 1–2.

7   American Social Medicine in the Shadow of Socialized Medicine

Jeremy A. Greene, Scott H. Podolsky, and David S. Jones

Speaking to an international audience of medical educators in 1953, Dr. John Perry Hubbard attempted to describe the stigma attached to social medicine in Cold War America. In the "all-out war" between the medical profession and proposals for national health insurance, the University of Pennsylvania Professor of Public Health and Preventive Medicine lamented that "socialized medicine was held up before the American public as a threatening evil. The average citizen – and many a physician, too – does not really know what he means by socialized medicine but he is sure that it is bad. And social medicine does not sound very different."[1] This confusion has been an enduring challenge.

Social medicine has a long and puzzling history in the United States. Several key figures in global social medicine worked in the US and won renown for their work. The Rockefeller Foundation provided substantial support that advanced the mission of social medicine worldwide – especially through the growing reach of early twentieth-century American imperialism. Yet social medicine achieved little institutional stature in the US, with a formal presence at only a handful of medical schools. This chapter examines this discrepancy. The obscurity of social medicine reflects in part the politics of the US in which "social medicine" was too often heard as "socialized medicine," a red-baiting tactic in US politics. Work that might otherwise have been called social medicine had to pass under other names, from hygiene to preventive medicine or community health. The near invisibility of social medicine poses a challenge for historians: what counts as "social medicine" in a profession whose dominant discourse denied its existence? Is it only those who self-identified as theorists or practitioners of social medicine or does it include people who self-identified differently but worked in the spirit of social medicine?

We take a hybrid approach. We begin with early invocations of "social medicine" in the US, its most visible theorists (e.g., Henry Sigerist), and an

---

[1] John Perry Hubbard, "Integrating Preventive and Social Medicine in the Medical Curriculum," *New England Journal of Medicine* 251 (1954): 513–19, quote at 514.

important patron, the Rockefeller Foundation. We then pause to examine several Black social theorists whose work can now unquestionably be recognized as social medicine yet who have been largely excluded from this pantheon. The Cold War put social medicine under great pressure in the US. Different threads, however, endured. The first, clinically oriented, focused on community health. The second, based in academic departments, applied the interpretive social sciences to explore the interspace between the clinical and the social. These threads converged in the 1990s and 2000s in new forms of social medicine-informed clinical practice which drew on both community health and critical social theory to define social medicine as healthcare committed to social justice and health equity. This recent synthesis, however, poses another puzzle: why, given growing consensus in US medicine about social justice and health equity, does social medicine remain on the margins?

Early Invocations and Advocates of Social Medicine

There are many ways to trace the histories of social medicine. One approach looks for recognizable intellectual antecedents, for instance theorists who insisted that medicine take social context or social justice seriously. This approach would acknowledge Henry Ingersoll Bowditch, chair of the first state board of health in the United States. In 1874, he called on Massachusetts to use its "moral power and material resources" in the service of preventive medicine, for instance making investments in housing and nutrition for the poor to combat tuberculosis.[2] Milton Rosenau, who became the first professor of preventive medicine at a US medical school, described tuberculosis in 1913 as a sociologic and economic problem and invoked justice and mercy to encourage investments in the health of vulnerable people.[3]

A more restrictive approach focuses on the term "social medicine." The phrase first appeared in the *Boston Medical and Surgical Journal* in 1876, in a review of medical education in Germany. It emerged sporadically over the next several decades, usually as a synonym for "preventive medicine."[4] In 1915, Richard Cabot described social medicine, "done on salary and for the

---

[2] Henry I. Bowditch, "Preventive Medicine and the Physician of the Future," *Fifth Annual Report of the State Board of Health* (Boston: Wright and Potter, January 1874), 30–60, quote at 33.

[3] Milton J. Rosenau, *Progress and Problems in Preventive Medicine* [Ether Day Address, 1913] (Boston: Jamaica Printing Company, 1913), quote at 28. At the same time, and illustrating the complexities of characterizing proponents of "preventive" or "social" medicine, Rosenau included a chapter (admittedly with caveats) on eugenics in multiple editions of his classic textbook on preventive medicine and hygiene; see, e.g., Milton J. Rosenau, *Preventive Medicine and Hygiene* (New York, NY, and London: Appleton and Company, 1913), 415–25.

[4] See, e.g., Theobald Smith, "Research into the Causes and Antecedents of Disease, Its Importance to Society," *Boston Medical and Surgical Journal* 153 (1905): 6–11; and Theobald Smith, "The Sphere of Social Medicine," *Boston Medical and Surgical Journal* 177 (1917): 299.

public benefit," as one of "the three great fields of medicine – medical science, medical practice and social medicine."[5] The *Journal of the American Medical Association* (*JAMA*) first printed the term "social medicine" in a 1910 review of a textbook of medical sociology that made the case for studying social conditions that threaten health.[6] In 1916, *JAMA* launched a column, variably titled "Social Medicine, Medical Economics and Miscellany" or just "Social Medicine."[7] Most of these essays, however, had nothing to do with a recognizable field of "social medicine." They instead explored myriad topics, from antivivisectionists to the merits of state medicine.

More progressive visions of social medicine emerged at the intersections of medicine and social work. Tuberculosis, housing, and occupational health drew particular attention. Francis Lee Dunham's 1925 *An Approach to Social Medicine* defined it as "a field of preventive science to which social science, psychology, psychiatry, and various other departments shall contribute ... Such a field functions more naturally as an attitude, a point of view, rather than as a specific department."[8] Such sentiments encountered increasing resistance in the US as conservatives recoiled from the Bolshevik revolution in Russia. As fears of "socialized medicine" began to circulate in *JAMA* and the *Boston Medical and Surgical Journal* in the late 1910s, social medicine was drawn into the debates.[9] In 1921, a concerned physician warned that, "If in the years to come social medicine has us enmeshed in its irksome bonds, let us blame only ourselves."[10] A 1927 review of "Group Practice" feared legislation that could socialize medicine: "State or social medicine, or compulsory health insurance, is intolerable. We must organize and be ready to strike it down."[11]

Henry Sigerist, who would become one of social medicine's most effective early advocates, arrived in the US in the midst of these debates. He had been invited by William Henry Welch, who played a decisive role in establishing the German vision of scientific medicine in the US.[12] But Welch was also committed to the idea that medicine should not be reduced to science alone.

[5] Richard C. Cabot, "Women in Medicine," *Journal of the American Medical Association* 45 (1915): 947–8.
[6] "Review of *Medical Sociology*," *Journal of the American Medical Association* 54 (1910): 154–5. This also mentioned the establishment of a new chair of social medicine in Vienna.
[7] "Social Medicine, Medical Economics and Miscellany," *Journal of the American Medical Association* 77 (1916): 1390–1. This ran sometimes weekly, sometimes less often, until 1936.
[8] Francis Lee Dunham, *An Approach to Social Medicine* (Baltimore: Williams & Wilkins, 1925), 14.
[9] For an early occurrence, see, Review of "Transactions of the American Surgical Association, Volume 36," *Boston Medical and Surgical Journal* 181 (1919): 749.
[10] J. R. Fowler, "Impending Dangers," *Boston Medical and Surgical Journal* 185 (1921): 217.
[11] Philemon E. Truesdale, "Group Practice," *Boston Medical and Surgical Journal* 196 (1927): 973–83.
[12] George Rosen, "William Henry Welch: 1850–1934," *Journal of the History of Medicine and Allied Sciences* 5 (Summer 1950): 233–5.

After retiring from his deanships at the Johns Hopkins School of Medicine and then the Johns Hopkins School of Public Health, he dedicated his efforts to founding the Institute of the History of Medicine at Hopkins and recruited Sigerist to direct it. Sigerist had studied medicine, and then history of medicine, in Zurich, and joined the faculty at Leipzig in 1925.[13] Working amidst Germany's post-war economic crises, he became interested in the social and political organization of medicine. As he veered toward socialism, he became increasingly critical of the rise of German fascism. Welch invited him to tour the US in 1931. Bewildered by the Depression-era US, he criticized fee-for-service healthcare and mocked American resistance to health insurance. Cultured and erudite, he charmed the leaders of academic medicine. Welch offered him the leadership of the new Institute in 1932.

Sigerist quickly became a successful academic and public intellectual in the US. He presented history as a space for scholarly reflection about the importance of social context in medical care and advocated for a sociological and policy-oriented approach to social medicine in medical education.[14] Sigerist applauded the establishment of chairs of Social Medicine in the UK and closely followed John Ryle's efforts to build an academic field that would guide the new National Health Service.[15] He published an enthusiastic account of Soviet medicine and advocated for national health insurance in the US (frequently butting heads with Morris Fishbein and the American Medical Association, AMA).[16] He used his proximity to Washington to advise President Roosevelt about health policy.

From his base at Hopkins, Sigerist also mentored many physician-scholars who in turn became key figures in American social medicine. George Rosen first contacted Sigerist in 1933, as a medical student studying history and then sociology. With Sigerist's encouragement, Rosen turned his attention to occupational health, a field which made especially visible the pathways through which the social world shaped health and disease on the basis of class, race, ethnicity, and labor. In 1939 Rosen wrote Sigerist seeking advice: "I would like to write my dissertation in the field of social medicine (in the broadest

[13] Elizabeth Fee, "The Pleasures and Perils of Prophetic Advocacy: Henry E. Sigerist and the Politics of Medical Reform," *American Journal of Public Health* 86 (1996) 1637–47. See also Elizabeth Fee and Theodore M. Brown (eds.), *Making Medical History: The Life and Times of Henry E. Sigerist* (Baltimore: Johns Hopkins University Press, 1997).

[14] Henry E. Sigerist "Trends in Medical Education: A Program for a New Medical School," *Bulletin of the History of Medicine* 9 (1941): 177–98; Leslie Falk, "Medical Sociology: The Contributions of Henry E. Sigerist," *Journal of the History of Medicine and Allied Sciences* 13 (1958): 214–28.

[15] Sigerist to Ryle January 28, 1944. The Henry E. Sigerist Collection at the Alan Mason Chesney Medical Archives of The Johns Hopkins Medical Institutions (hereafter, SigH), 3.1R. The pair kept up a lively exchange of letters and students and visited each other when possible.

[16] Emily Ann Harrison, "Indicating Health: Leona Baumgartner, Global Development, and the Metrics of Infant Mortality (1950–1980)," PhD, Harvard University, 2017, 43–4.

sense of that term)."[17] Rosen continued to seek Sigerist's help and advice as he moved onto his next projects, a history of public health and his essay, "What is Social Medicine?," which established Virchow as an icon for the field – as discussed in Carsten Timmerman's contribution to this volume.[18]

Enthusiasm in the US for the USSR cooled quickly after the Soviet–Nazi pact and the Soviet invasion of Finland in 1939. Sigerist, however, continued to push for socialized medicine in the early 1940s. By 1944, though, rising anti-communist sentiment ended his advisory work for the US government. He participated in analyses of healthcare in Canada and then in India, serving with Ryle on the Bhore Commission.[19] He invited Ryle to visit the US to help evangelize for social medicine. "Your presence," he explained, "would give an enormous stimulus to the development of social medicine in this country which is still in its early beginnings."[20]

Sigerist also strategized with Iago Galdston, a psychiatrist and historian at the New York Academy of Medicine (NYAM). In 1947, NYAM hosted an Institute on Social Medicine, a three-day conference that included, among others, Sigerist, Rosen, Ryle, other prominent historians (e.g., Richard Shryock, Ludwig Edelstein, and Owsei Temkin), and Alan Gregg, the Associate Director of Medical Sciences for the Rockefeller Foundation.[21] "In this country social medicine is everybody's business but nobody's responsibility," NYAM President George Baehr reflected, "We know that poverty, food, housing, conditions of work – all have an important bearing upon the prevalence of certain diseases; but we have not yet proceeded very far in investigating and eliminating the specific causative factors that have the greatest social import."[22] Sigerist congratulated Galdston on a "superb Institute," and hoped social medicine might play an important role in progressive postwar social reforms.[23]

---

[17] This led to George Rosen, *The History of Miners' Diseases: A Medical and Social Interpretation* (New York, NY: Schuman's, 1943).

[18] Rosen to Sigerist, October 21, 1944, SigH 3.1R; George Rosen, *A History of Public Health* (New York, NY: M.D. Publications, 1958); George Rosen, "What Is Social Medicine? A Genetic Analysis of the Concept," *Bulletin of the History of Medicine* 21 (1947): 674–733.

[19] For the Bhore Commission, see Sunil S. Amrith, *Decolonizing International Health: India and Southeast Asia, 1930–65* (New York, NY: Palgrave Macmillan, 2006); Kiran Kumbhar, "Healing and Harming: The 'Noble' Profession of Medicine in Post-Independence India, 1947–2015," PhD, Harvard University, 2022.

[20] Sigerist to Ryle, February 6, 1945, SigH, 3.1R. This letter is the first we have found arguing explicitly for the field of "social medicine" in the US.

[21] "Institute on Social Medicine – March 19, 20, and 21, 1947," Archives, New York Academy of Medicine. Centennial. Institute on Social Medicine [Correspondence and miscellaneous papers. New York, 1946–47. 26 letters and 16 miscellaneous items]. The meeting was sponsored jointly by NYAM's Committee on Medicine and the Changing Order and its Committee on Medical Information.

[22] George Baehr, "Foreword," in Iago Galdston (ed.), *Social Medicine: Its Derivations and Objectives* (New York, NY: Commonwealth Fund, 1949), v–vi.

[23] Galdston to Sigerist, March 28, 1947, SigH, 3.1R.

But his impact in US health policy had already waned and as Sigerist retired to Switzerland that year, he became increasingly disillusioned with both social and socialized medicine in the US and USSR, while Galdston in New York tried to find new futures for the field.[24]

Globalizing American Social Medicine

As they worked to theorize and foster social medicine in the US, Sigerist, Rosen, Galdston, and like-minded colleagues had gained substantial moral and financial support from the Rockefeller Foundation. In the first half of the twentieth century, the Foundation was the most important philanthropic institution for medical research and international health. Internal tensions between its two poles – reductionist biomedicine and social medicine – were pervasive.[25]

John D. Rockefeller established the Rockefeller Institute for Medical Research in 1901 but interests soon expanded from basic science to public health. The Rockefeller Sanitary Commission for the Eradication of Hookworm found partial success in the American South with programs that targeted doctors, schools, newspapers, and legislatures. This experience inspired the Rockefeller Foundation, founded in 1913, to establish its International Health Board (renamed the International Health Division in 1927) to pursue hookworm programs in other countries whose geographical reach meshed closely with changing forms of US imperialism.[26]

The International Health Division (IHD), with its mix of health workers, Christian charity, and public health interventions, soon expanded beyond hookworm to tackle tuberculosis, malaria, yellow fever, and other diseases of poverty.[27] It focused particularly on what would later be termed the social determinants of health in rural areas, from the American South to France, Eastern Europe, China, and India. The Rockefeller Foundation facilitated an international commerce in rural health expertise. It supported the work of Andrija Štampar, a socialist public health reformer, in Yugoslavia, and then sent him as an advisor to China. It sent another socially minded medical consultant, D. L. Hydrick, to Java to advise the Dutch on rural health. Victor Heiser, who led Rockefeller Foundation efforts in the US-occupied Philippines, used the opportunity to test theories of ecological intervention

[24] Iago Galdston, *The Meaning of Social Medicine* (Cambridge, MA: Harvard University Press, 1954), 1–30.
[25] Angela Matysiak, *Health & Well-Being: Science, Medical Education, and Public Health* (New York, NY: Rockefeller Foundation, 2014), 11.
[26] Warwick Anderson, *Colonial Pathologies: American Tropical Medicine, Race, and Hygiene in the Philippines* (Durham, NC: Duke University Press, 2006).
[27] John Ettling, *Germ of Laziness: Rockefeller Philanthropy and Public Health in the New South* (Cambridge, MA: Harvard University Press, 1981).

and race uplift.[28] As Laurence Monnais and Hans Pols describe in Chapter 4 in this volume, this Rockefeller vision of social medicine had a significant impact on the health programs of the League of Nations, especially as seen in the 1937 Bandung Conference.[29]

As Anne-Emanuelle Birn and Elizabeth Fee have shown, the IHD "befriended dozens of governments around the world by tackling diseases deemed to cause underdevelopment, helping build and modernize health institutions, promoting the importance of public health among countless populations, and preparing vast regions for investment and increased productivity."[30] It also helped found schools of public health across Europe, Asia, and the Americas. Birn and Fee describe how, by 1951, "the IHD had spent the current-day equivalent of billions of dollars on scores of hookworm, yellow fever, and malaria campaigns, as well as on more delimited efforts against tuberculosis, yaws, influenza, rabies, schistosomiasis, malnutrition, and other health problems in some 93 countries and colonies."[31]

Deep tensions ran through these programs. On the one hand, the Foundation supported reductionistic, "magic-bullet" approaches to public health.[32] Birn and Fee critique how its narrowly focused disease control campaigns "tended to be run with business-like efficiency: specific interventions were planned with measurable goals and results regularly reported to the central office, serving to hold field officers accountable as well as to quantify progress in quarterly reports reviewed by trustees, who were leading men from the worlds of medicine, education, and banking."[33] On the other hand, the Foundation (or at least factions within it) explicitly supported social medicine. Birn and Fee describe how the Rockefeller Foundation "diverged at times from its own principles, funding studies of universal health insurance and supporting certain social medicine efforts that integrated the sociopolitical conditions underlying health with overall public health work."[34] Birn later explained that "the RF remained tolerant and even intellectually open to alternatives to its techno-medical focus and afforded long-time RF officers the leeway and independence to pursue

---

[28] Anderson, *Colonial Pathologies*, 217.
[29] See also Amrith, *Decolonizing International Health*, 26–46; Patrick Zylberman, "Fewer Parallels than Antitheses: René Sand and Andrija Stampar on Social Medicine, 1919–1955," *Social History of Medicine* 17 (2004): 77–92.
[30] Anne-Emanuelle Birn and Elizabeth Fee, "The Rockefeller Foundation and the International Health Agenda," *Lancet* 381 (11 May 2013): 1618–19, quote at 1618. See also Matysiak, *Health & Well-being*, 11.
[31] Birn and Fee, "Rockefeller Foundation," 1618.
[32] Amrith, *Decolonizing International Health*, 18; Zylberman, "Fewer Parallels than Antitheses"; E. Richard Brown, *Rockefeller Medicine Men: Medicine and Capitalism in America* (Berkeley: University of California Press, 1979).
[33] Birn and Fee, "Rockefeller Foundation," 1618.
[34] Birn and Fee, "Rockefeller Foundation," 1619.

these interests, albeit under financial, time-horizon, and other constraints."[35] It provided funding for academic programs, for instance establishing the Institute of Human Relations, led by Milton Winternitz, at Yale University in 1929, designed "to bridge the gap between medical and social knowledge of human behavior," to create "clinical sociology" and medicine for the "whole person."[36] It supported Sigerist, Štampar, Ryle, and René Sand, who became Professor of Social Medicine at the University of Brussels in 1945.[37] It supported progressive public health programs in Latin America in the 1930s as part of US State Department efforts to counter growing German influence. And it collaborated with the League of Nations Health Organization on a series of social medicine projects.[38]

Rockefeller officials became key players in social medicine on a global stage. John Grant began his career working with the Rockefeller Sanitary Commission's campaigns against hookworm in North Carolina. He then studied public health at Hopkins. The Foundation sent him to China in 1921, where he worked for many years to support Peking University Medical College. He adapted ideas from European social medicine to design prevention campaigns there.[39] For instance, he worked with C. C. Chen to implement a sophisticated healthcare system for the rural villages in the Tinghsien region. He served for several years in India in the 1940s, introducing social medicine there through his work (with Sigerist and Ryle) on the Bhore Commission, and then through the establishment (via grants from Rockefeller Foundation) of professors of Preventive and Social Medicine at Indian medical colleges. He also supported the work of Sidney and Emily Kark in South Africa (see below and Chapter 9 by Abigail H. Neely in this volume).[40]

The Second World War disrupted this work. The Rockefeller Foundation, however, remained integrally involved in global social medicine. Many people with ties to the Foundation participated in the international health conference in New York City (NYC) in 1946 that led to the establishment of the

---

[35] Anne-Emanuelle Birn, "Philanthrocapitalism, Past and Present: The Rockefeller Foundation, the Gates Foundation, and the Setting(s) of the International/Global Health Agenda," *Hypothesis* 12 (2014):e8, doi:10.5779/hypothesis. v12i1.229: 6.

[36] Matysiak, *Health and Well-being*, 153; Harrison, "Indicating Health," 63; Dorothy Porter, "How Did Social Medicine Evolve, and Where Is It Heading?" *PLoS Medicine* 3, no. 10 (October 2006): e399, 1667–72; A. J. Viseltear, "Milton C Winternitz and the Yale Institute of Human Relations: A Brief Chapter in the History of Social Medicine," *Yale Journal of Biology and Medicine* 58 (1984): 869–89.

[37] Porter, "How Did Social Medicine Evolve"; Andrew Seaton, "The Gospel of Wealth and the National Health: The Rockefeller Foundation and Social Medicine in Britain's NHS, 1945–60," *Bulletin of the History of Medicine* 94 (2020): 91–124, at 99.

[38] Birn, "Philanthrocapitalism"; Porter, "How Did Social Medicine Evolve."

[39] Matysiak, *Health and Well-being*, 100; Socrates Litsios, "John Black Grant: A 20th-Century Public Health Giant," *Perspectives in Biology and Medicine* 54 (2011): 532–49.

[40] Litsios, "John Black Grant," 540–4; Seaton, "Gospel of Wealth," 102.

WHO in 1948. Rockefeller social medicine shaped the preamble of the WHO through the influence of Štampar, who served on the preparatory committee.[41] As Dorothy Porter has argued, the "international social medicine movement," stoked by the Foundation, "aimed to create a new social role for medicine in order to grapple with the epidemiological transition created by economic and social developments in the twentieth century."[42] With the establishment of the WHO, the Rockefeller Foundation wound down some of its own operations, for instance closing its IHD in 1951. However, it remained active in various ways. Some were narrow and technocratic, whether its support of Fred Soper's work on DDT and malaria eradication or its advocacy for family planning in the global south.[43] Other work preserved its interests in social medicine, especially its social medicine programs in India. Yet overall, there was less and less room for social medicine in the increasing economic rationality of international health in the 1950s.[44]

Excluded Voices

As social medicine developed in the United States, scholars and physicians of color were excluded from the field, despite having considerable expertise in what we would now call social medicine. Traditional histories of social medicine have perpetuated this by failing to recognize their contributions to the genealogy of social medicine. We must understand the structural processes by which minoritized voices (whether by race, sex, gender, or other markers of difference) have been systematically excluded from genealogies that emphasize its white men.[45]

The polymath W. E. B. Du Bois is an important starting point. In 1899, Du Bois published what is now recognized as a landmark study in sociological theory and method: a radically different take on "the Negro question" entitled *The Philadelphia Negro*. Du Bois drew on extensive, almost ethnographic, interviews with families in Black neighborhoods and a rich analysis of quantitative economic and demographic data. He showed how every aspect of African American life in the US was shaped by racism, segregation, and the legacies of slavery. He hoped that his scholarship would

---

[41] Amrith, *Decolonizing International Health*, 74.

[42] Porter, "How Did Social Medicine Evolve," 1668.

[43] Amrith, *Decolonizing International Health*; Mathew Connelly, *Fatal Misconception: The Struggle to Control World Population* (Cambridge, MA: Harvard University Press, 2010); Nancy Leys Stepan, *Eradication: Ridding the World of Diseases Forever?* (London: Reaktion Books, 2011).

[44] Amrith, *Decolonizing International Health*, 93.

[45] This section draws on Alexandre White, Rachel L. J. Thornton, and Jeremy A. Greene, "Remembering Past Lessons about Structural Racism: Recentering Black Theorists of Health and Society," *New England Journal of Medicine* 385 (2021):850–5.

fuel activism: it should "act as a spur for increased effort ... and not as an excuse for passive indifference, or increased discrimination."[46] He followed this with his 1903 *Souls of Black Folk*.[47] Du Bois demanded that goals of social analysis must shift away from blaming social ills on those oppressed by economic or racial degradation. It should instead seek a more complex understanding of the myriad ways in which power relations shape everyday life and health outcomes.

Only recently has Du Bois's work been recognized as foundational for US sociology writ large and it deserves similar stature within social medicine.[48] Du Bois demonstrated that racial disparities in mortality from tuberculosis, "the most fatal disease for Negroes,"[49] were themselves a product of social forces: the racial disparities in health so evident in the streets of Philadelphia were the products of a social force, racism, rather than any inherent biological difference between the races. He detailed the pathways by which the health of middle-class, working-class, and unemployed Black Philadelphians alike were affected by the racial segregation of housing, economic opportunity, and access to healthy food and environments. Du Bois grounded his social theory in data visualization, charts, survey data, and careful statistical analysis. As he explained, to compare the health of White Philadelphia and Black Philadelphia was not only to view "side by side and in intimate relationship in a large city two groups of people, who as a mass differ considerably from each other in physical health," but to apprehend the social, economic, historical, and legal structures that produced racial disparities in health.[50]

By linking tuberculosis and other health inequities to these social forces, Du Bois extended his work to become a study of power relations, what we now term structural violence and racism, and the ways these become historically constituted inequalities. Du Bois painted a nuanced picture of communities that were further impoverished because of their disproportionate burden of illness. They suffered from inadequate housing made worse by landlords' refusals to repair racially segregated housing. This demonstrated both the general effects of living conditions on individual health and the specific, pervasive, and toxic role of racism as a structural and organizing social force.

Du Bois was not alone in this endeavor. Howard University's Kelly Miller produced detailed analyses of the pathways by which the sociology of racism – and not some predetermined biology of racial differences – determined the

---

[46] W. E. B. Du Bois, *The Philadelphia Negro: A Social Study* (Philadelphia: University of Pennsylvania Press, 1899).

[47] W. E. B. Du Bois, *The Souls of Black Folk* (Chicago, IL: A.C. McClurg & Co., 1903).

[48] See, e.g., Aldon Morris, *The Scholar Denied: W. E. B. Du Bois and the Birth of Modern Sociology* (Oakland, CA: University of California Press, 2015).

[49] Du Bois, *Philadelphia Negro*, 107.   [50] Du Bois, *Philadelphia Negro*, 114.

stark health inequities between Black and white Americas.[51] Yet the work of Miller, Du Bois, and other Black scholars of race and health in the early twentieth century was largely sidelined by mainstream medical and scholarly journals. Instead, physicians and social scientists looked to figures like the University of Chicago's Robert Park to define the new field of American sociology and its health consequences. Park and his colleagues assumed that racial differences were fixed and health disparities therefore inevitable.[52]

Du Bois, Miller, and others forcefully insisted that Black people were not a "problem" to be explained or solved by social-scientific or medical expertise, but human beings deserving of full personhood. Yet their calls were ignored by (mostly white) physicians for far too long. That is not surprising, especially in a medical profession that routinely excluded Black physicians from membership in local, state, and national medical societies from Reconstruction until the era of Medicaid and Medicare.

Although W. E. B. Du Bois lived in Baltimore during the Sigerist years, we have found no evidence of the two meeting. When Sigerist attended the first NYAM Institute on Social Medicine in 1947 on the eve of his departure from Johns Hopkins, he had taught no Black physicians, historians, or sociologists while serving on the faculty. The school, which ran a segregated hospital, had to date categorically denied entrance to every applicant of African or African American heritage.

Social Medicine and Socialized Medicine in the Cold War

As advocates worked to revitalize social medicine in the US after the Second World War, they took the problem of race more seriously. This was, in part, an outgrowth of the field's new focus on urban health. Following the 1947 NYAM Institute for Social Medicine, organized by Galdston and Sigerist, NYC became an important center for US social medicine. One key figure was René Dubos.

Dubos, a French microbiologist, joined Oswald Avery's laboratory at the Rockefeller Institute in 1927. His work on enzymes produced by soil microbes led to the discovery of several antibiotics in the 1930s and 1940s. This work epitomized the "magic-bullet" tradition of biomedical science. However, Dubos's interests soon broadened to include the interplay between organisms and their environments. In 1952, he and his wife, Jean Dubos, published a

---

[51] Samuel Kelton Roberts, *Infectious Fear: Politics, Disease, and the Health Effects of Segregation* (Chapel Hill, NC: University of North Carolina Press; 2009); Lundy Braun, *Breathing Race into the Machine: The Surprising Career of the Spirometer from Plantation to Genetics* (Minneapolis, MN: University of Minnesota Press, 2014).

[52] Morris, *The Scholar Denied.*

history of tuberculosis.[53] While this book did not use the phrase "social medicine," it has been adopted as a work of social medicine. They saw the tuberculosis pandemic as the result of mismanaged industrialization and urbanization.
Produced by social forces, tuberculosis could be addressed through social
action: "We need to develop a new science of social engineering," Dubos concluded, "that will incorporate physiological principles in the complex fabric of
industrial society."[54]

If *The White Plague* was a study of social disease, Dubos's 1959 *Mirage
of Health* described social medicine as a space for exploring the relations of
disease, medicine, and society. Dubos traced how enlightenment scholars pursued "a scientific philosophy of public health which emphasized complex relationships between social environment and the physical well-being of man."[55]
The epidemics of cholera and tuberculosis in nineteenth century motivated
communities to grant power to health departments "for the regulation of community life."[56]

Dubos influenced many New York physicians who would go on to shape the
practice of social medicine. Walsh McDermott led clinical trials of antibiotics
at New York Hospital in the 1930s and 1940s. He was drawn to the Navajo
Reservation in 1952 because of the opportunities it offered to test new antibiotics for tuberculosis.[57] While there, he found that tuberculosis was the tip
of the iceberg: antibiotics alone could not address the stark health disparities
suffered by a community mired in rural poverty. He teamed up with Dubos in
1953 and 1954 to conduct health surveys of the Navajo. They found terrible
problems with infant and child mortality, especially from diarrhea, pneumo-
nia, and tuberculosis. Much of this burden of disease could be prevented by
proper medical and public health systems. McDermott credited Dubos with
envisioning a new model of medicine, a "hospital without walls" that would
manage the "total health" of the population.[58] This became McDermott's
healthcare experiment at Many Farms.[59]

---

[53] René Jules Dubos and Jean Dubos, *White Plague: Tuberculosis, Man, and Society* (Boston: Little, Brown, and Company, 1952).

[54] Dubos and Dubos, *The White Plague*, 228; see also vii–viii.

[55] René Dubos, *Mirage of Health: Utopias, Progress, and Biological Change* (New York, NY: Harper, 1959), 23.

[56] Dubos, *Mirage of Health*, 234.

[57] David S. Jones, "The Health Care Experiments at Many Farms: The Navajo, Tuberculosis, and the Limits of Modern Medicine, 1952–1962," *Bulletin of the History of Medicine* 76 (2002): 749–90; David S. Jones, *Rationalizing Epidemics: Meanings and Uses of American Indian Mortality since 1600* (Cambridge, MA: Harvard University Press, 2004).

[58] John Adair and Kurt W. Deuschle, *The People's Health: Medicine and Anthropology in a Navajo Community* (New York, NY: Meredith Corporation, 1970), 144.

[59] Walsh McDermott, Kurt Deuschle, and Clifford Barnett, "Health Care Experiment at Many Farms," *Science* 175 (January 7, 1972): 23–31.

McDermott's interest in community, ecology, and disease was influenced by others in the NYC medical scene at the time, including Galdston, Alexander Leighton, and Lawrence Hinkle. While McDermott and his team did not use the phrase "social medicine," their work was very much in that spirit. Many alums of the project applied its insights throughout their careers. Kurt Deuschle, for instance, worked at Many Farms from 1954 to 1960. This experience led him to reorient his career toward the emerging field of community medicine. He recognized that medical interventions required both technical knowledge and human considerations – a comprehensive, holistic approach to medicine, a "united effort by modern medicine and social science in the translation of technical knowledge into improved and expanded health services that are medically sound, economically feasible and capable of reaching entire communities."[60] He left Many Farms to become chair of the Department of Community Medicine at the new School of Medicine at the University of Kentucky (the first such department in the US).[61] At Kentucky, he continued to work to achieve Dubos's vision of a hospital without walls. In 1968, he moved to New York to lead community medicine at Mount Sinai Hospital and its new medical school.

Another New York hospital took a lead role in reimagining social medicine at an urban hospital. Montefiore Hospital had long focused on the social and community aspects of care delivery.[62] By 1950, Montefiore's director, Ephraim Bluestone, had founded the country's first explicit hospital-based program in social medicine. Interested in the social organization of medical practice and the social factors impacting care, he saw social medicine as a way of situating care in the community, both before and after hospitalization. The Division of Social Medicine oversaw the hospital's social work services, home care, a prepaid medical group practice, and relevant teaching and research.[63] As Bluestone explained in *Modern Hospital*, the social medicine division would

---

[60] Donald L. Hochstrasser, G. S. Nickerson, and Kurt W. Deuschle, "Sociomedical Approaches to Community Health Problems," *Milbank Memorial Fund Quarterly* 44 (July 1966): 345–59, quote at 346.

[61] Alan L. Silver and David N. Rose (guest eds.), "Urban Community Medicine: The Mount Sinai Experience Honoring the Work of Kurt W. Deuschle," *Mount Sinai Journal of Medicine* 59 (1992): 439–68.

[62] Victor W. Sidel, "Social Medicine at Montefiore: A Personal View," *Social Medicine* 1 (2006): 99–103; Dorothy Levenson, *Montefiore: The Hospital as Social Instrument, 1884–1984* (New York, NY: Farrar, Straus & Giroux, 1984). Ernest Boas (son of Franz Boas) directed the hospital in the 1920s. With Sigerist's support, he asked the Rockefeller Foundation in 1947 to fund a *Journal of Social Medicine*; the Foundation declined. See Dorothy Levenson, "The Origins of the Department of Social Medicine at Montefiore," *Montefiore Medicine* 5 (1980): 49; George Rosen, "In Memory of Henry Ernest Sigerist," *Bulletin of the History of Medicine* 13 (1958): 126.

[63] E. M. Bluestone, "Social Medicine Arrives in the Hospital," *Modern Hospital* 75 (August 1950): 59–62.

be the "conscience of the hospital ... which will continuously draw attention to the human being as an individual during sickness and near-sickness, psycho-somatically and in relation to his family and his environment, and which will care for him completely, comprehensively and continuously."[64] Any conscientious physician, he continued, must include the social world when thinking of a patient's history, physical examination, assessment, and therapeutic plan:

> The study of the signs and symptoms of disease is vital to the practice of medicine, but additional vital factors must be studied with equal diligence, such as the living quarters of the patient, his food, his family, the climate in which he lives (literally and figuratively), the way in which he makes a living, as well as the pressures, the resistances and the tensions that characterize his struggle for existence and survival.[65]

When Montefiore Hospital affiliated with the Albert Einstein College of Medicine in the 1960s, the Division became a Department of Social Medicine. Victor Sidel became its chair in 1969.[66]

Yet few schools or hospitals followed Montefiore's lead. Part of the problem was the ongoing politics of socialized medicine. As Bluestone lamented in *JAMA* in 1952, "'social medicine,' which is the finest flower of modern medical practice, has been tarred of late with the brush of 'socialized medicine.'"[67] Hubbard, quoted at the outset of this chapter, explained to international social medicine educators that US medical schools "avoided" the term, though he considered that in the "broad sense there is little difference between the meaning of preventive medicine in the United States and the meaning of social medicine."[68] Each, he related, "recognizes the relation between man and his environment; each implies the importance of social factors as they influence health."[69] But the Cold War was heating up and red-baiting reached to new heights.[70] The AMA furiously opposed President Truman's efforts to enact national health insurance, labeling it as a dangerous form of "socialized medicine." This limited the space in which proponents of social medicine could work.

The American Association of Medical Colleges (AAMC), meanwhile, turned to "preventive medicine," mandating its teaching at all US medical schools

---

[64] Bluestone, "Social Medicine Arrives," 60.

[65] Bluestone, "Social Medicine Arrives," 61.

[66] Sidel, "Social Medicine at Montefiore," 100–1. By 1985, the department would merge with the Department of Community Health to become the Department of Epidemiology and Sociology; by 2004, it would become the Department of Family and Social Medicine.

[67] E. M. Bluestone, "'Socialized Medicine' and 'Social Medicine' [Letter to the Editor]," *Journal of the American Medical Association* 148 (1952): 1358.

[68] Hubbard, "Integrating Preventive and Social Medicine," 514; see also George A. Silver and William Kissick, "A Social Medicine Residency Program," *Journal of Medical Education* 37 (1962): 1217.

[69] Hubbard, "Integrating Preventive and Social Medicine," 514.

[70] Levenson, "Origins of the Department," 52.

in 1945. Students were to consider: "the general and specific relationship of social environment on community and individual health; housing in relation to public health; the correlation of morbidity and mortality with low income; ... the social order, its effect upon public health and practices, and its influence on the practice of medicine."[71] In this vision, preventive medicine could cover the ground of social medicine without the baggage of socialized medicine.

Social Medicine As Community Practice

As the AAMC pushed schools to adopt preventive medicine, other schools turned to "community medicine" instead. The movement had many origins. The most famous began in South Africa. Inspired by the work of Rudolf Virchow and Henry Sigerist, Sidney and Emily Kark established a health center for Black South Africans in Pholela, Natal, in 1940. This work was funded by the Rockefeller Foundation. The Karks recognized that it was necessary to change the social order to improve health. This required interventions at both the individual and community level.[72] As Neely describes in Chapter 9 in this volume, the clinic's success depended on the work of the women and other community members in Pholela.[73] After a 1942 National Health Services Commission recommended expanding their model across South Africa, the government opened 44 community health centers. However, the movement lost support after the 1948 elections cemented the ascension of the National Party and the establishment of the Apartheid regime. The community clinics, and the academic units that had supported them, had all closed by 1960.[74]

Though short-lived, the community-oriented social medicine developed in Pholela had a far-reaching legacy. While a medical student at Case Western in 1957, Jack Geiger traveled to South Africa and worked for four months with the Karks. Inspired by that experience, he dedicated his career to developing community health centers in the United States. Geiger studied with John Grant at the Rockefeller Foundation. He then completed his medical training in Boston

---

[71] H. S. Mustard, Jean A. Curran, Hugh R. Leavell, and Charles E. Smith, "Final Report of the Committee on the Teaching of Preventive Medicine and Public Health," *Journal of the Association of American Medical Colleges*, 20 (1945): 152–65, quote at 164.
[72] For a detailed description of their model, see Sidney Kark and Emily Kark, "A Practice of Social Medicine," in Sidney L. Kark and Guy W. Steuart (eds.), *A Practice of Social Medicine: A South African Team's Experiences in Different African Communities*, (Edinburgh: E&S Livingstone, Ltd., 1962), 3–40, reprinted in *Social Medicine* 1 (August 2006): 115–38.
[73] See Abigail H. Neely, Chapter 9, this volume. See also, Abigail H. Neely, *Reimagining Social Medicine from the South* (Durham, NC: Duke University Press, 2021).
[74] Mervyn Susser, Zena Stein, Margaret Cormack, and Michael Hathorn, "Medical Care in a South African Township," *Lancet* 268 (1955): 912–15; Shula Marks, "South Africa's Early Experiment in Social Medicine: Its Pioneers and Politics," *American Journal of Public Health* 87 (1997): 452–9.

and joined the faculties at Harvard and Tufts. Active in the civil rights movement, he worked on the "Freedom Summer" in Mississippi in 1964. He joined other physicians to establish the Medical Committee for Human Rights.[75] He pitched his plan for community health centers to the Office of Economic Opportunity (OEO), which had been created by the Economic Opportunity Act of 1964 as part of President Johnson's "War on Poverty." The OEO awarded its first grant, in June 1965, to Geiger and his colleague Count Gibson, to create two health centers. Geiger and Gibson opened the first in renovated apartments in the Columbia Point housing project in South Boston. Geiger opened the second in Mound Bayou, in Bolivar County on the Mississippi Delta.[76] Community members set the clinics' priorities. The clinics provided health education, prevention, and healthcare. They developed community partnerships to break the cycles of poverty, ill-health, and unemployment. The OEO funded six other community health centers in 1966.

Geiger's work in South Boston caught the attention of Massachusetts Senator Edward Kennedy, who visited Columbia Point in August 1966 and spent the afternoon speaking to staff, patients, and community leaders. Impressed by what he saw, Kennedy pushed through legislation to create the Office of Health Affairs within the OEO to create a national network of neighborhood health centers. Kennedy hoped that the $50 million in funding would establish 800 clinics and restructure the US healthcare system. Alice Sardell has called this attempt the only serious attempt to implement social medicine in the US.[77] Opposition from the Nixon and Ford administrations soon stymied progress; only 150 clinics were established.[78] The surviving clinics and neighborhood health centers struggle to maintain their commitment to community-centered healthcare within a larger healthcare system that does not prioritize community interests.

While Geiger is often identified as a foundational figure for community health in the US,[79] his was not the only model. Several minoritized communities also took matters into their own hands. For example, the Black Panther Party was established in 1966 to take a stand against police violence.

[75] Bonnie Lefkowitz, "The Health Center Story: Forty Years of Commitment," *Journal of Ambulatory Care Management* 28 (2005): 295–303; H. Jack Geiger, "The First Community Health Centers: A Model of Enduring Value," *Journal of Ambulatory Care Management* 28 (2005): 313–20; John Dittmer, *The Good Doctors* (Jackson, MS: University Press of Mississippi, 2017).

[76] Thomas J. Ward, *Out in the Rural: A Mississippi Health Center and Its War on Poverty* (New York, NY: Oxford University Press, 2016); Judy Schader Rogers, "Out in the Rural," film, 1970, at: https://vimeo.com/9307557.

[77] Alice Sardell, *The US Experiment in Social Medicine: The Community Health Center Program, 1965–1986* (Pittsburgh, PA: University of Pittsburgh Press, 1988).

[78] Lefkowitz, "The Health Center Story"; Geiger, "The First Community Health Centers."

[79] Denise Grady, "H. Jack Geiger, Doctor Who Fought Social Ills, Dies at 95," *New York Times*, December 28, 2020.

Its mission expanded to include community empowerment and social welfare programs. Party leaders argued that urban Black communities had been excluded from or abused by the healthcare system. They demanded access to care and "emancipation from 'medical apartheid.'"[80] They drew inspiration not from the traditional icons of social medicine, but from Mao Zedong, Che Guevara, and the Martinique-born French psychiatrist Franz Fanon, whose work documented the harms of colonialism and racism. The party established its first Peoples' Free Medical Clinics in 1968, in Kansas City, Chicago, and Seattle. In April 1970, party president Bobby Seale called on all party chapters to open their own clinics.

By 1971, the Panthers had established a network of thirteen health clinics nationwide. In Alondra Nelson's telling,

the Party brought to the efforts of the radical health movement its own social health perspective. This agenda, reflecting the formative influence of the social medicine tradition, assumed a holistic view of disease and illness and incorporated antiracism, Marxist-Leninist ideology, and a critique of medical authority. Conceived as sites of social change, Party medical clinics attended to more than just narrowly defined health needs.[81]

A parallel movement of Latinx activism, most evident in the work of the Young Lords, also pursued a radical vision of community health. They commandeered health services, including a brief takeover of a New York hospital, to demand healthcare that prioritized community needs.[82] These health revolutionaries faced a difficult choice: to rely on the community's own expertise (since doctors were part of the problem/system) or to accept allies from within a healthcare system dominated by white doctors and nurses.

These "bottom-up" radical community health campaigns also carefully negotiated federal and state efforts to establish neighborhood health centers and alternately depended on and critiqued the limitations of existing antipoverty measures, such as the "ghetto medicine" programs of the late 1960s. The state of New York, for instance, enacted a "Ghetto Medicine Law" in 1968 that made funds available for academic medical centers to provide care to minoritized residents in nearby neighborhoods.[83] These partnerships struggled to overcome long-standing mistrust that was often made worse by the programs' limited and short-term funding.

---

[80] Alondra Nelson, *Body and Soul: The Black Panther Party and the Fight against Medical Discrimination* (Minneapolis, MN: University of Minnesota Press, 2011), 20.

[81] Nelson, *Body and Soul*, 114.

[82] Joshanna Fernandez, *The Young Lords: A Radical History* (Durham, NC: University of North Carolina Press, 2020).

[83] Betsey J. Bernstein, "What Happened to Ghetto Medicine In New York State?" *American Journal of Public Health* 61 (1971): 1287–93.

Harlem became an iconic site for both demonstrating the health disparities of the "medical ghetto" and for imagining solutions to resolve them. In
their time working with the Navajo, McDermott and Deuschle had come to see
the Navajo Reservation as a "Third World country within the United States,"
underdeveloped economically, socially, and medically.[84] When Deuschle
arrived in NYC to establish community medicine at Mount Sinai, he saw a similar situation in Harlem.[85] Deuschle sought ways to provide appropriate medical technology in ways that would benefit the community. He found a key ally
in Carter Marshall, an African American physician and East Harlem resident.
Marshall envisioned a neighborhood health program that would stretch directly
from Mount Sinai Hospital into Harlem's public housing. He used cable televi-
sion technology to establish a video link between the Wagner Homes Projects
and the hospital. "There are two ways you can look at problems that involve the
delivery of health services," Marshall told the *New York Times*. One of them
was to fix the structure of the healthcare system itself. The other was to use
technology to circumvent these fundamental problems. "Our interest here," he
continued, "is how we can adapt technology to the delivery of health services,
regardless of the organizational framework."[86]

Marshall, whose *Dynamics of Health and Disease* placed health in its social
contexts, joins Du Bois as an underrecognized African-American theorist of
social medicine.[87] Yet despite writing more than 400 pages that documented
the social determinants of disease, he scarcely mentioned the term "race" and
did not use "racism" once. Later scholars faced substantial pushback when
they tried to make racism a valid category of academic analysis. When David
Williams conducted his far-reaching Detroit Area Study in the 1990s, a pioneering work of health disparities research, he likewise faced critics who
argued that racism could not be measured and was not a valid subject for public health or medical research.[88]

Social Medicine As an Academic Field

After the establishment of social medicine as a division at Montefiore Hospital
and community medicine as a department at Mount Sinai, two other medical

[84] Kurt Deuschle, "Cross-Cultural Medicine: The Navajo Indians as Case Exemplar," *Daedalus* 15 (1986): 175–84, quote at 176.
[85] Hugh S. Fulmer, Anthony C. I. Adams, and Kurt W. Deuschle, "Medical Student Training in International Cross-Cultural Medicine," *Journal of Medical Education* 38 (1963): 920–31.
[86] "Child Clinic Gets Physicians via TV: Mt. Sinai Doctors Examine Patients in East Harlem," *New York Times*, June 6, 1973, p. 94.
[87] Carter L. Marshall, *Dynamics of Health and Disease* (New York, NY: Appleton-Century-Crofts, 1972).
[88] David R. Williams and Michelle Sternthal, "Understanding Racial–Ethnic Disparities in Health Sociological Contributions," *Journal of Health and Social Behavior* 51, suppl 1 (2010): S15–27.

schools in the United States established academic departments of social medicine in the 1970s and 1980s: Harvard Medical School (HMS) and the University
of North Carolina (UNC).[89] These demonstrated diverse visions of what social
medicine was or could be.

When HMS inaugurated its Department of Preventive and Social
Medicine in 1971, it built on a century of work under the mantle of hygiene
and then preventive medicine. The school had periodically offered lectures
on social medicine but had no formal programs under that name. Political
unrest in the 1960s, and especially the assassination of Martin Luther
King, Jr. in 1968, prompted Dean Robert Ebert to rethink the long-standing
Department of Preventive Medicine and the relationships between medicine
and society. A faculty committee deemed that "Preventive Medicine" had
become an "anachronism."[90] It preferred "Social Medicine," explaining that
the societal upheaval and self-reflection of the previous decade had made
it important not only to teach anatomy, pathophysiology, and diagnostics
to medical students, but "something of the anatomy, physiology, and even
pathophysiology of the medical care system of which they will soon become
a part."[91]

Wanting to broaden the mandate to include "the relationship of medicine
to society as a whole," HMS initially grafted "Social Medicine" onto its
Department of Preventive Medicine in 1971.[92] Students pushed for more and
demanded that they be prepared for careers of social and political activism:
"Where alleviation of a health problem requires political action, as in housing
and lead poisoning, some physicians must be prepared to participate effectively in the political process."[93] HMS respected this vision. Ebert recruited
pediatrician Julius Richmond, whose career moved back and forth between
government and academia, to be the inaugural chair.[94] Conceptions of social
medicine itself also shifted, with a growing interest in bioethics and the

---

[89] University of California San Francisco (UCSF) established its Department of History,
Anthropology, and Social Medicine in 1998 by merging long-existing programs in history
and anthropology; it never developed the social medicine component. See "History of the
Department of History & Social Sciences," University of California San Francisco, 2022, at:
https://humsci.ucsf.edu/history-department-history-social-sciences.

[90] "Minutes of Meeting of Ad Hoc Committee on Department of Preventive Medicine, 7/16/69,"
p. 5, in Box 31, ff 5, HMS Archives 00154.

[91] Charles Lewis, "Why Social Medicine?" p. 4, Box 31, ff 5, HMS Archives 00154; "Minutes of
Meeting of Ad Hoc Committee on Department of Preventive Medicine, 7/16/69," p. 6, in Box
31, ff 5, HMS Archives 00154.

[92] "Report of the Ad Hoc Committee on the Future of the Department of Preventive Medicine,"
pp. 3, 8, Box 31, ff 5, HMS Archives 00154.

[93] Don Berwick, Howard Graves, Mark Chassin, Gordon Mosser, David Calkins, Bob Kirkman,
Diana Petitti, and Andy Vernon, "Teaching of Preventive and Social Medicine at Harvard
Medical School," p. 6, March 1972, Box 31, ff 1, HMS Archives 00154.

[94] Richmond had initiated Project Head Start and would later be recruited to become Surgeon
General.

medical humanities.[95] A new dean, Daniel Tosteson, finally split the department in 1980 into the Department of Preventive Medicine and Clinical Epidemiology and the Department of Social Medicine and Health Policy, chaired by psychiatrist Leon Eisenberg.[96] That department, in turn, split – in 1990 – into two separate departments of Social Medicine and of Health Policy. Under the leadership of Eisenberg and then Arthur Kleinman, social medicine at Harvard adopted an academic orientation, focused on "the social sciences basic to medicine," especially anthropology, sociology, history, and economics. Its faculty pursued studies of the social production of disease, the social meanings of disease, and the social responses to disease.

A similar vision developed in parallel at the University of North Carolina. As early as the 1920s, sociologists at UNC had studied the health outcomes of the South's economic and social problems.[97] The Department of Epidemiology hired both Rosenau (who had retired from Harvard in 1946) and John Cassel, who had worked with the Karks in Pholela. When UNC upgraded its medical school in 1952, it established the Department of Preventive Medicine, led by Cecil Sheps. Sheps had studied social medicine with Rockefeller's John Grant.[98] This department taught epidemiology and preventive medicine to medical students and supported research in social and community medicine.

In the 1970s, UNC implemented reforms to foster community medicine, family medicine, and hospital administration. These were reorganized in 1980 as the Department of Social and Administrative Medicine. Glenn Wilson, who led the department, argued that "the best science and technology in the world will be of little value if it is applied without an understanding, or with misunderstanding, of the social situations of those it aims to benefit."[99] His successor, Donald Madison, articulated a vision of social medicine that included five

---

[95] Dieter Koch-Weser, "Present and Desirable Activities of the Department of Preventive and Social Medicine," addressed to Deans Adelstein, Federman, Meadow, Spellman, and Tosteson, 7/24/78, Box 53, "Preventative and Social Medicine, 1977–1981," HMS Archives 00154. See also: Jeremy A. Greene and David S. Jones, "The Shared Goals and Distinct Strengths of the Medical Humanities: Can the Sum of the Parts Be Greater than the Whole?" *Academic Medicine* 92 (2017): 1661–4.

[96] "Departmental Fission" [In "The Dean Reports"], *Harvard Medical Alumni Bulletin* 54 (December 1980): 2; "Two New HMS Departments Created from Partition of Preventive & Social Medicine," *Harvard Medical Area Focus*, 10/23/80, pp. 6–7.

[97] Donald L. Madison, "Introduction," in *Social and Administrative Medicine, 1987–1988* (Chapel Hill, NC: Department of Social and Administrative Medicine, University of North Carolina at Chapel Hill, 1988), 1–3, at: www.med.unc.edu/socialmed/about/department-field/.

[98] Donald L. Madison, "Introduction: Where Medicine and Society Meet," in *Social Medicine, 1998* (Chapel Hill, NC: University of North Carolina, Chapel Hill, 1998), 7–18, at 8, 10, at: www.med.unc.edu/socialmed/about/department-field/.

[99] I. Glenn Wilson, "From the Chair," in *Social and Administrative Medicine, 1987–1988* (Chapel Hill, NC: Department of Social and Administrative Medicine, University of North Carolina at Chapel Hill, 1988), 4–7, quote at 6. Wilson offered UNC's expansive definition of social medicine:

ideas – community, political action, organization of healthcare services, prevention, and epidemiology – with attention to the social sciences and humanities more broadly.[100] Social medicine would, by necessity, be "a polyglot admixture."[101] The faculty showcased its vision by producing a series of social medicine readers.[102]

Yet many of the most important developments for the field again took place outside academic medicine. In the 1970s and 1980s, Black feminist theorists Audre Lorde and Kimberlé Crenshaw demonstrated how socially inscribed forms of difference such as race, class, gender, and sexual orientation did not inhabit separate planes. These forces, instead, intersected in powerful and synergistic ways. Understanding intersectionality is crucial to elucidating how power relations produce social disparities. These perspectives have now become part of the basic toolkit for understanding health disparities. Not only did mainstream medicine fail to acknowledge their contributions for decades, but genealogies of social medicine have continued this erasure as well.

Social Medicine at the Bedside: Resurgence and Persistence in Twenty-First-Century American Medicine

Despite its small institutional footprint in the 1990s, at just Mount Sinai, Harvard, and UNC, and despite the ongoing political liability of "socialized medicine," the idea of social medicine has remained alive in the US. Clinicians have repeatedly been drawn to its theories and practices as they sought solutions to health threats facing their communities. Just as tuberculosis, the "social disease," had motivated social medicine theorists in the nineteenth and twentieth centuries, HIV/AIDS demanded social medicine in the late twentieth century.

When Paul Farmer, then a young medical student, first traveled to work in rural Haiti, he struggled – like so many before him – to imagine how to provide healthcare for people living in rural poverty. Trained in Harvard's mode of medical anthropology and biosocial analysis, he offered diagnoses of structural violence and social suffering.[103] For treatment, he turned to liberation

---

Nearly every sector of society has has [sic] some influence upon our understanding of illness, disease and health. All human activity – art, literature, theatre, cultural symbols, history, the economic system, the system of government, the moral values, the entire way of life of a people – contributes to the understanding of health, illness, and the role of the physician.

[100] Madison, "Introduction," 11.   [101] Madison, "Introduction," 12.

[102] Gail Henderson, Nancy M. P. King, and Ronald P. Strauss (eds.), *The Social Medicine Reader* (Durham, NC: Duke University Press, 1997). Revised editions have been published in 2005 and 2019.

[103] Paul Farmer and Arthur Kleinman, "AIDS as Human Suffering," *Daedalus* 118 (Spring 1989): 135–61; Paul Farmer, *AIDS and Accusation: Haiti and the Geography of Blame* (Berkeley: University of California Press, 1992); Paul Farmer, "On Suffering and Social Violence: A View from Below," *Daedalus* 125 (Winter 1996): 261–83.

theology's call for a preferential option for the poor. He argued that physicians must not blame poor people for their plight. Instead, physicians had a moral obligation to develop programs that could provide them with care and work toward health equity. He teamed up with like-minded health activists and philanthropists to found Partners in Health (PIH) in 1987. PIH began by creating health services based around community health workers and accompaniment, an idea adopted from liberation theology and Latin American social medicine.[104] But simply bringing medical care to individuals was not enough. PIH addressed its patients' social and economic needs by providing food, housing, and education. It intervened against global health policy to challenge the logics of cost-effectiveness analysis and drug pricing to change what was possible for healthcare for the poor. And it has worked with governments to pursue health systems strengthening in order to ensure that the needed space, staff, stuff, and systems are available.[105]

PIH was not alone in this work. The call to take social suffering seriously drew in scholars who had worked in many parts of the world.[106] Nancy Scheper-Hughes, for instance, authored a devastating ethnography of urban poverty in Brazil.[107] She and Farmer became leaders of the new movement of critical medical anthropology that called on anthropologists to intervene to aid the communities they studied. In the 2010s, two scholars in the next generation of MD–PhD social scientists, Helena Hansen and Jonathan Metzl, formulated "structural competency."[108] They argued that social medicine had to be a basic component of medical education so that physicians could recognize – and engage with – the structural forces that determine who gets sick and who gets access to care. Another group linked analyses of structural violence and a commitment to health equity to build a global community of healthcare provider–activists, the Social Medicine Consortium (SMC).[109] Established in 2015 by Michele Morse and Michael Westerhaus, the SMC offers a new definition of social medicine: social medicine is what happens when medicine commits itself to social justice and health equity.

Recent decades have seen a resurgence of social medicine at places old and new. The group at Montefiore founded the journal *Social Medicine* in 2000.

[104] Heidi L. Behforouz, Paul E. Farmer, and Joia S. Mukherjee, "From Directly Observed Therapy to Accompagnateurs: Enhancing AIDS Treatment Outcomes in Haiti and in Boston," *Clinical Infectious Diseases* 38, suppl 5 (2004): S429–36.
[105] Paul E. Farmer, *Fevers, Feuds, and Diamonds: Ebola and the Ravages of History* (New York, NY: Farrar, Straus and Giroux, 2020).
[106] Arthur Kleinman, Veena Das, and Margaret Lock, *Social Suffering* (Berkeley: University of California Press, 1997).
[107] Nancy Scheper-Hughes, *Death without Weeping: The Violence of Everyday Life in Brazil* (Berkeley: University of California Press, 1992).
[108] Jonathan M. Metzl and Helena Hansen, "Structural Competency: Theorizing a New Medical Engagement with Stigma and Inequality," *Social Science and Medicine* 103 (2014): 126–33.
[109] Social Medicine Consortium, at: www.socialmedicineconsortium.org/.

The City University of New York (CUNY) Medical School has founded a Department of Community Health and Social Medicine.[110] The Department of Medicine at UCSF founded a Social Medicine Core.[111] Berkeley established a Center for Social Medicine in 2013.[112] The University of California Los Angeles (UCLA) opened a Center for Social Medicine and Medical Humanities in 2015.[113] Johns Hopkins founded its Center for Medical Humanities and Social Medicine in 2017.[114] Zuckerberg San Francisco General Hospital established a social medicine program in 2017.[115] Columbia University started the Division of Social Medicine and Professionalism in 2018.[116] The activity across different geographies and institutions suggests that "social medicine" still has useful work to offer in motivating progressive commitments to social justice and health equity.

This resurgent interest in social medicine has been invigorated and validated amidst the pandemics of the present. The Covid pandemic may have been caused by a new virus, but it echoed old analyses of tuberculosis in the nineteenth century and AIDS in the 20th. Covid struck hardest at the most vulnerable, revealing deep fault lines in American society and profound failures in our systems of care and caregiving. The murder of George Floyd a few months

---

[110] "Community Health and Social Medicine Department," CUNY School of Medicine, at: www .ccny.cuny.edu/csom/communityhealthandsocialmedicinedept.

[111] "Social Medicine Core," UCSF Hospital, Department of Medicine. "The goal of Social Medicine Core is to develop a group of DHM faculty and staff to engage in dialogue, identify gaps, and design solutions around issues of equity, advocacy, diversity, and inclusion that impacts our patients, learners, and ourselves," at: https://ucsfhealthhospitalmedicine.ucsf .edu/social-medicine-core. It was established "Years ago": "Message from the Chief – August 2020," at: https://ucsfhealthhospitalmedicine.ucsf.edu/about-us/message-chief#Message-from-the-Chief--August-2020.

[112] Berkeley Center for Social Medicine, "About," University of California, Berkeley, available at: https://issi.berkeley.edu/centers/bcsm/about-bcsm:

Founded in 2013, BCSM links to the discipline of social medicine internationally by bringing together Bay Area scholars from the social and historical sciences who are working on questions related to medicine, the health sciences, public health, global health, the social structuring of suffering, violence and the body. BCSM brings together faculty and students with expertise in the social sciences of health from across campus and beyond, primarily from the fields of medical anthropology, medical sociology, medical history, and critical public health. The Center promotes research, interdisciplinary writing and publication, graduate and undergraduate training, as well as conferences, colloquia and other events that engage broad publics.

This program "critically engages the intersection of social systems, social difference, health and health care in the United States and across the globe."

[113] Center for Social Medicine and Medical Humanities, UCLA, at: https://socialmedicine.semel .ucla.edu/.

[114] Center for Medical Humanities & Social Medicine, at: https://hopkinsmedicalhumanities.org/.

[115] Natalia Gurevich, "SF General Treats Patients by Considering 'Whole Life Story'," *San Francisco Examiner*, May 20, 2024 (updated May 23, 2024).

[116] Division of Social Medicine and Professionalism, Department of Medical Humanities and Ethics, Columbia University, at: www.mhe.cuimc.columbia.edu/division-social-medicine-and-professionalism.

later made visible once again the bodily costs of another, intersecting pandemic of structural racism. Social medicine had much to offer as physicians worked toward solutions of both sets of problems.

But social medicine has a complex legacy in the US, simultaneously marginal and vibrant, at both elite medical centers and neighborhood clinics. It remains a field in flux. If early twentieth-century American social medicine was not as egregiously racist as its Australian counterpart (see Anderson, Dunk, and Musolino, Chapter 12 in this volume) it has nonetheless had a mixed tracked record, both eliding or drawing attention to racism as a social driver of health and illness. In contrast to Norway or the UK (see Kveim Lie and Haave, Chapter 6 in this volume), in which the state played a central role in defining social medicine, American social medicine practitioners tended to see themselves as operating from the margins: social medicine picked up where the state left off. This definition, however, has allowed subsequent iterations of American social medicine to elide and ignore those unsavory histories where medically informed social policy *was* picked up by the state, especially with the eugenics movement.

Adherents of social medicine today – as in the 1940s – remain divided over the relationship of social medicine to politics. On the one hand, it could be apolitical: a set of empirically justified theories and practices – a basic science of medicine – that all physicians should understand. On the other hand, it is deeply political, led by its social analyses to call for the fundamental restructuring of healthcare, and of society more broadly. It is a mode of academic analysis and a call for engagement through medical and political action.

Yet it is not clear that social medicine needs to resolve its internal inconsistencies to be relevant. Throughout the variety of forms it has taken over the past century, social medicine in the United States has remained a field that is not easily intelligible to those who do not already consider themselves to be part of it. Perhaps too many people simply do not know what the term "social medicine" means for it to have become a commonplace term. Perhaps too many still hear social medicine as "socialized medicine." Despite these obstacles, the basic ideas of social medicine have repeatedly resurfaced and been developed and deployed by physicians working in many settings – and their patients have benefited. The most essential challenge lies in translating the relevance of the work that social medicine *does* in a world of unequal health and steep social disparities into the critical and clinical tools that it can provide to future generations.

8 A "Counter-Hegemonic" Social Medicine
Leftist Physicians during the Latin American Cold War

Sebastian Fonseca

> If dependency theory, liberation theology, decolonial theory and participatory action research can be said to have been the most original contributions of Latin American critical thought in the twentieth century, the (Latin American social medicine) emerges as heir to this tradition and makes major contributions to the field, which can and should no longer be ignored or undervalued.
>
> Borde and Hernandez, "Global South," 857–8.[1]

Social medicine is a field fundamentally devoted to unfolding the social basis of health and disease. It argues that health cannot be understood exclusively in biomedical terms but requires different concepts and methodologies to apprehend the relationship between health and society. For this reason, social medicine integrates work from various disciplines, particularly the social sciences in health and the medical humanities.[2]

The attempts to tackle social processes and conditions to better population health have an extensive history in Latin America. Scholars of the field characterize two different waves of regional social medicine during the twentieth century. On one side, the first wave of physician activists and politicians emerged in close relationship with early populist governments.[3] Scattered and seemly unconnected, these actors were affiliated with all sorts of ideologies

---

[1] Elis Borde and Mario Hernández. "Revisiting the Social Determinants of Health Agenda from the Global South," *Global Public Health* 14, nos. 6–7 (2019): 847–62.

[2] Michelle Pentecost, Vincanne Adams, Rama Baru, Carlo Caduff, Jeremy Greene, Helena Hansen, David Jones, Junko Kitanaka, and Francisco Ortega. "Revitalising Global Social Medicine." *The Lancet* 398, no. 10300 (2021): 573–4, Doi: 10.1016/S0140-6736(21)01003-5; Vincanne Adams, Dominique Behague, Carlo Caduff, Ilana Löwy, and Francisco Ortega. "Re-imagining Global Health through Social Medicine," *Global Public Health* 14, no. 10 (2019): 1383–400.

[3] Eric D. Carter. *In Pursuit of Health Equity: A History of Latin American Social Medicine* (Chapel Hill, NC: University of North Carolina Press, 2023); Maria Eliana Labra, "Política e medicina social no chile: Narrativas sobre uma relação difícil," *História, Ciências, Saúde: Manguinhos* 7, no. 1 (2000): 23–46; Christopher Hartmann, "Postneoliberal public health care reforms: Neoliberalism, social medicine, and persistent health inequalities in Latin America," *American Journal of Public Health* 106, no. 12 (2016): 2145–51.

and political movements, from Catholic conservatism to hardcore communism. They commonly advocated for social reforms that broadly impacted health, including labor rights and better working conditions, land liberation and food security, and the establishment of social nets like public education and healthcare services. An example of the first wave is physician, Minister of Health, and former president of Chile, Salvador Allende.[4]

On another side, linked to the era of right-wing authoritarianism in Latin America, the second wave of social medicine emerged from the Cold War turmoil. Preceded by the so-called Latin American Social Medicine Network (ALAMES) in the late 1960s,[5] the new wave was made up of social scientists of health and physicians seeking impact beyond the clinics and adhered to leftist, anti-colonial, and anti-US ideals.[6] Members of the network were based at schools of medicine, most of which were integral parts of public universities and their intellectual environments. Their endeavors focused on a comprehensive critique of "scientific medicine" – an approach that radically reformed medical education since the mid 1950s, constituting a subsidiary element of the Developmentalist agenda in attempts to sway governments and local population away from the "communist threat." By 1984, the social medicine network formalized its internationalism into the Latin American Social Medicine Association (ALAMES).

Existing histories about the second wave of Latin American social medicine differ in extent and scope. The ALAMES collective has produced the most prominent narrative, which attributes the origins of the wave to leftist physician Juan César García and his team at the Pan-American Health Organization's (PAHO) Department of Human Resources.[7] This version portrays Garcia as a Marxist leader who recruited scattered groups of political dissenters across public universities in Latin America, unifying their ideas under the umbrella term of "social medicine." Within the PAHO, Garcia and

[4] Tanya Harmer, *Allende's Chile and the Inter-American Cold War* (Chapel Hill, NC: University of North Carolina Press, 2011); Howard Waitzkin, *Medicine and Public Health at the End of Empire* (London: Paradigm Publishers, 2011).

[5] Sebastian Fonseca, "Latin American Social Medicine: The Making of a Thought Style," PhD, King's College London, GHSM/KCL, 2020.

[6] Howard Waitzkin, C. Iriart, A. Estrada, and S. Lamadrid. "Social Medicine Then and Now: Lessons from Latin America," *American Journal of Public Health* 91, no. 10 (2001): 1592; Oscar Feo, Carlos Feo, and Patricia Jimenez. "Pensamiento contrahegemónico en salud," *Revista Cubana de Salud Pública* 38, no. 4 (2012): 602–14; Jaime Breilh. *Critical Epidemiology and the People's Health* (New York, NY: Oxford University Press, 2021).

[7] Saul Franco, Everardo Duarte-Nunes, Jaime Breilh, and Asa Cristina Laurell, *Debates en medicina social* (Quito: OPS, 1991); Miguel Marquez, "Formacion del espiritu cientifico en salud pública," in Miguel Marquez (ed.), *Escenarios epistémicos en la formación del espíritu científico en salud: Una antología* (La Habana: Impresión Palcograf, 2013), 3–18; Ana Lucia Casallas "La medicina social-salud colectiva Latinoamericana: Una visión integradora frente a la salud pública tradicional," *Revista Ciencias De La Salud* 15, no. 3 (2017): 397–408.

the team are said to have acted as "leftist moles," supporting developmentalist programs while surreptitiously strengthening "counterhegemonic" social science research in health.[8]

This chapter reimagines the history of social medicine beyond Garcia and the team, shedding new light on the PAHO's role as a place for pragmatic possibilities linked to medical education and technical assistance programs. I argue that the second wave emerged partly due to international health organizations and not despite them, problematizing the over-emphasis on Garcia in ALAMES's accounts. The PAHO's role as a mere conveyor belt of US foreign policies is put into question, presenting the regional organization as an ideologically diverse space in need of nuanced interpretations.

I will start the chapter by introducing Juan César García, underscoring his intricate political background vis-à-vis the myth created in ALAMES literature. The second section discusses the PAHO's research project on medical education (1966–72) and medical library Programa Ampliado de Libros de Texto y Materiales de Instruccion/Biblioteca Regional de Medicina PALTEX/BIREME (1967–), reassessing Garcia and the team's role in connecting leftist scholars at public universities. Finally, I offer concluding remarks on the role of the PAHO in paradoxically enabling the development of leftist networks amidst the anti-communist sentiment of US foreign policy during the Cold War.

Juan César García, the Opportunistic Scholar

The ALAMES idea of Garcia is constructed in parallel to the rise of the North American medical education reforms in Latin America, beginning in the early 1950s "medical missions" in Colombia.[9] Under the banner of modernization, multiple international health organizations like the PAHO, the Milbank Memorial Fund (MMF), the Kellogg, and the Rockefeller Foundation, and Truman's Point IV program collaborated to tackle the "scientifically retrograde," "disintegrated," and "methodologically anachronistic" education

---

[8] Everardo Duarte-Nunes, *Ciencias sociales y salud en america latina: Tendencias y perspectivas*, ed. Everardo Duarte-Nunes, 1st ed. (Montevideo: Organizacion Panamericana de la Salud/CIESU, 1986); Mario Rovere, "Mario Rovere y la tarea de Juan César García," paper presented at the ALAMES course on Social Medicine and Collective Health, Universidad Nacional de Lanus, 2015, at: https://youtu.be/V8jEyX036fo; Howard. Waitzkin, Alina Perez, and Matthew Anderson, *Social Medicine and the Coming Transformation* (New York, NY: Routledge, 2021).

[9] Carlos Gil Yepez, "Bases y doctrinas para una reforma de la educacion medica en Venezuela," in Emilio Quevedo and Juliana Perez (eds.), *De la restauracion de los estudios de medicine en el colegio mayor de nuestra señora del rosario 1965–1969* (Bogota: Universidad del Rosario, 2009); Howard Waitzkin, "Social Medicine: Home and Abroad," in Anne-Emanuelle Birn and Theodore Brown (eds.), *Comrades in Health: U.S. Health Internationalists, Abroad and at Home* (London: Rutgers University Press, 2013): 153–67.

in the region.[10] The reforms are said to have met their highest point with the advent of the so-called preventive medicine approach via two PAHO international conferences: the Seminars in Viña del Mar, Chile (1955), and Tehuacán, Mexico (1956).[11]

Despite the rhetoric of comprehensiveness encountered in the PAHO reports,[12] ALAMES members argue that the events did more to boost the expansion of a biology-centered education in the region than the actual goals it set out to complete. Mario Rovere, former ALAMES general coordinator and head of the Health Sciences Department at the Universidad de Lanus in Argentina, argued that the North American reforms aligned with US medical education in its foundational features: the predilection of disease-specific practices, the fragmentation of medical knowledge, and the preference for laboratory research, amongst others.[13] According to Sérgio Arouca, leader of the Brazilian *Sanitarismo* movement and ALAMES founding member, "preventivism" morphed the original concern for the social basis of health into the management of individual risk factors, making medical education individualistic in method, mechanistic in explanation, and closely attached to emerging quantitative approaches like biostatistics and epidemiology. He explained: "To find its specificity, Preventive Medicine distinguished itself from Social Medicine and Public Health by affirming its identity attached to Clinical Medicine. Preventive Medicine became a new form of private medicine, whilst the other two represented state involvement."[14] As the reforms settled throughout the 1960s, Arouca concluded, biological reductionism took precedence in practice at the expense of comprehensiveness in health.[15]

Juan César García is situated at the crossroads between the preventivist reforms, Juan Domingo Peron's populist government, and US McCarthyism.[16] Garcia was born in 1932 in Necochea, Argentina), completed clinical training in Community Paediatrics at rural La Plata, and became head of the Berisso

[10] Juan César García, "Juan César García entrevista a Juan César García," *Medicina Social* 2, no. 3 (2007): 151.
[11] Franco et al., *Debates*.
[12] PAHO, Seminarios sobre la enseñanza de medicina preventiva. Reporte final de Viña del Mar, Chile (10–15 de octubre, 1955); y Mexico Tehuacan, (23–28 de abril, 1956) (Washington, DC: PAHO/WHO, Publicaciones Cientificas No. 28, 1957), 16.
[13] Rovere, "Mario Rovere y la tarea."
[14] Sérgio Arouca, "O dilema preventivista: Contribuçao para a compreensao e crítica da medicina preventiva," PhD, Universidade Estadual de Campinas (State University of Campinas), 1975, 177–8.
[15] Duarte-Nunes, *Ciencias Sociales*.
[16] Mario Rovere, Maria Isabel Rodriguez, Maria Laura Passareli, and Carlos Gallego, "Homenaje a Juan César García" (Conference Proceedings at the Semana de Salud Internacional, Escuela de Gobierno en Salud Floreal Ferrara, September 23, 2021), at: https://youtu.be/4oZAJbFmat8.

Health Centre in the province of Buenos Aires during the late 1950s.[17] By 1960, developmentalist policies promoted by the first Cold War military Junta in the country granted Garcia a scholarship to study sociology at the Latin American Faculty of Social Sciences (FLACSO) in Santiago de Chile – where he also became a lecturer in Social Theory shortly after.[18] In 1965, Garcia was awarded a fellowship at Harvard University to train in research methods, which also led to his appointment as a research assistant at the MMF-financed project to survey the quality and impact of medical schools in Latin America. Garcia was also recruited for the PAHO's Department of Human Resources while leading the MMF project, where he remained until a premature death in 1984 (aged 52). The research, belonging to the US modernizing push across the region, facilitated Garcia's seminal book *La Educación Médica en la América Latina* (*The Latin American Medical Education*), published in 1972.[19]

Contrasting the ALAMES idea of Garcia's life-long commitment to Marxism, his trajectory as "the main actor of the social sciences in the field of health,"[20] makes evident a changing political ethos that followed different stages. According to Galeano and colleagues, Garcia first trained in the growing biological reductionism of the 1950s, attuned with his medical education.[21] Only in the following decade did the scholar turn toward leftist

---

[17] Everardo Duarte-Nunes, *Juan César García: Pensamento social em saúde na América Latina. Colecao pensamento social e saúde* (Sao Paulo: Cortez Editora/Abrasco, 1989); Everardo Duarte-Nunes, "O pensamento social em saúde na América Latina: Revisitando Juan César García," *Cadernos de Saúde Pública* 29, no. 9 (2013): 1752–62.

[18] FLACSO was a UNESCO-funded institution established in Santiago de Chile to support the social sciences in Latin America. Its creation followed the First Regional Conference on the Social Sciences at Rio de Janeiro (1957), founding the Latin American School of Sociology ELAS – the first of its kind in the region and home to Garcia's sociological training. The FLACSO–ELAS complex enabled ideas from across the ideological spectrum, dominated by US functionalism and conservative politics (i.e., Talcott Parsons, Robert Merton, and Gino Germani), but pervasive to leftist social theory. The pluralism, in fact, prompted its forced closure following dictator Augusto Pinochet's political persecution of the left in the 1970s. For details on FLACSO, see A. Abarzua Cutroni, "The North–South Circulation of Experts and Knowledge in Latin America: The Asymmetric Impact of UNESCO Missions between 1945 and 1984," in P. Duedhal (ed.), *A History of UNESCO: Global Actions and Impacts* (Basingstoke: Palgrave Macmillan, 2016), 181–98; Rolando Franco. *La FLACSO clásica (1957–1973): vicisitudes de las ciencias sociales Latinoamericanas* (Santiago de Chile: FLACSO, 2007); G. Sorá and A. Blanco, "Unity and Fragmentation in the Social Sciences in Latin America," in J. Heilbron, G. Sorá and T. Boncourt (eds.), *The Social and Human Sciences in Global Power Relations: Socio-historical Studies of the Social and Human Sciences* (Basingstoke: Palgrave Macmillan, 2018), 127–52.

[19] Juan César García, *La educación médica en la América Latina.* (Washington, DC: PAHO/WHO, 1972).

[20] PAHO, "In Memoriam – Juan César García," *Educacion Medica y Salud* 18, no. 3 (1984): 236–38.

[21] Diego Galeano, Lucia Trotta, and Hugo Spinelli, "Juan César García and the Latin American Social Medicine Movement: Notes on a Life Trajectory," *Salud Colectiva* 7, no. 3 (2011): 300.

ideas, presumably connected to his encounters with sociological thinking.[22] Dr. Hugo Spinelli, Professor of Sociology and Director of the Collective Health Institute at the Universidad Nacional de Lanus, Argentina, explained that the most significant problem in studying Garcia is apprehending "when and how he radicalised."[23] He suggested that Garcia's wife, Carlota Rios, introduced him to historical materialism while working at FLACSO in 1960–4. For Duarte-Nunes, the institution itself was the critical enabler of his radicalization, as Garcia met renowned scholars of Latin American leftism, including Anibal Quijano, Hugo Zemmelman, and Cecilia Muñoz.[24] Scholars also point at FLACSO's ideological pervasiveness to Marxist student groups as the driving force of Garcia's exposure to "radical politics."[25] It may be that Garcia's relationships and his immediate, yet surreptitious, academic context were instrumental in the turn he began from a positivist background to leftist ideology from the FLACSO period onward.

Garcia's publications shed light on his journey navigating political views. His early work at FLACSO featured debates around the doctor–patient relationship and the elite status of physicians, in line with the dominant US functionalism of the institution. It was not until 1964 that Garcia invested in the critique of medical positivism and utilitarian healthcare to "increase the historic-dialectic perspective" in population studies. The critique revealed an initial inclination to Marxism to help clarify "the relationship between health and socio-cultural factors,"[26] albeit not fully embracing it.[27] Instead, his publications highlighted the relevance of objectivity in scientific research and emphasized the study of human behavior – two features that evoke the central tenets of preventivism.[28] Moreover, Garcia's references in the texts include scholars like Talcott Parsons and David Mechanic – making no mention of Marxist literature or leftist theory. Even as late as 1971, Garcia still relied on Leavell and Clark's natural history of disease as a central "paradigm in

---

[22] Asa Cristina Laurell, "Social Analysis of Collective Health in Latin America," *Social Science & Medicine* 28, no. 11 (1989): 1183–91; Adolfo Sanchez-Vasquez, *De Marx al marxismo de América Latina*. (México: Itaca, 2012); Nestor Kohan, "Sociología académica y marxismo Latinoamericano: Historia de una polémica," *Utopia y Praxis Latino Americana* 24, no. 85 (2019): 117–39.

[23] Hugo Spinelli, "Interview," by Sebastian Fonseca, May 2022.

[24] Duarte-Nunes, "Revisitando," 1754–5.

[25] Miguel Marquez, "Juan César García y la medicina social durante la década de 1960 y 1970: Entrevista," by Hugo Spinelli, Centro Pensar en Salud, Universidad de Lanus, 2015, at: https://youtu.be/OIr2doQsjiU; Everardo Duarte-Nunes, "Juan César García: Social Medicine as Project and Endeavour," *Ciência & Saúde Cletiva* 20, no. 1 (2015): 139–44.

[26] Juan César García, "Sociología y medicina: Bases sociológicas de las relaciones médico-pacientes," *Cuadernos Médico Sociales* 4, nos. 1–2 (1963): 14–15.

[27] Duarte-Nunes, *Pensamento social*, 14.

[28] Arouca, "O dilema"; Naomar Almeida-Filho and Jairnilson Silva-Paim, "La crisis de salud pública y el movimiento de la salud colectiva en América Latina," *Cuadernos Medicos Sociales* 75, no. 1 (1999): 5–30; Jairnilson Silva-Paim, *Desafios para la salud colectiva en el siglo XXI* (Buenos Aires: Lugar Editorial, 2011).

the teaching of social science" in health,[29] despite the paradigm's centrality for preventive medicine education. Though publications from the mid 1970s reveal the change in Garcia toward Marxism, the researcher never actually discarded his functionalist background for approaching population health.

As best depicted by Galeano's work,[30] Garcia's profile corresponds to a pragmatic and opportunistic researcher, activist, and international health representative who, rather than dogmatically adhering to an ideology, utilized different approaches to make sense of and act upon his immediate reality. For instance, Garcia integrated community-based health research in peripheral regions of Argentina while training in pediatrics, making attempts to impact structural determinants of health while remaining bound to preventivist medical education. Even Garcia's "radicalization" at FLACSO is intimately attached to the context unfolding around him. The opportunity to study sociology abroad was the result of developmentalist policies during the Argentinian regime of 1955, supported by US foreign aid. Beyond reflecting ideas about Garcia's politics, his studies show a level of shrewdness in taking advantage of extraordinary opportunities, regardless of the ideological underpinnings. Garcia's concern for the social basis of health ran parallel to a practical approach to life, finding more fruitful opportunities in keeping a flexible (and changing) affiliation to politics – rather than living by the strict Cold War dichotomy arising at the time.

By the time Garcia joined the MMF-funded research, he had established his academic and political legacy around the development of human resources in health, focusing on the inclusion of critical social sciences in medical studies. In the next section, we turn to this work and the relationship with the PAHO Department of Human Resources.

Leftist Physicians in the PAHO during the Cold War

The PAHO was a central player in international health throughout the Cold War, creating regional professional networks via technical assistance programs. The networks were multiple – from centers for national health planning (the CENDES-PAHO method)[31] to international biomedical research.[32]

---

[29] Juan César García, "Innovations in Medical Education in Latin Americ," paper presented at the III Annual Meeting of the Health Sciences Education Information Center, Washington, DC, 1971).

[30] Galeano, Trotta, and Spinelli, "Juan César García."

[31] L. Gutiérrez, "Health Planning in Latin America," *American Journal of Public Health* 65, no. 10 (1975): 1047–9; Lígia Giovanella, "As origens e as correntes atuais do enfoque estratégico em planejamento de saúde na américa latina," *Cadernos De Saúde Pública* 7, no. 1 (1991): 26–44; Mario Testa, "Historia de vida y la salud pública en américa latina: Interview," by L. Trota, Federico L., Centro Pensar en Salud, Universidad de Lanus, 2015, at: https://youtu.be/rLN3zZasVKI.

[32] Miguel Bustamante, Carlos Viasca Treviño, Federico Villaseñor, Alfredo Vargas, Roberto Vastañon, and Xochitl Martinez, *La salud pública en México 1959–1982*, (Mexico: Secretaria

Less known is the PAHO's contribution to *leftist* groups concerning the work of Garcia and staff at the Department of Human Resources since the 1960s. The exploration of the PAHO programs involved in Latin American social medicine during the Cold War shifts the emphasis from exalting the role of Juan César García (as is found in ALAMES's narrative) toward analyzing the context underlying the social medicine network at the time. The context reveals that the origins of social medicine at the time, rather than the ALAMES story of the field "despite" US foreign policy, may be reinterpreted precisely due, parallel, or in relation to developmentalism. The 1960s Alliance for Progress agreement guides the argument in this section.

The Alliance for Progress was an agreement of cooperation signed at Punta del Este, Uruguay, in 1961 between the US Government and governments of Latin America, prompted by the call for social reforms at the international level (and reacting against the success of the Cuban Revolution).[33] The agreement constituted a unified effort to better the region's social welfare and economic growth, with a keen awareness that "health programs are part of – not separate from – general development planning."[34] According to the charter, the PAHO was summoned to function as a technical support organization, providing expertise on health-related concerns.[35] Derived from Resolution A-2, the organization convened ministers of health from signatory governments to form the "Task Force on Health," meeting for the first time in Washington, DC, in April 1963.[36] Resulting from the meeting, the PAHO's Advisory Committee devised a Ten-Year Public Health Program, placing human resources at the forefront,[37] and supporting two essential programs: the medical library for the region of the Americas PALTEX/BIREME (based in Sao Paulo, Brazil) and

de Salubridad y Asistencia, 1982); Roberto Bazzani, Eduardo Levcovitz, Soledad Urrutia, and Christina Zarowsky. "Building Bridges between Research and Policy to Extend Social Protection in Health in Latin America and the Caribbean: A Strategy for Cooperation," *Cadernos de Saúde Pública* 22 (2006): S109–12; Nevin Scrimshaw, "The Origin and Development of INCAP," *Food and Nutrition Bulletin: Food Nutr Bull* 31, no. 1 (2010): 4–8.

[33] Jeffrey Taffet, *Foreign Aid As Foreign Policy: The Alliance for Progress in Latin America* (New York, NY: Routledge, 2007); Thomas Allcock, *Thomas C. Mann: President Johnson, the Cold War, and the Restructuring of Latin American Foreign Policy* (Lexington, KY: University Press of Kentucky, 2018); David Johnson Lee, *The Ends of Modernization: Nicaragua and the United States in the Cold War Era* (Ithaca, NY: Cornell University Press, 2021).

[34] PAHO, *Task Force on Health at the Ministerial Level: Meeting of Health Ministries of the America*, 15–20 April, 1963 (Washington, DC: PAHO/WHO, 1964), 3–4.

[35] Organizacion de Estados Americanos, "Declaración a los pueblos de América: Carta de Punta del Este. Plan decenal de educación (anexo I) y Plan Decenal de salud pública de la alianza para el progreso (anexo II)," *Boletín De La Oficina Sanitária PanAmericana* 5, no. 5 (1961): 134–62; PAHO. *Needs in research training and medical education in Latin America. First meeting of the advisory committee on medical education. Held in June 18–22, 1962.* (Washington DC: PAHO/WHO, RES1/4, 1962).

[36] PAHO, *Reunión de ministros de salud: Grupo de estudio* (Washington, DC: PAHO/WHO, CE48.R3 Es, 1963).

[37] PAHO, *Task Force.*

the survey of medical education in Latin America (led by Harvard associate, Juan César García).

Following the incoming investment, the PAHO established the first bureau's Advisory Committee on Medical Research (ACMR) in 1962,[38] which partnered with the MMF to evaluate the impact of medical education reforms in Latin America – approved by the council in September 1963.[39] By the end of the year, the two organizations arranged the Conference on Health Manpower and Medical Education, specifying the "research design, methodology, parameters and emphasis of the study" and approving the first survey of medical education in Colombia during 1964–7.[40] The report served as a pilot and methodological background for future work in the region,[41] including a study to "evaluate the results of the seminars in the teaching of preventive medicine a decade ago" (referring to the seminars at Viña del Mar and Tehuacán) and designating Juan César García as the principal investigator of the research.[42]

It is essential to consider that, at this stage of the Cold War, technical assistance programs were functional for multiple objectives in the global ideological struggle. To lure Latin American governments away from communism, the US agenda often defined the knowledge circulated, the content discussed, the technology utilized, and practices replicated in fields like agriculture, nuclear power, and communications.[43] At the core of the strategy laid a standard

[38] PAHO, *Final Report of the 46th Meeting of the Executive Committee of the Pan-American Health Organisation. Held from the 23–27 April 1962 in Washington, DC* (Washington, DC: PAHO/WHO, CE46/15, 1962): 18–31.

[39] PAHO, *Minutes of the XIV Meeting of the Directing Council of the Pan-American Health Organisation* (Washington, DC: PAHO/WHO, CD14/28, 1963b), 121–30.

[40] PAHO, *Research Activities of PAHO in Selected Fields (1963–1964): Document Presented for the Third Meeting of the Advisory Committee on Medical Research, Held 15–16 June 1964* (Washington, DC: PAHO/WHO, RES3/3, 1964); PAHO, *Minutes of the XV Meeting of the Directing Council, Pan-American Health Organisation, Held in August–September 1964, Mexico D.F.* (Washington, DC: PAHO/WHO, CD15/33, 1964), 106; Milbank Memorial Fund, "Health Manpower and Medical Education in Latin America: Report of a Round Table Conference," *Milbank Memorial Fund Quarterly* 42, no. 1 (1964): 11 and 16–66. According to the records, Colombia was chosen as the site for the pilot mainly due to the advanced education infrastructure it had developed via the national association of medical faculties – Asociacion Colombiana de Facultades de Medicina (founded in 1959 and the first of its kind in Latin America).

[41] Robin F. Badgley, Carlos Agualimpia, Richard V. Kasius, Alfonso Mejia, and Marjorie Schulte, "Illness and Health Services in Colombia: Implications for Health Planning," *Milbank Memorial Fund Quarterly* 46, no. 2 (1968): 146–64; D. K. Zschock, "Health Planning in Latin America: Review and Evaluation," *Latin American Research Review* 5, no. 3 (1970): 35–56.

[42] PAHO, *Minutes of the XVII Pan-American Sanitary Conference, Held in September–October 1966, Washington, DC* (Washington, DC: PAHO/WHO, CSP17/36, 1966), 821.

[43] Gabrielle Hecht, *Entangled Geographies: Empire and Technopolitics in the Global Cold War* (Cambridge, MA: MIT Press, 2011); Audra Wolfe, *Competing with the Soviets: Science, Technology, and the State in Cold War America* (Baltimore: Johns Hopkins University Press, 2013); Simone Turchetti and Peder Roberts, *The Surveillance Imperative:*

set of principles related to control and discipline, swaying regional politics toward Western capitalism. The fact that the PAHO considered Colombia's pilot survey to establish "a method that can be used in other Latin American countries to obtain data for a more rational planning of health personnel,"[44] should be read with surveillance goals in mind. Garcia's involvement in the research was likely enabled by his functionalist background from early studies. It remains to be established whether the joint venture was made with little consideration of Garcia's leftist inclinations – or precisely because of it (and why this was so).[45]

Despite the overarching control that international health agencies intended through the programs, in practice, the survey of medical education became the means through which a growing international social science community, critical of the dominant medical education, developed in Latin America. The process of data collection during the survey of medical education provides crucial insights into the social medicine leftism running parallel to the PAHO's research.

The survey included over a hundred medical schools registered by the PAHO that Garcia traveled to between 1967–8, directly interviewing staff and students or hiring local researchers to complete questionnaires. Through the travels, Garcia met and empathized with many leftist physician dissenters at public universities that served as the basis for the Latin American social medicine network. Dr. Miguel Marquez, ALAMES co-founder and Professor of Public Health at the public *Universidad de Cuenca*, recounted that: "(Garcia) completed a journey very similar to 'Che' Guevara's ... not just appreciating the development of preventive medicine in Latin America, but understanding the context of public universities, and the ruptures that differentiated the social sciences in health in the region."[46] According to Marquez, when staff at Cuenca found out Garcia was supported by a US-based institution that the CIA financed (the MMF), they "decided to give him 24 hours to explain – and, in the meantime, he was declared *persona non-grata*." Garcia responded that he had "no business" with the finance of the research and that his only objective was to "bring down the empire." For Marquez, it became clear that he was

Geosciences during the Cold War and Beyond (London: Palgrave Macmillan, 2014); Naomi Oreskes and John Krige, *Science and Technology in the Global Cold War* (Cambridge, MA: MIT Press, 2014).

[44] PAHO, *Biomedical Research Policy in Latin America: Report Prepared for the Fourth Meeting of the Advisory Committee on Medical Research, PAHO, Held in June 14–18, 1965* (Washington, DC: PAHO/WHO, RES4/6B, 1965), 34.

[45] During my time exploring Latin American social medicine in the US National Security Archives, I did not find mentions of Juan César García or his endeavors. This suggests that either the US national intelligence did not consider Garcia a threat to their model of democracy or that Garcia's leftist inclinations were never noted in the surveillance agencies.

[46] Marquez, Interview.

encountering an extraordinary moment of PAHO pervasiveness to Garcia's politics, which motivated him to join the research.

Marquez also highlighted Garcia's political changes whilst traveling Latin America. Although Garcia might have been inclined toward historical materialism by the start of the research, Marquez remarked that he adopted a firm commitment to leftist politics through multiple encounters with colleagues at public universities that persuaded the researcher to take different perspectives into account. Rather than the diffusion of Western ideology from Garcia to physicians on the ground, the growing critique of dominant medical education from social medicine groups in the region consolidated a definitive stance in Garcia's thinking.

Garcia's 1972 book bears the changes undergone by the author after his fieldwork. Announced in 1967, the survey's initial objective was a "detailed description of the teaching of preventive and social medicine in medical schools of Latin America,"[47] including the conditions that promote, delay, or impede changes and innovation. According to Garcia, two innovations were made to the original ideas of the project in the late 1960s: the use of an explanatory, rather than descriptive, research design; and the broad study of medical education that expanded the analysis beyond preventive and social medicine.[48] The changes enabled Garcia to face medical education beyond the institutional cloister of universities, coming to terms with the "subordination of clinical training to the economic structure" à la Marx.[49] The book's epilogue, written at the end of the research, worked a retrospective analysis linking medical education to the "structures of society" – making use of Althusserian ideas to argue against the "hegemonic socioeconomic system" (capitalism) permeating society.[50] In other words, Garcia did not conceive the project as a Marxist endeavor from his initial involvement in 1966 but only after fieldwork encounters – as suggested by Marquez.

However accurate, in recognizing the transformation process generated by regional social medicine dissenters, the ALAMES narrative tends to skew the field's history by lionizing Garcia and his contributions. ALAMES co-founder Professor Dr. Saul Franco explained that Garcia, following his entry to the PAHO, was able to "travel all of Latin America" to identify the people who were "open-minded" in the search for alternative views on population health and to support the work on social science in health.[51] For Rovere, Garcia was conscious of the need for changes in medical education and invested in Marxist scholars to challenge the dominant positivist medical epistemology.[52] Given

---

[47] PAHO, *XVII Conferencia*, 340.   [48] Garcia, *Educación Medica*, 2.
[49] Duarte-Nunes, *Pensamento social*, 17.   [50] Garcia, *Educación Medica*, 390.
[51] Saul Franco, "Latin American Social Medicine Association: Interview," by Sebastian Fonseca, Bogota, DC, Colombia, 2018.
[52] Rovere, "Mario Rovere y la tarea."

the leftist intellectualism at public universities during his research, Garcia found favorable conditions to link the groups together over aligning goals and theoretical focus. Nevertheless, the move to advance a network of anti-US scholars was enabled only through a US-funded program.[53] The need to incorporate *another* social science, one that was critical of the standing biological reductionism, sparked the beginning of the *Latin American social medicine network* on the shoulders of PAHO's research project.

The case of the University of El Salvador is exemplary of the contrast above. Professor Dr. Maria Isabel Rodriguez, former ALAMES general coordinator and renowned public health expert, commented that Garcia arrived in late 1967 at the university – when the Faculty of Medicine was undergoing "late" reforms to integrate the US medical education model.[54] The reforms happened late due to a combination of factors. First, the cycles of military dictatorships in the country since the 1940s delayed reforms in higher education until the late 1960s, when Rodriguez was appointed Dean of the Faculty of Medicine. And second, the reforms were late because of the mounting critiques against preventivism that grew parallel to their introduction. "So, we had an interesting overlap of reforms," Rodriguez elaborated, "when the first reform (preventivism) was advancing, we already had a response." Garcia entered the scene precisely during this ambivalence. According to Rodriguez, he "supported" the critique of biological reductionism by summoning the local group of social science scholars into international forums. In so doing, Rodriguez concluded, Garcia associated like-minded people across Latin America to engage in dialogues and weave transnational relations that gave way to many "social science applied on health" meetings in the subsequent year.[55] Indeed, this was an extraordinary achievement in the era of anti-communist repression, which used foreign aid as a stepping stone for leftist internationalism.[56]

In May 1972, Garcia and social science colleagues organized the social medicine network's first international meeting, known as the Reunión Sobre la

[53] Hugo Mercer, "La incorporación de las ciencias sociales a la medicina social: Interview," by L. Federico and J. Librandi, Centro Pensar en Salud, Universidad de Lanus, 2015, at: https://youtu.be/at77qTvI91o.
[54] Maria Isabel Rodriguez, "Entrevista PALTEX/BIREME, Juan César García, y reformas universidad de el salvador," by Sebastian Fonseca, April 6, 2022; and Maria Isabel Rodriguez, "Reflexiones con la Dra. María Isabel Rodríguez, ministra de salud de el Salvador: Interview," by PAHO, 2018, at: https://youtu.be/iO8tAjkzf_k.
[55] Galeano et al., "Juan César García," 296. Rodriguez, *Entrevista*; Jose Roberto Ferreira, "Juan César García como precursor de innovaciones en la cooperacion tecnica internacional," Paper presented at the Instituto Juan César García, Quito, Ecuador, 1986, 23–4.
[56] Anne-Emanuel Birn and Raúl Necochea López, *Peripheral Nerve: Health and Medicine in Cold War Latin America* (Durham, NC: Duke University Press, 2020); Birn and Brown (eds.), *Comrades in Health*.

Enseñanza de las Ciencias Sociales en las Facultades de Ciencia de la Salud.[57] The meeting, sponsored by the PAHO and funded by the MMF, took place in Cuenca, Ecuador, and was later renamed the "Cuenca I" meeting.[58] The survey on medical education and the Cuenca I meeting are considered the epistemological and organizational background that made possible the establishment of ALAMES in the 1980s.[59]

The PALTEX/BIREME Program

Other institutional processes overlapping the PAHO and the *Latin American social medicine network* remain unexplored in ALAMES' accounts of its origins. According to Rodriguez, though Garcia's efforts enabled connections that otherwise would have been difficult, the network of social science scholars was already under development years before the survey on medical education. Crucially, the PALTEX/BIREME program "identified many people working on alternative approaches to medical education, generating a tremendous shock to many sectors that considered medical education exclusively constituted by the basic sciences like physiology or pharmacology."[60] Rodriguez's remarks are unique in that no other account in ALAMES flags the involvement of the PAHO's regional library of medicine in the development of Latin American social medicine during the Cold War. Despite the newness, Rodriguez's narrative does not feature prominently in the social medicine association.

The Expanded Textbook and Instructional Material program PALTEX/ BIREME was a PAHO-centralizing regional library of medicine established in 1967 as part of the ACMR developmentalist agenda. The assistance program was charged with supplying medical literature to physicians, healthcare institutions and medical schools through loans or through their acquisition at rates lower than market value.[61] Devised in the early 1960s, the proposition to establish the regional library was made by a panel of US representatives based at organizations like the National Library of Medicine (NLM), the Department of State, the Book Exchange, and Ivy League universities.[62] The board argued that the chronic scarcity of funds and the faulty medical education in Latin America "operated to inhibit the development of comprehensive collections of

---

[57] PAHO, "Aspectos teóricos de las ciencias sociales aplicadas a la medicina," *Educación Medica y Salud* 8, no. 4 (1974): 354–9.

[58] Duarte-Nunes, *Ciencias Sociales.*   [59] Franco et al., *Debates.*   [60] Rodriguez, *Reflexiones.*

[61] PAHO, *Regional Library of Medicine: Pan-American Health Organization: Advisory Committee on Medical Research, Sixth Meeting on 12–16 June, Item 4.4 of the Agenda* (Washington, DC: PAHO/WHO, RES6/20, 1967).

[62] Table II in PAHO, *Proposed Regional Medical Library Centre for Latin America: Pan-American Health Organization: Advisory Committee on Medical Research, Fourth Meeting on 14–18 June* (Washington, DC: PAHO/WHO, RES4/12, 1965), 19.

world journal literature," making medical libraries in the region "small, insufficient, and under-supported."[63] Similarly to the medical education problem, the library program aimed to enhance the provision of "necessary information" as a matter of medical training, fulfilling multiple objectives in the modernization of Latin America that underpinned the US policies during the Cold War.[64] "The high-quality, low-cost textbooks and library consultation service" devised for the PALTEX/BIREME constituted a "planned development of manpower" essential for the "socioeconomic progress" of the region.[65]

During the fourth Conference of the Latin American Faculties of Medicine in 1964 at Poços de Caldas (Brazil), an agreement between the PAHO, the Brazilian military regime, and the Escola Paulista do Medicina was struck to establish the physical center of the library in Sao Paulo.[66] Funded by the Commonwealth Fund and the Inter-American Developmental Bank,[67] the PALTEX/BIREME was boosted by mounting requests that PAHO member states made for a "program of modern texts that could be offered to students in conditions adapted to their financial possibilities."[68] The endeavor utilized the PAHO's administrative tools, including their network of schools aggregated under the Pan-American Federation for Medical Faculties or Schools FEPAFEM, to begin operations in 1969 under the directorship of Chilean physician Amador Neghme.

When Garcia became part of the PAHO in 1966, the PALTEX/BIREME program had completed two preliminary journeys exploring Latin American medical resources. The first trip, involving Dr. David Kronick and Mortimer Tauber, approached medical faculties and their libraries in Uruguay, Colombia, Brazil, Argentina, and Venezuela.[69] Though the main objective was to verify the viability of installations for a regional library, the report summarized the research and teaching difficulties in the region. The second journey, completed by Hugo Trucco and Alejandro Jimenez, visited thirty-two faculties and interviewed over a hundred people across nine countries, including Mexico and

---

[63] PAHO, *Proposed Regional Medical Library*, 1.

[64] PAHO, *XVI Meeting*, 4. For details on the PALTEX/BIREME program, see F.A. Pires-Alves, "A biblioteca da saúde das américas: A BIREME e a informação em ciências da saúde 1967–1982," PhD, História das Ciências e da Saúde, Fiocruz, 2005.

[65] PAHO, *Special Meeting of Ministries of Health of the Americas: Final Report and Speeches, Held in 14–18 October 1968, Buenos Aires, Argentina* (Washington, DC: PAHO/WHO, 1968): 46–7.

[66] Associação Brasileira de Escolas Médicas, *Abem. Anais da II Reunião Anual da associação brasileira de escolas médicas* (Rio de Janeiro: Abem, 1964).

[67] PAHO, Noticias; PAHO, *Report on Medical Education: Provisional Agenda Item 25, Completed by the Directing Council of the Pan-American Health Organization on the XIX Meeting 26th August 1969* (Washington, DC: PAHO/WHO, CD19/16, 1969).

[68] CSP17/55, 28 in PAHO, *XVII Pan-American Sanitary Conference*, 769.

[69] PAHO, *Regional Medical Library*.

various countries in Central America.[70] The trip sought to identify the bibliographic material lacking at medical schools and surveyed the best way to approach the problems for local staff.

The mobilization of science through a centralizing library was a fundamental element instrumental in the Cold War's ideological struggle. The program followed similar patterns of practice to other technical assistance programs, including the diagnosis of a country's knowledge infrastructure, a grand narrative of a struggling process, and the salvific alternatives in the form of cooperation.[71] Though the programs' initial development was typically one-sided (US officials), the adaptation of the library on the ground uncovered the regional autonomy at play. For instance, during the mid 1960s planning, the NLM took charge of the library's bibliography, the operational infrastructure, and the training expertise in ways that displayed political and economic dependency.[72] Local voices, knowledge, and practices were never included at this stage – if they were ever considered. However, in practice, the maintenance and expansion of the program heavily relied on the Latin American workforce. They surreptitiously utilized the resources and professional opportunities to accomplish parallel and sometimes conflicting political objectives, mainly strengthening a growing critique of dominant medical education.[73] The adaptation of foreign programs locally enabled interstices of resistance where minority groups, like the *Latin American social medicine network,* emerged as alternative players in the history of social medicine.

Though the ALAMES collective makes Garcia the fundamental father of the so-called second wave of social medicine, programs like the PALTEX/ BIREME underscore other mechanisms through which the network was established and maintained independently of Garcia. As recounted by Maria Isabel

---

[70] PAHO, *Programa de libros de texto para estudiantes de medicine. Presented at the XVII conferencia sanitaria panamericana, XVIII reunión del comité regional. Septiembre–Octubre* (Washington, DC: PAHO/WHO, CSP17/27, 1966).

[71] This pattern is found in various cases where science, technology and medicine were used to further US political objectives internationally. See, for instance, Erez Manela, "A Pox on Your Narrative: Writing Disease Control into Cold War History," *Diplomatic History* 34, no. 2 (2010): 299–323; John Agar, *Science in the Twentieth Century and Beyond* (Cambridge: Polity Press, 2012); Young-sun Hong, *Cold War Germany: The Third World and the Global Humanitarian Regime* (New York, NY: Cambridge University Press, 2015).

[72] PAHO, *Proposed Regional Medical Library*; PAHO, Regional Library of Medicine: Present Status, *Pan-American Advisory Committee on Medical Research, Eighth Meeting, 9–13 June, 1969, Item 10.2 of the Agenda* (Washington, DC: PAHO/WHO, RD8/3, 1969); Wyndham Miles, *A History of the National Library of Medicine: The Nation's Treasury of Medical Knowledge* (Bethesda, MD: USDHHS, 1982).

[73] Márcia Regina Silva, Ferla Luis Barros, and Marcello Claramonte, "Uma 'biblioteca sem paredes': História da criação da bireme," *História, Ciências, Saúde: Manguinhos* 13, no. 1 (2006): 91–112; F. A. Pires-Alves and C. H. Assunção-Paiva, *Recursos críticos: História da cooperação técnica opas-brasil em recursos human os para a saúde (1975–1988)* (Rio de Janeiro: Fiocruz, 2006).

Rodriguez, parallel to assisting Garcia in the survey during the late 1960s, she also participated in the PALTEX/BIREME Scientific Committees that reported to the PAHO the literary and infrastructural necessities of medical schools across the region.

As early as 1965, the PALTEX/BIREME program established a series of Scientific Committees composed of experts from Latin America, who met in Washington, DC, to determine the library's primary literature.[74] The reports of the meetings and agreed textbook titles, journal archives, and teaching material were published in the PAHO's medical education journal in 1968 on topics like anatomy, physiology, pharmacology, and preventive medicine.[75] In summoning local expertise, the program provided the PAHO with a map of scholars developing various types of health research in Latin America – including critical social science in health. As such, before Garcia's recruitment process, the library program had already developed an early database, a regional cartography even, of medical knowledge that included emerging social medicine groups. Central figures in the development of social medicine appeared in PALTEX/BIREME's reports, including Maria Isabel Rodriguez, Raul Paredes, and Gabriel Velazquez-Palau.[76] In fact, according to Rodriguez, Garcia utilized this preliminary matrix to visualize the scattered pool of social science scholars across public universities and connect groups via data collection during the survey of medical education.[77] Rather than Garcia's effort in creating the network, the researcher enhanced the pre-existing connections established by the PALTEX/BIREME program years before the PAHO-MMF research.

Moreover, the library program helped build the Latin American social medicine network by "enabling a space of constant exchange and interactions … promoting permanent working groups that supported scholars in developing strong critiques of medical education."[78] Though PALTEX/BIREME did not create a critical mass of scholars in the social sciences of health, the program prompted vital conversations during "committee discussions, report agreements, and even coffee breaks."[79] Rodriguez explained that public universities across Latin America experienced the exponential rise of study groups critical of the dominant medical education in the faculties, which largely focused on

[74] CSP17/27 Annex III, 11 in PAHO, *Programa de libros*, 19 and 34; PAHO, *Provision of Books for Medical Students: Pan-American Health Organization: Advisory Committee on Medical Research, Sixth Meeting on 12–16th June, Item 7 on the Agenda* (Washington, DC: PAHO/ WHO, RES6/10, 1967): 7.
[75] PAHO, *Report to the Director: Pan-American Health Organization, Advisory Committee on Medical Research, Seventh Meeting 24–28 June* (Washington, DC: PAHO/WHO, RES7/22, 1968).
[76] PAHO, *Programa de Libros*, 9–14.
[77] María Isabel Rodríguez, "96 años: Interview," by Alberto Arene for FOCOS TV at El Salvador, 2018, at: https://youtu.be/yRF0LtbI34E.
[78] Rodriguez, "96 años."   [79] Rodriguez, "96 años."

biological science and its dependency on foreign technology. These groups used the PALTEX/BIREME committees as a platform to exchange ideas, share literature, and deepen the regional pedagogy. "We were like a family," Rodriguez concluded.[80]

PAHO's reports and publications uncover the emergence of the social medicine network and internationalism in between the cracks of developmentalist programs, as members conducted key roles throughout both the library and the survey of medical education.[81] For instance, Dr. Hesio Cordeiro was a leader of the Brazilian *Sanitarismo* movement, an attendee of the Cuenca I meeting, co-founder of ALAMES, was listed as a collaborator in Garcia's research, and was a permanent member of the Advisory Committee on preventive medicine for PALTEX/BIREME. Dr. Jose Manuel Alvarez Manilla was a PAHO delegate to Mexico during Garcia's research, integrated the executive secretary of the PALTEX/BIREME Morphology, Microbiology, Parasitology, and Internal Medicine for their corresponding first reports in 1969, joined the PAHO's Department of Human Resources in the early 1970s, and became a member of the Advisory Committee for the second report on preventive medicine in 1975. He was also the Mexican representative at the Cuenca I meeting on social sciences in health. Finally, Dr. Gustavo Molina was chairman of the first reports on preventive and social medicine for the PALTEX/BIREME, a member of the Advisory Committee on Medical Education that supervised Garcia's research, and a strong supporter of the socialist president Salvador Allende in Chile before going into exile following the military coup.

Several figures already discussed in this chapter feature prominently in the PAHO's reports as well. Rodriguez appears extensively in the PALTEX/BIREME, met and collaborated with Garcia in medical education research, has been a prominent figure in ALAMES since its foundation, and, though she could not attend Cuenca I due to El Salvador's military anticommunism, she was involved in the planning and organizing of multiple social medicine events throughout the 1970s. Marquez followed suit in ways already described and engaged in numerous reports on morphology and pathology for PALTEX/BIREME. Ramon Villareal was virtually in every account of PALTEX/BIREME. He heavily assisted Garcia in his research while directing the PAHO's Department of Human Resources and was co-founder of the Master's in Social Medicine at UAM-X (Mexico).

In this way, though Garcia's efforts during the medical education survey were pivotal in connecting scholars, it was the aggregation of various circumstances that led to the establishment and growth of the social medicine

---

[80] Rodriguez, "96 años."
[81] PAHO, *Report on Medical Education*; PAHO, *Educación medica: Informes de los comités del programa de libro de texto de la OPS 1968–1977* (Washington, DC: PAHO/WHO, 1978).

network. The PAHO, as an institution representing developmentalism, experienced a period of openness whereby US-funded programs became means for Cold War critique and resistance. Likewise, leftist scholars across Latin American public universities, though critical of the medical science programs in education, gathered and grew together through projects embodying the very principles they scrutinized. Beyond the ideological divide typical of the Cold War, the advancement of alternatives in health throughout Latin America was a pragmatic endeavor that sought opportunities within the borders of rigid politics – within the grey areas of developmentalism and the interstices of partisan struggles.

Conclusion

Juan César García was certainly a figure that rose above the circumstances during the mid Cold War in Latin America to become a pivotal actor in the development of the Latin American social medicine network. As such, social medicine collectives like ALAMES point to Garcia to narrate the movement's origins and establish a distinctive identity against the backdrop of developmentalism, preventive medicine, and medical reforms. Following his death in 1984, the Latin American social medicine network came together at Ouro Preto (Brazil) to realize the last wish of such an influential figure: the establishment of a regional association integrating practitioners, researchers, and activists around a culture of socialist health. This marks the birth of ALAMES,[82] an association that furthered the pre-existing network of scholars commonly advocating for reforms in medical education and the comprehensive transformation of technocratic health epistemology.

Garcia's networking influence even goes beyond the limits of ALAMES's origins. Beginning with Guatemala's coup against socialist president Jacobo Arbenz in the 1950s, the list of *Juntas Militares* embodying an anti-communist sentiment grew across Latin America, aided by the Condor Operation that reigned since the 1970s across the Southern Cone (Brazil, Chile, Argentina, Paraguay, Uruguay, and Bolivia). The Condor Operation, a CIA-directed program supporting right-wing authoritarianism to guarantee the success of Western capitalism (against the backdrop of emerging national liberation armies),[83] directly impacted regional social medicine – driving the circulation

---

[82] Asociación Latinoamericana de Medicina Social, "Acta de Ouro Preto: Constitución de la Asociación Latinoamericana de Medicina Social (22 de noviembre, 1984)," *Medicina Social* 4, no. 4 (2009): 263–4.

[83] J. Dinges, *The Condor Years: How Pinochet and His Allies Brought Terrorism to Three Continents* (London: New Press, 2004); J. P. McSherry, *Predatory States: Operation Condor and Covert War in Latin America* (Oxford: Rowman and Littlefield, 2005); Francesca Lessa, *The Condor Trials: Transnational Repression and Human Rights in South America* (London: Yale University Press, 2022).

of texts, ideas, and personnel into hiding. For many, ALAMES members persecuted for their political affiliation in Argentina, Chile, and Colombia, for instance, their only means of survival emerged from the network of social science scholars that Garcia's recruitment process made possible.

Though a history worth telling, ALAMES's narratives tend to exalt Garcia into a myth that runs the risk of ignoring the multiple ways in which the PAHO, thought to be an auxiliary organization of US interests, also became a site for medical pluralism and the growth of leftist physician's internationalism. Without disregarding Garcia's contribution through networking, moving science, and organizing bureaucracy in the age of the Iron Curtain, this chapter provided a more comprehensive approach to the history of social medicine in Latin America by integrating elements that transpired during the 1960s and 1970s. Particularly, the chapter focused on the much more intricate political development in Garcia's thinking, the underlying processes involved in the PAHO–MMF survey of medical education (overlapping Garcia's work), and the PAHO's PALTEX/BIREME program (independent of Garcia). Subsequent phenomena in Latin American social medicine and health, such as the rise of community health programs, the impact of indigenous and feminist movements, and the crisis of the socialist camp globally are topics of research explored in different publications.[84]

---

[84] Notably, the Latin American social medicine network criticized the rise of community health programs during the 1970s. Associated with the consolidation of developmentalism, central actors in the regional movement paradoxically considered these programs as a type of "medical police" or auxiliary to consumerism, despite community health's history connected to key social medicine figures such as Sydney and Emily Kark (South Africa's Pholela Community Health Centre, in what is today KwaZuly-Natal). For details on the ALAMES critique, see, Maria Cecilia Donnangelo, *Saúde e Sociedade* (Sao Paulo: Libraria Duas Cidades, 1976); Jaime Breilh, "La Medicina Comunitaria, una nueva policia medica?," *Rev Mex Ciencias Pol y Soc*, 84 (1976): 57–81; Jairnilson Silva-Paim, "Medicina comunitaria: introducción a un análisis critico," *Salud Colectiva* 5, no. 1 (2009):121–6.

9   The African Roots of Community-Oriented Primary Care

Abigail H. Neely

"They were nice. They cared about us."

For the past seventeen years, I have heard this over and over as I talk with elderly people about the work of the Pholela Community Health Centre (PCHC) in the middle of the twentieth century. Located in the rural, mountainous Pholela region of what is today KwaZulu-Natal, South Africa, the PCHC was an experiment in social medicine carried out in the 1940s and 1950s. One of social medicine's most important origin sites, the PCHC married clinical care with an attention to what are today called the social determinants of health at the household and community scales to improve the health of the entire region. In Pholela, doctors, community health workers, and residents worked together developing a brand of social medicine called Community-Oriented Primary Care (COPC). Within ten years, infant and crude mortality had plummeted, malnutrition had all but disappeared, and communicable diseases like syphilis had decreased markedly.[1] The PCHC was a resounding success. It was so successful, in fact, that it has been referred to as a model for the world.[2]

The PCHC and the social medicine pioneered there looms large in the history of social and community health. Not only has it served as a model for the world, taken up in places like Uganda, Israel, Chile, the United States, and Canada, but even to this day it is pointed to as the kind of practice the world needs to alleviate health disparities. Central to the stories and legacies of COPC is Sidney Kark, founder of the PCHC and world-renowned social medicine practitioner. Kark got his start in Pholela and from there went on to found the Institute for Family and Community Medicine at the first Black medical school in South Africa at the University of Natal. Through this work, he brought COPC to urban South Africa, first in Durban and later to cities across the country. As apartheid hardened in

---

This chapter draws on material from my book, Abigail H. Neely, *Reimagining Social Medicine from the South* (Durham, NC: Duke University Press, 2021), which has a more complete list of references as well.
[1] Mervyn Susser, "Pioneering Community-Oriented Primary Care," *Bull World Health Organization* 77, no. 5 (1999): 436–8.
[2] "Community Health: A Model for the World," *Against the Odds*, accessed October 21, 2016, at: https://apps.nlm.nih.gov/againsttheodds/exhibit/community_health/model_world.cfm.

the 1950s and his work became impossible, Kark left South Africa, taking positions at Harvard University and the University of North Carolina, Chapel Hill (UNC), in the United States, before settling in Jerusalem, where he founded the Department of Community Medicine at the Hebrew University and helped reorient the Israeli health system around community health centers and the practice of COPC. Kark even went on to contribute to the WHO's Alma-Ata Declaration of Primary Health Care for all in 1978. A storied and important career by any measure, Kark had a tremendous impact on social medicine worldwide.

But Kark was not alone in Pholela. The "they" in the quote that opens this chapter tells us as much. Sidney Kark arrived in Pholela with his wife Emily, who was also a medical doctor and who accompanied him in his medical practice and his academic career. Together, they pioneered COPC and co-authored some of the most important texts on social medicine in the twentieth century.[3] But they did not do so alone, Edward and Amelia Jali, a Zulu health aid (one step below a doctor) and nursing sister, and a team of Zulu-speaking community health workers joined them in Pholela where together they worked to develop COPC. While the legacy of Sidney Kark is well documented through his own writings and writings about his work,[4] the legacy of Emily Kark, Edward and Amelia Jali, the community health workers at the PCHC, and Pholela's residents is harder to find. Drawing on over seventeen years of ethnographic research and conversation in Pholela with its residents, this piece offers an alternative history of COPC and by extension social medicine, one which decenters Sidney Kark (though he was very important), and focuses instead on the work and lives of his team, the communities in which they implemented their programs, and the things they used in that implementation. So doing, it shifts understandings of the production of science and social medicine away from (mostly white, mostly male) doctors and offers alternative explanations of how and why with their social medicine practices become important, meaningful, and successful.

Sidney and Emily Kark met at the University of Witwatersrand (Wits) in Johannesburg, where they were medical students. At Wits, they blended a typical biomedical education with classes in the critical social sciences.[5] From

---

[3] Sidney L. Kark, *Epidemiology and Community Medicine* (New York, NY: Appleton-Century-Crofts, 1974); Sidney L. Kark, *The Practice of Community-Oriented Primary Health Care* (New York, NY: Appleton-Century-Crofts, 1981).

[4] H. Jack Geiger, "Community-Oriented Primary Care: The Legacy of Sidney Kark," *American Journal of Public Health* 83, no. 7 (July 1993): 946–7; Sidney L. Kark and John Cassel, "The Pholela Health Centre: A Progress Report," *South African Medical Journal* 26, no. 6 (1952): 101–4; Sidney L. Kark and Guy W. Steuart, *A Practice of Social Medicine: A South African Team's Experiences in Different African Communities* (Edinburgh: E. & S. Livingstone, 1962).

[5] In addition to their classroom teaching, a number of the faculty from the university's Medical School held important posts in the South African government and the Ministry of Health in particular. It was these men who would champion Sidney's early career.

a number of well-known, progressive faculty members they learned about Marxist interpretations of South Africa's class structure and political-economy, what the Karks later called "socio-economic historical analysis."[6] They learned about the problems created by the country's racial divides and the realities of life for the majority of South Africa's poor Africans. Connecting these lessons with their medical education, they learned that the difficult lives and ill health of many Africans could be attributed to a long history of oppression, disenfranchisement, and race-based economic inequality, or what is today called "racial capitalism."[7] The professors at Wits taught that improving the lives of South Africans living in poverty could only happen by addressing systemic issues: oppression, disenfranchisement, economic inequality, and racism at national and local scales.[8] When applied to health, this approach addressed what we call today the "social determinants of health," recognizing the role of racial capitalism in setting the terms of what is possible. At Wits, the Karks also learned anthropological and historical methods like surveys, participant observation, and analysis trained on structural rather than individual forces. These methods were key to their approach to social medicine and their understanding of Pholela and where the health problems there originated. During their hands-on training, they had opportunities to visit parts of South Africa they had never seen before, witnessing what they had learned in their classes playing out in the lives of the country's majority African population. This experience and education helped lay the foundation for the work Sidney and Emily would do in Pholela and for the relationships that made that work so successful and important.

The professors at Wits also pushed their students to act, insisting that they had a responsibility to do so. Through these professors, the Karks learned about the work of the nascent South African Institute for Race Relations (SAIRR). The SAIRR is an organization dedicated to research and awareness about racial inequality in South Africa and the political struggle to end segregation and oppression.[9] It provided the Karks with a model for a marriage between

---

[6] Sidney Kark and Emily Kark, *Promoting Community Health: From Polela to Jerusalem* (Johannesburg: University of Witwatersrand Press, 1999), 7.
[7] A term most famously coined by Cedric Robinson, "racial capitalism" recognizes the inextricability of capitalism and racism, with specific attention to anti-Black racism. While Robinson's analysis unpacks the Atlantic slave trade, he also offers a general history of capitalism. Cedric J Robinson, *Black Marxism: The Making of the Black Radical Tradition* (Chapel Hill, NC: University of North Carolina Press, 2000). The relationships around both race and class that make up racial capitalism make particularly strong impressions in settler states. South Africa, especially under apartheid, offers one of the most obvious and striking examples of this. Indeed, the term "racial capitalism" was first coined in South Africa.
[8] Their most influential professors included William Macmillian, R. D. Rheinallt Jones, and Alfred and Winifred Hoernlé.
[9] The South African Institute for Race Relations, established in 1929, was the first national multiracial organization to conduct socioeconomic research about race relations in South Africa. To this day, it is known for its liberal politics and rigorous research.

research and theory on the one hand, and political action on the other.[10] The ideas they encountered in classrooms and from the SAIRR were radical in a country with a long history of racist ideology codified into law (culminating in apartheid, which formally began in 1948). These experiences transformed the Karks from medical students occupied with anatomy, pathology, and other components of a biomedical education, to future physicians dedicated to social change and concerned with the broad social and cultural factors that shape both health and healthcare delivery. Thanks to connections he made as a student, in the years immediately after graduating, Sidney began working at the Ministry of Health and with Edward Jali conducted a large-scale survey of the nutrition of African school children throughout South Africa. This survey offered Kark and Jali hands-on training in the social science methods that would come to underpin COPC as well as an understanding of the depth of malnutrition in South Africa and its links to poverty.

Sixty years after the Karks had left Pholela, in 2008, I sat in a neat, red-brick home at the top of a hillside community I call Enkangala in the catchment of the former Pholela Community Health Centre.[11] In the corner of a spare bedroom lay Gogo Heni (*gogo* is the Zulu word for grandma). In the 1940s and 1950s, she had worked as a community health worker for the PCHC. Community health workers had been the backbone of the PCHC's efforts in Pholela. They worked primarily in communities, gathering data on households to both guide health center programs and evaluate their efficacy. It was through this work that the PCHC measured its remarkable success.[12] They also visited home-steads, helped to build demonstration gardens, met with community groups, and assisted with health education, school lunch, and other programs at area schools. These health assistants were largely from and lived in the communi-ties that surrounded the health center, which meant that educated community members could be employed at home investing the money they earned there. It also meant that the health center would have a workforce that knew the com-munity intimately. It was through people like Gogo Heni and their interactions with community members in Pholela that COPC first took its form.

---

[10] In addition to their studies, the Karks were heavily involved in student politics and activism, including through the National Union of South African Students (NUSAS), an inclusive, non-racist and non-sexist student organization, with chapters at a number of universities. Kark and Kark, *Promoting Community Health*.

[11] In accordance with the IRB, all names of residents are pseudonyms and all specific community names are pseudonyms. Because the doctors at the PCHC are well known and published exten-sively on their experiences there, I use their real names.

[12] For a full explanation of this work and a critical take on how the PCHC produced and mea-sured its success, see Neely, "Chapter 1: Seeing Like a Health Center," in *Reimagining Social Medicine*.

By the time I met Gogo Heni she was in the last months of a long life and suffering from dementia. I sat in the dim, cold room on wobbly blue-green plastic chairs with Enkangala's current community health worker, Zanele, a woman who would go on to become a cherished friend. Zanele and I talked about the passage of time and how long it had been since the Karks were at the PCHC. Zanele arrived in Pholela after the Karks had left the country. She came to Enkangala because she married a man from this place. She had heard about the Karks' work and knew that things were different now. There were fewer gardens in homes, more young people migrated for work (which was saying something, since Pholela had the second-highest levels of out-migration in South Africa in the 1940s), and there was much less investment in the community and care from the health center. Though Zanele visited individual households to offer treatment support and health education, the health center's program in the early 2000s was far different than it had been "in the time of the Karks," as residents called the period when "they" (Sidney and Emily Kark) were there caring for them.

As I got to know the community more, I began to see the remnants of the PCHC's work everywhere. On another afternoon, I was wandering with a woman I call Gogo Ngcobo in her garden. I learned that the health assistants had taught her to plant vegetables and staples like maize and sorghum in neat rows and in separate beds so that she could easily spot where beetroot, maize, or peppers would grow. They taught her to fertilize with cow manure and rotate her garden beds periodically so as not to exhaust the soil. She explained that these vegetables were important for her health because of their nutrients and that to preserve those nutrients one needed to boil instead of fry them. As our conversation made clear, she had learned from the health center to sure up her health through nutrition by tending to everything from the soil to food preparation. Gogo Ngcobo's garden and her knowledge were particularly striking because her neighbors had neither gardens as diverse nor such a sophisticated understanding of nutrition and how it affected health. Gogo Ngcobo had grown up in the catchment of the PCHC and had only moved to Entabeni when she was an adult, bringing with her the lessons she learned as a girl. Her neighbors had had none of this experience as children.

In another community I call Ethafeni, which was closer to the PCHC, Mkhulu Vilakazi (*mkhulu* is the Zulu word for grandfather) took me on a tour of the mountains that sat above his home. Long known to the nomadic pastoralist ancestors of today's residents because of the nutritious sourveld that grew there, the mountains of Pholela served as pastureland for the communities' livestock. As Mkhulu and I walked slowly up the mountain, we paused to step over a fallen wire fence and looked at a wooden fence post in the distance weathered by the sun and rain. Mkhulu explained that fencing was crucial for the rotational grazing that agricultural extension workers taught residents they needed because it allowed large sections of the pasture to rest while livestock grazed in other places. As we continued, he pointed out three subtle indentations in the hillside. These were cattle dams, he explained, or they had been. The government workers had built these dams for the livestock to drink as they grazed in this pasture. As he talked, his expression betrayed a wistfulness for a time when the government cared about Pholela and its residents. These ghosts in the landscape offer reminders of the past, of things that are there but not there, much like Gogo Heni who lay on her deathbed occupying a place between past and present. The landscapes and the people of Pholela offer reminders of the work of the PCHC in the time of the Karks and the lasting power of COPC in this place.

In 1940, when the Karks established the PCHC, Pholela was part of the African Reserve area of KwaZulu in the province of Natal. Nestled in the foothills of the southern Drakensberg Mountains, the district sits in a messy patchwork where communally held African land is mixed in amongst European farms and small European (white)-occupied towns. Though apartheid would not officially begin until 1948, there had long been policies and practices of dispossession of and discrimination against African populations, part of what Patrick Wolfe refers to as the apparatus of settler colonialism.[13] In the nineteenth and early twentieth centuries, economic and minority interests coalesced into policies that forced native Africans onto smaller and smaller pieces of land called "Reserves," forcibly settling nomadic and semi-nomadic peoples like the ancestors of Pholela's residents. The most significant early legislation was the 1913 Natives Land Act, which made it illegal for Africans to own or lease land in white areas. When the PCHC was established, African Reserves comprised 11.7 percent of the land in South Africa and housed the vast majority of Africans, who made up 69 percent of the country's population.[14] This dispossession meant that whites gained access to extensive parcels of land for agricultural production, mining, and other natural resource extraction. The industrial development that followed was key to making South Africa the biggest economy on the continent. It also meant that most rural Africans had only limited space for agriculture and few or no opportunities to expand their production. As a result, African men were compelled into wage labor because they could no longer make a living from the land. And as African men migrated to urban, industrial, mining, and agricultural areas to work, they left their families behind because of laws requiring Africans to carry passes for work in white areas.[15]

---

[13] Patrick Wolfe, *Settler Colonialism* (London and New York, NY: A&C Black, 1999).

[14] Leonard Monteath Thompson, *A History of South Africa*, 3rd ed., Yale Nota Bene, (New Haven, CT: Yale University Press, 2001), 297.

[15] Dorrit Posel, "How Do Households Work? Migration, the Household and Remittance Behaviour in South Africa," *Social Dynamics* 27, no. 1 (2001): 165–89; Cherryl Walker, *Women and Gender in Southern Africa to 1945* (Cape Town: New Africa Books, 1990).

Stolen land and compulsory labor together enabled huge profits for white people in South Africa. This stratified landscape and stratified wealth is what racial
capitalism had wrought.

Pholela exemplified this political reality. Women remained at home growing what little they could on too-small patches of marginal lands while men
sent remittances from the meager wages they earned as unskilled laborers in
cities and on farms. The combined livelihood approach meant that families
barely survived and that their health often suffered. Indeed, malnutrition was
one of the most remarkable features of the population when the PCHC began
its work in 1940. In addition, when they returned home, the men brought new
diseases like syphilis and tuberculosis with them, which took root in their mal-
nourished families and neighbors. It was this political, economic, and health
context that would help shape the possibilities and limitations of the social
medicine that developed in this place.

Many of the gogos I work with in Pholela had been girls or young women
when COPC began. Take one woman who I have spent a lot of time with
over the years, Gogo Sithole. Affable and open, Gogo Sithole was an important presence in Pholela in the early 2000s, as well as fun and easy company.
She was also energetic and hard-working, well into her nineties, often running
around Enkangala, working in her garden, and helping out friends at a pace
that tired me out. This plus the little bit of English she had learned made her a
perfect candidate to be a domestic servant for the Karks sixty-five years before
I met her. After the Karks arrived, Gogo Sithole took care of their house and
their children and came to know a bit about social medicine from that experience. She also loved and appreciated the Karks in a way I found common for
those who lived in Pholela in the 1940s and 1950s – she even named her first
child after theirs, Carol.

In the early 1940s, Gogo Sithole was a young woman. She had grown up
in Enkangala and was recently married. She had little formal schooling, but
lots of experience caring for children, working in fields and gardens, taking
care of livestock, and generally contributing to her household's livelihood.
She would go on to have eleven children, the first out of wedlock. Her husband, who also came from Enkangala, migrated for work for most of their
life together, sending money home on occasion and keeping the company of
"girlfriends" in the city, on the farms, and along the railroad where he found
employment. To make ends meet, Gogo Sithole worked as well, first for the
Karks and the doctors who followed. Later, she opened up a small stand to sell
food and drinks to patients and employees at the health center. She combined
this income and the money her husband sent home with what she could grow in
her garden and in her fields to provide for her family. By the time I met Gogo
Sithole, she was already in her eighties and lived at a ramshackle homestead
that was always teeming with several generations. Six of her eleven children

had predeceased her due to accidents and disease, both HIV and untreated chronic conditions like diabetes. While Gogo Sithole was uncommon, her experience was not.

The importance of the work of the PCHC was present in Gogo Sithole's homestead and her long life, as well as in her stories. As I got to know her better and as I got to know the work the PCHC had done in the 1940s and 1950s, I began to notice various elements of her homestead like the vegetable garden, pit latrines, and rubbish pit that I had learned about in the archives. These things had been key to the health center's vision of a healthy homestead and by extension social medicine. One day, soon after I had returned to Pholela from two months in the archives, Gogo and I ambled around her homestead chatting. I looked down and right in front of us was a new water tap. I asked Gogo about it. She told me that the family had collected its money to buy a new tap because their other one had run dry. Access to protected water was important, as Gogo Sithole and her neighbors had explained to me, because it ensured that they would not get sick from bacteria (and other things) in the water they drank. In the years before the PCHC, there were no protected water sources in Pholela, nor were there pit latrines, rubbish pits, compost pits, or diverse gardens. As I walked around Gogo Sithole's homestead that afternoon, it suddenly dawned on me that many of the homestead elements I had taken for granted were actually products of the health center's social medicine program. They remained in Pholela's homesteads thanks to the upkeep and work of area residents.

The importance of the PCHC's work was also evident in the way she participated in my research. Months before, as I conducted my first major interview with her to better understand what life was like in "the time of the Karks," it became clear that Gogo Sithole was an old hand at research. I used a printed questionnaire I had based on Sidney and Emily Karks' publications and the annual reports they and others produced about the PCHC. I was hoping to gather similar data so that I could trace change over time. As we moved through the questions, Gogo Sithole sat straight up and the wrinkles in the space between her eyebrows deepened as she concentrated in order to be sure that she fully understood what I was asking. The answers she gave were both accurate and comprehensible, two good qualities for research it seemed to me.

After a few questions, Gogo Sithole stopped me. She told me she knew exactly what we were doing. She explained that in the "time of the Karks," community health workers and researchers would come around and ask many of the same kinds of questions. And then she pointed out that I was not doing it very well because I did not know the right order of the questions and I did not phrase them correctly. In addition, I fumbled a bit and appeared unprepared (which was true, it being my first interview).

To be the kind of researcher Gogo Sithole was expecting, I needed to ask the right types of questions – about specific illnesses, crop yields, and hygiene practices in the household – and I needed to do so quickly, efficiently, and confidently, using the correct phrasing, all in the right order. In return, Gogo would answer those questions "correctly," concisely, and efficiently. According to Gogo, those were our roles in the research process.[16]

Like the fruit trees that lined her garden and the waste-disposal pits in her yard, Gogo Sithole's commentary on my research was a reminder of the impact of the PCHC on this place and its people. More importantly, however, it offered a lesson about her role and that of her neighbors in the work that the PCHC did in Pholela. Soon after the Karks and their team had established the PCHC, they set out to get to know the communities that surrounded the health center. In addition to meeting with the *Inkosi* and his *Ndunas* (the local power structure), the PCHC began with a household survey carried out by community health workers to gather information on basic household demographics, garden and field inventories, and health. This allowed them to get to know the conditions of life in the communities and in households, and it provided baseline data against which to measure progress. Focusing on the household had an added benefit of introducing the health center's staff to Pholela's residents, a first step in the relationships that would be so important to the PCHC's success and the development of COPC.

From the information it gathered in those surveys and in discussions with residents, the PCHC developed a social medicine program that was rooted in the homesteads of Pholela, reflecting both the needs of the communities and the possibilities for health and healing in this place. In practice, this meant a major health education and health improvement campaign. To make this happen, health assistants went door to door bringing lessons on hygiene and nutrition as well as plans for how to improve homesteads. To make the homestead a healthy place, the PCHC believed that residents needed to add new elements, rearrange existing components, and keep everything neat and tidy; they needed to reshape the landscape. In practice, successfully remaking the homestead required that health assistants and residents work together and learn from each other. It also required new relationships between people and things, as community health workers, Pholela's residents, and the things of homestead transformation reconfigured homesteads, health, and relationships together.

To promote health, the PCHC focused on the home vegetable garden. The health center saw vegetables packed with vitamins and minerals (micronutrients) as key to improving baseline health. The homestead vegetable garden, like the one Gogo Ngcobo showed me around in her homestead, became an important component of COPC because it provided an easy way to supply

---

[16] For more on my process of learning to be a researcher and on the role of research participants in the work of the PCHC, see Neely, "Chapter 2: Relationships and Social Medicine," in *Reimagining Social Medicine.*

nutrients to residents' diets, a way that was not deemed communist and therefore illegal as prescriptions of fresh vegetables were. Building gardens and growing new crops required new seeds, new tools and techniques, new knowledge, and labor, especially at first. As a result, health assistants and Pholela's residents built these home vegetable gardens together with seeds and tools provided by the health center and tips and techniques offered by agricultural extension workers in the area, the same agricultural extension workers who built the cattle fences and dams on the mountain top that Mkhulu Vilakazi and I visited.

Once they began growing, residents consumed the vegetables from their gardens. The micronutrients in those vegetables helped to counteract some of the most pernicious aspects of malnutrition and led to significant drops in overall rates. This was a biomedical solution to a health problem. But this biomedical solution was an intervention in the biology of the landscape as well as the body. And just as in the case of the new waste-disposal system, it was an intervention that necessarily involved people. Vegetables, people, nutrients, cells, and science all worked together to improve health. These improvements motivated residents to continue planting vegetables as they felt their positive effects and saw them in their children. Thanks to the impact that increased nutrients in diets had on residents, the non-human components of gardens, like soil, seeds, and shovels, became integral to the relationships between health center staff and area residents that underpinned the COPC developing in Pholela. Through new vegetable gardens (as well as other elements), the homestead landscape and the bodies of Pholela's resident were transformed.

Of course, the Karks and the PCHC understood ill health to be rooted in social structures as well as biology and the environment. For them, South Africa's system of racial capitalism, which kept Africans in the Reserves and ensured that they would remain destitute, was the ultimate social cause of illness. But these broad-scale political-economic processes were harder, if not impossible, to intervene in. As a result, the PCHC saw efforts to remake homesteads as a winnable stopgap measure (an intervention in the biological world) that could improve health, even if they did not reduce poverty (the most important aspect of the social world). This approach of focusing on the biological was quite successful and it was built on a bedrock of relationships among health center staff, residents, and the stuff of homestead transformation.

The transformation of homesteads catalyzed even more new relationships. Soon after they began planting new vegetables in their home gardens, Pholela's women formed seed cooperatives to share seeds and knowledge as they worked to improve their gardens in terms of both taste and nutrition. As women traded seeds, their gardens grew more diverse, and their yields improved. Together, they selected vegetables and seeds for taste and productivity. These seeds, the vegetables they would become, and the nutrients they would supply led to a new social formation and more influence for the women of Pholela. The seed cooperatives became the basis for a woman's advisory group first at the health center and later for the area chief, giving women a voice in official politics. The new social organization around seeds mattered beyond Pholela, too. As the women who were members of the seed cooperatives interacted with health center staff, the PCHC began to see the positive impact that these cooperatives offered to garden variety and yields. Seeing this as an excellent community solution to a health problem (malnutrition), the Karks and others incorporated cooperatives into COPC. By the 1970s, seed and other cooperatives had become a hallmark of this brand of social medicine as they traveled beyond Pholela to places like Mound Bayou, Mississippi. In Mound Bayou, the site of the first rural health center modeled on Pholela in the US, the farmer's cooperative was one of its most important and distinctive features.[17]

The PCHC staff's ability to recognize the value of seed cooperatives and their subsequent incorporation into COPC was thanks to the staff's relationships with Pholela's women. Relationships that Emily Kark played a central role in creating. It was Emily, not Sidney, who one woman asked about when I had just arrived in Pholela in 2008. She had not heard from her in a while and was worried. Emily sent a Christmas card every year. She loved them and they loved her, the women explained. She had been the one who studied them and their children, who cared about them and their health.[18] After all those years and across thousands of miles, the ties that bound these women together remained strong. But that was not all; the value of the seed cooperatives came in part through the seeds the women shared, the vegetables that grew from them, and the nutrients they contained. After all, it was the improvements in health that the PCHC and the Karks are best known for. The seeds these women shared led to new configurations of human social relationships that would extend beyond Pholela to other sites of COPC and beyond gardens to broader political structures. It would not be a stretch to say that thanks to the flexibility of the seed cooperative model, residents like Gogo Sithole have left a mark on places like Mound Bayou, Mississippi, and Jerusalem.[19] It was the non-humans – the things that could travel and adapt – that made it possible for

[17] "Community Health: A Model for the World."
[18] For example, see: Emily Kark, "Menarehe in South African Bantu Girls," *South African Journal of Medical Sciences* 8, no. 1 (1943): 35–40; Emily Kark, "The Growth and Nutritional State of Bantu Girls in Durban," *South African Journal of Medical Sciences* 18 (1953): 109–24; Emily Kark, "Puberty in South African Girls: I. The Menarche in Indian Girls of Durban," *South African Journal of Clinical Science. Suid-Afrikaanse tydskrif vir kliniese wetenskap* 4, no. 1 (1953): 23–35.
[19] I think with Marianne de Laet and Annemarie Mol's concept of fluidity here to understand seed cooperatives as a fluid technology. Marianne De Laet and Annemarie Mol, "The Zimbabwe Bush Pump: Mechanics of a Fluid Technology," *Social Studies of Science* 30, no. 2 (2000): 225–63.

Pholela's women to leave this mark. And it was in part their relationship with Emily Kark, that amplified their work through COPC.

As the example of vegetable gardens reveals, the relationships between Pholela's residents and health center staff and between people and the environment underlie the dramatic improvements in the health and the groundbreaking innovations the PCHC offered social medicine. These relationships are obscured by the aggregate data that fill annual reports, articles, and books written about the PCHC, rendered invisible in official accounts of COPC and in the publications of the Karks and their colleagues. In their role as research subjects and in their relationships with researchers and the things of social medicine, Pholela's residents and their knowledge, experience, and social world had a tremendous impact on how the PCHC, the government, and the rest of the world would understand Pholela and replicate the social medicine developed there. And it was these relationships – relationships between health center staff and area residents and between people and things – that provide the lasting imprint of COPC in Pholela. "They were nice. They cared about us." This is one of the lasting legacies of the PCHC in this place.

The value of writing from Pholela, from the perspective of this place and its people, is that it centers relationships. It reveals that COPC emerged just as much from the people of Pholela as it did from Sidney and Emily Kark, John Cassel, the second medical director and father of social epidemiology, and the nurses and community health workers they worked with. My experience in Pholela and my relationships with residents taught me this. As Marilyn Strathern writes, "it is through their relations with others that [researchers] understand relationships."[20] And as Gillian Rose writes, one of the consequences of these relationships is that "neither the researcher nor the researched remains unchanged through the research encounter."[21] As the stories of my time with Gogo Sithole makes clear, the woman I met and worked with was forever shaped by her relationships with the people who worked at the PCHC. The PCHC's practice produced research subjects. Its work in communities also produced researchers, as the health center's staff learned how to be social medicine practitioners through their work with Pholela's residents. Just as I learned to be a researcher from Gogo Sithole. In her study of the Rhodes Livingston Institute, Lynn Schumaker asserts that relationships between British researchers and African researchers ensured that anthropology would be "an activity done by and meaningful to Africans."[22] Likewise, thanks to

---

[20] Marilyn Strathern, "Don't Eat Unwashed Lettuce," *American Ethnologist* 33, no. 4 (2006): 532–4, 523.

[21] Gillian Rose, "Situating Knowledges: Positionality, Reflexivities and Other Tactics," *Progress in Human Geography* 21, no. 3 (1997): 305–20, 315.

[22] Lyn Schumaker, *Africanizing Anthropology: Fieldwork, Networks, and the Making of Cultural Knowledge in Central Africa* (Durham, NC: Duke University Press, 2001), 249.

the long-term relationships developed in Pholela, social medicine was deeply meaningful to communities, to the homestead landscape, and to the individuals whose health improved. But the PCHC's social medicine was not just meaningful to Pholela's residents, it was also the *product* of their relationships with the staff at the PCHC and the things of social medicine. And the impact of those relationships can be seen in the work of many of the social medicine doctors and pioneers highlighted in the other chapters of this book.

Science studies scholars have long sought to uncover the social relationships that underpin science. As Sandra Harding writes, science is "co-constituted with [its] social [order]."[23] Through insights like this one, feminist and postcolonial scholars have challenged often unspoken assumptions that science is a white, male endeavor. In doing so, they question ideas of universality and objectivity – ideas that are entangled with the practices of legibility, standardization, replicability, and consistency that were so important in the PCHC's work in Pholela. These scholars demonstrate that objectivity and universality are partial and particular, and that science is as much about the places in which research is conducted and the people it is conducted by and with as it is about the subjects researched and knowledge produced.[24] In Pholela and in many places in the Global South, the relationships that formed the basis of the practice of science are obscured. The result is that people like Gogo Ngcobo and Gogo Heni are written out of the stories of scientific achievement. Twenty minutes sitting on a bench in Gogo Sithole's yard taught me how important that silence is. But sitting in her yard and standing on the mountain with Mkhulu Vilakazi taught me that things matter too. Donna Haraway and others demonstrate that non-humans play an important role in the practices of science, the production of knowledge, and everyday life more generally. Taken together, these scholars demonstrate that knowledge, practices, landscapes, and people are the products of people, plants, animals, and things.[25]

Centering Pholela's residents and its landscape forces us to rethink what constitutes social medicine. While the doctors who implemented and helped develop COPC are key to its spread – after all, it was Sidney Kark who helped lay the foundation for the Alma-Ata Declaration – they were not the only ones who were important to the development of social medicine in Pholela.

[23] Sandra Harding, "Postcolonial and Feminist Philosophies of Science and Technology: Convergences and Dissonances," *Postcolonial Studies* 12, no. 4 (2009): 401–21, 403.

[24] Donna Haraway, "Situated Knowledges: The Science Question in Feminism and the Privilege of Partial Perspective," *Feminist Studies* 14, no. 3 (1988): 575–99; Sandra G Harding, *The Science Question in Feminism* (Ithaca, NY: Cornell University Press, 1986); Anne Pollock and Banu Subramaniam, "Resisting Power, Retooling Justice: Promises of Feminist Postcolonial Technosciences," *Science, Technology, and Human Values* 41, no. 6 (2016): 951–66.

[25] Karen Barad, *Meeting the Universe Halfway: Quantum Physics and the Entanglement of Matter and Meaning* (Durham, NC: Duke University Press, 2007); Donna Haraway, *Simians, Cyborgs, and Women: The Reinvention of Nature*, 1st ed. (New York, NY: Routledge, 1991).

As the unkempt fences, the pit latrines, the vegetable gardens, Gogo Sithole's efforts to teach me how to conduct research, and Gogo Heni's ruminations reveal, Pholela's people and landscapes were integral to the social medicine developed there and exported around the world. And following Schumaker, it was residents' work with internationally recognized doctors like Sidney and Emily Kark and John Cassel that would make what developed in Pholela valuable to the science of social medicine – to the project of universal science. After all, Pholela's residents already knew it was valuable. They could feel it in their bodies and see it in their children. It was the rest of the world that needed to be convinced.

The global importance of Pholela's residents and the things of social medicine came into sharp relief as I sat in the archives at the University of North Carolina, Chapel Hill, in the summer of 2021. A particularly prescient site given that Sidney Kark and John Cassel had founded the Department of Epidemiology there. I was reading through the files of the Delta Health Center in Mound Bayou, Mississippi, as well as the files of H. Jack Geiger, social medicine icon and founder of the Delta Health Center. In the 1950s, Geiger was a medical student at Case Western Reserve University and traveled to South Africa to train with the Karks in Pholela and Durban. There he learned about COPC and social medicine, which became foundational to his life's work. In 1968, after Freedom Summer, he advised Sargent Shriver, the architect of US President Lyndon Johnson's War on Poverty, about how to extend healthcare to end poverty. His model was based directly on what he had learned in South Africa and centered on community health centers. Thanks to Geiger, the first two health centers of the Great Society Program were in Mound Bayou, MS, and Columbia Point, a housing project in Boston, MA, where Geiger lived and worked. As I read through the Delta Health Center's papers and through Geiger's correspondence, the lessons of Gogo Sithole and her neighbors came through. In his papers, the needs and wants of Mound Bayou's residents were front and center, just as they had been in Pholela. The structure of the health center and in the specific programs taken up bore striking resemblance to that of the PCHC where health center staff and residents had worked together to develop COPC. One need look no further than the Bolivar Country Farming Cooperative, so important for nutrition, which was a key component of the health center's efforts. Modeled in part on the seed cooperatives of Pholela's women and in part on the larger practice of collective action and organizing among rural Black people in the US South, the Bolivar County Farming Cooperative, like Pholela's women's seed cooperatives, offers evidence of the centrality of Mound Bayou's residents to the social medicine practiced there. A medicine made visible through the white doctors who practiced it but always meaningful to the African and African American women who were so important to its development.

After a long and storied career, Geiger passed away in December 2020. Obituaries ran in publications from *The New York Times* to the *New England Journal of Medicine*, chronicling a truly remarkable life. Geiger was a decorated professor of social medicine, started two organizations that would go on to win Nobel Peace Prizes, and had a hand in bringing social medicine all over the world. His legacy is everywhere in the US, from Mound Bayou to Boston, from the US–Mexico border to King County, WA. Community health centers that were built thanks to Geiger's efforts serve over 23 million people who have no other access to healthcare. This is Geiger's legacy. But it is also Gogo Sithole's legacy, it is also Gogo Heni's legacy. That we know about Geiger and not about these gogos tells us something profound and important about the stories we tell about social medicine.

Emily Kark shows us this, too. She was Sidney's partner in life and in Pholela but as the memories of Pholela's women attest, she was the one they had such strong bonds with. As they told me, she was also a mother, she understood them and their children. They had something in common. They could work together. And, indeed, Emily produced a number of chapters and articles about women and children and the work she was doing in Pholela, offering evidence of the importance of these bonds (as well as the health impacts of gender).[26] And yet, it is Sidney whom scholars tend to write about when writing about the history of social medicine. And all of this is to say nothing about the non-humans – the vegetables and their nutrients, the household waste, and the germs it allowed to procreate – that made up the landscapes of social medicine in Pholela.

As the archives I visited at UNC made clear, underlying the legacy of COPC and its founders was a profound willingness to learn and to listen, to be in community with the people social medicine is there to serve, to recognize the role of Gogo Sithole, Gogo Heni, Gogo Ngcobo, and Mkhulu Vilakazi in the practice of social medicine. This is the lesson of Emily and Sidney Kark. This is the legacy articulated by Pholela's women: "They were nice. They cared about us." A legacy made plain not only through drops in infant and crude mortality rates and the end of malnutrition, but also in the worried look and desperate request for help to find Emily to be sure she was OK. While none of Pholela's residents were memorialized in print when they died, their work and legacy live on in part through the life's work of people like Sidney and Emily Kark and H. Jack Geiger profoundly shaping both social medicine and the health of the people it serves all over the world.

---

[26] See n. 19.

10   Barefoot Doctors and Social Medicine in China

Xiaoping Fang

In the sociopolitical discourse of twentieth-century China, the core topics of medicine and health as a crucial part of nation-building were reflected in either the original blueprint design or through work principles such as "state medicine for all" and "serve the workers, peasants, and soldiers." "Medicine and healthcare" and "social medicine" were essentially interchangeable terms during this process, as both highlighted social relations of health and illness and pursued social equity. Since 1949, the Chinese Communist government further justified its political legitimacy by criticizing the political and medical incapacity of the preceding Nationalist government and it delivered medicine and health services in alignment with social restructuring brought about by continuous political campaigns. It mainly focused on addressing sociopolitical and economic institutional determinants of health, disease, and the delivery of medical cares.

During this process, China's social medicine had been predominantly shaped by changing sociopolitics, including political ideologies, institutional structures, governance capacity, and resources distribution. Further, because of ongoing epidemiological transitions, the shift of medical official discourse, and the change of the economic developmental model, social medicine in China demonstrated its specific characteristics. The barefoot-doctor scheme in rural areas, which was first promoted during the Cultural Revolution of 1966–76 was a synonym for China's social medicine policy. This program aimed to provide a low-cost solution to the huge population's medical and health provision with limited medical resources and had attracted social and medical attention inside and outside China from the outset.

This chapter aims to show the unique path of social medicine in China based on analysis of the history of the barefoot-doctor program over the past seven decades. It investigates how barefoot doctors transformed social medicine in rural China and how the government clarified and addressed the contradiction between ideological equity and structural inequity in social medicine. It discusses how epidemiologic transitions both facilitated and challenged the barefoot doctor program and how they impacted on social medicine. This chapter further investigates how the evolution of community medicine impacted on social medicine due to the changing roles of barefoot doctors. It discusses how the barefoot doctors echoed the themes of social medicine in developing and developed countries, where its inspirations and legacies were left. By revisiting the state's role in the barefoot-doctor program, it is possible to contribute to a new understanding of the global history of social medicine in the twentieth century and beyond when sociopolitics, disease, and medical technologies have shaped both the social determinants of health and the relationship between medicine and social equity.

Barefoot Doctors: Transformation of Social Medicine in Rural China

In the 1930s, the governmental and non-governmental blueprints and practices of the rural medical and the health system aimed to serve peasants who counted for 85 percent of China's total population and train sufficient medical staff for rural areas in the state medicine framework.[1] However, this structural design did not change the social relations of health and illness as the sociopolitical system remained intact. After 1949, restructuring the medical and health system and the sociopolitical structures developed concurrently. This was evidenced by the establishment of healthcare stations at agricultural co-ops, which were established following the progress of the Agricultural Collectivization campaign of 1953–6. Healthcare workers, with ten to fifteen days of training, assisted the Health Department to publicize medical and health policies and provided basic services to peasants, such as bandaging wounds and first aid. During the Great Leap Forward of 1958–62, the People's Commune established a relatively complete medical and health system, in which production brigades temporarily had their own healthcare workers in some areas. In the suburban counties of the Shanghai Municipality, villagers usually called these healthcare workers "barefoot doctors" because they labored barefoot in rice paddy fields but were ready to do medical and health work as needed.[2]

On September 14, 1968, the *People's Daily*, an organ of the Central Committee of the Chinese Communist Party, published an investigative report about the work of barefoot doctors in Jiangzhen Commune, Chuansha

---

[1] AnElissa Lucas, *Chinese Medical Modernization: Comparative Policy Continuities, 1930s–1980s* (New York, NY: Praeger, 1982).

[2] He Gongxin, "Pinxiazhongnong shengzan zhege chijiao yisheng: ji jinshanxian youxiu weishengyuan Hu Lianhua" (Poor and Lower-Middle Peasants Applaud This Barefoot Doctor: The Story of Excellent Health Care Worker Hu Lianhua), *Xinmin wanbao* (*Xinmin Evening News*), September 5, 1965.

County, Shanghai Municipality.[3] Soon the barefoot doctor program was promoted nationwide, together with cooperative medical services during the Cultural Revolution. They formed the lowest level of a three-tiered state medical system that comprised the county, people's commune, and production brigade levels. Each production brigade implemented "cooperative medical services" to cover the costs of establishing these medical service stations, which would be presided over by barefoot doctors. By the collapse of the People's Commune system in 1983, 87 percent of the production brigades had cooperative medical stations presided over by barefoot doctors.[4] As a new medical and healthcare scheme, barefoot doctors significantly changed the delivery method of healthcare and transformed social medicine in rural China. Indeed, the Cultural Revolution restructured the rural medical world and altered the social relations of medicine and health.

In terms of knowledge transmission, the healers that made up the Chinese rural medical world prior to 1949 followed longstanding family-based or apprenticeship-based traditions and in both cases, medical knowledge and healing experiences were not readily shared with others. However, the new selection criteria for barefoot doctors emphasized age, gender, and educational background. This ensured that barefoot doctors came from ordinary rural families rather than village elites as with traditional practitioners. The scheme therefore quickly increased the number of people with medical knowledge in the villages. Gender was particularly significant as this feature set barefoot doctors apart from existing professional Chinese medicine doctors and folk healers.[5]

The large-scale medical publications also facilitated knowledge dissemination. This program needed a unified body of knowledge to promote a health program nationwide at the quickest possible pace. With the advent of the barefoot doctors, all of whom were at least partly literate, textbooks such as *Textbooks for Barefoot Doctors* that specifically targeted them were soon widespread. There were two series of barefoot doctor textbooks during the 1970s: one for southern China and another for northern China because of the variations in climatic and geographic conditions, which in turn had a bearing on disease.[6]

---

[3] "Cong 'chijiao yisheng' de chengzhang kan yixue jiaoyu geming de fangxiang: shanghaishi de diaocha baogao" (Fostering a Revolution in Medical Education through the Growth of the Barefoot Doctors: An Investigative Report from Shanghai Municipality), *Renmin ribao* (*The People's Daily*), September 14, 1968.

[4] Zhongguo weisheng nianjian bianzhuan weiyuanhui (Editorial Board of China Health Yearbook) (ed.), *Zhongguo weisheng nianjian 1984 (China Health Yearbook 1984)* (Beijing: Renmin weisheng chubanshe, 1985), 23.

[5] Charlotte Furth, *A Flourishing Yin: Gender in China's Medical History, 960–1665* (Berkeley: University of California Press, 1999).

[6] Xiaoping Fang, *Barefoot Doctors and Western Medicine in China* (Rochester, NY: University of Rochester Press, 2012), 58–60.

Barefoot doctors also demonstrated a unique trajectory of professional development. In the 1970s, barefoot doctors were mainly responsible for the medical and public health work of their own production brigades and they did not intervene in each other's geographical domains, which minimized competition between colleagues in neighboring villages. Inside the medical stations, the non-profit orientation of cooperative medical services and salary-calculation methods also minimized conflicts among the barefoot doctors in terms of personal income and professional prestige during the 1970s. All of these contributed to the formation of their sense of group identity.

For villagers, after the advent of the barefoot-doctor program, access to pharmaceuticals significantly changed. The main pharmaceuticals consumed in rural China had been herbal medicines that were primarily gathered from the fields. After 1968, the cooperative medical stations and kits extended the pharmaceutical sales network throughout rural China at an unprecedented pace. Western pharmaceuticals – mainly antibiotics and vaccines – began to enter the countryside.[7] Meanwhile, the consumption of Chinese herbal medicines and folk medical practices were promoted to meet the demands of the national health program in view of its low economic cost. Western medicines and Chinese herbal medicines circulated simultaneously in Chinese villages for the first time in the history of medicine in China. Villagers could access pharmaceuticals much more easily than before, while self-medication became more common among villagers.

In the meantime, the proximity of the personal relationships in these tightly knit communities made a positive impact on doctor–patient power relations. The villagers felt quite relaxed about communicating with "one of their own" about their diseases.[8] As for barefoot doctors, they primarily treated commune members in their own production brigades under the policy of "medical regionalization" – they basically treated their fellow villagers. As they gained experience, the barefoot doctors became increasingly familiar with the health problems of the local people.

All in all, the significance of the barefoot doctor program for social medicine lay in that it created a new, relatively equal relations of medicine and health through the changes in knowledge transmission, professional identity, pharmaceutical consumption, and relationships between doctors and patients following the sociopolitical restructuring of the Cultural Revolution. As the program covered basic medical service, public health, preventive medicine, and environmental hygiene, it facilitated preliminary but comprehensive health delivery to villagers and contributed to the improvement of basic health indicators.

[7] Liu Xiaoxing, "Change and Continuity of Yi Medical Culture in Southwest China," PhD, University of Illinois at Urbana-Champaign, 1998, 17.
[8] Fang, *Barefoot Doctors*, 162–6.

Ideological Equity, Structural Inequity: Legitimacy and Practice of Social Medicine

The transformation of social medicine brought about by barefoot doctors occurred in broader, complicated sociopolitical contexts which shaped social determinants of health and the relationship between medicine and social equity. As the Communist Party claimed, the People's Republic of China was a socialist country ruled by a people's democratic dictatorship under the leadership of the working class, based on the union of workers, peasants, and soldiers.[9] The commitment of the Communist Party reflected in the medicine and health work principles proposed in 1950, including "serve workers, peasants and soldiers" and "combine health work with a mass campaign."[10] The political discourse of the Cultural Revolution claimed, barefoot doctors, and cooperative medical services were "great inventions made by poor and lower-middle peasants to combat diseases by depending on collective forces" because they "solved the problems of poor and lower-middle peasants seeking medicine and health care."[11] In this sense, barefoot doctors justified the revolutionary commitment to the social equity of medicine and health.

The political legitimacy of barefoot doctors was buttressed by top-down administrative and medical systems composed of the county, people's commune, and production brigade in the new central and local relationship promoted by the Cultural Revolution. Barefoot doctors and cooperative medical stations were operated by production brigades. Medical station funds were collected from brigades, teams, and commune member individuals.[12] However, the barefoot doctor program was implemented nationwide in the context of a Chinese urban–rural dual sociopolitical structure from the 1950s, in which structural inequity in terms of medical resource allocation across urban–rural areas and social classes was predominant. In all, the governmental expenditure on medicine and health did not correspond to its ideological claim. Throughout Mao's era from 1949 to 1976, health expenditure accounted for less than 1.39

---

[9] Qian Xinzhong, "Woguo weisheng shiye shengli fazhan de huigu" (Review of Great Development in Medicine and Health of Our Nation), in Zhongguo weisheng nianjian bianzhuan weiyuanhui (Editorial Board of China Health Yearbook) (ed.), *Zhongguo weisheng nianjian 1983 (China Health Yearbook 1983)* (Beijing: Renmin weisheng chubanshe, 1983), 10.

[10] Qian, "Woguo weisheng shiye shengli fazhan de huigu," 11–12.

[11] "Shenshou pinxia zhongnong huanying de hezuo yiliao" (Cooperative Medical Service Warmly Welcomed by Poor and Lower-Middle Peasants), *Renmin ribao (The People's Daily)*, December 5, 1968.

[12] Fang Xiaoping, "Zhongguo nongcun de chijiao yisheng yu hezuo yiliao zhidu: zhejiangsheng fuyangxian de gean yanjiu" (Barefoot Doctors and Cooperative Medical Services in Rural China: A Case Study of Fuyang County, Zhejiang Province), *Ershiyi shiji (Twenty-First Century)* 5 (2003): 90.

percent of fiscal expenditure on average.[13] Furthermore, a huge gap existed between urban and rural areas. For example, clinic beds and professional medical staff per 1,000 urban residents in 1965 were 7.4 and 3.7 times those for rural residents, respectively.[14] In this year, the rural population was 4.6 times that of the urban population.[15]

The other closely associated issue is the distribution of resources across different sociopolitical groups. In 1951 and 1952, the government implemented free medical services and labor medical insurance. The former applied to staff of the Party and governmental agencies, while the latter covered employees in railway, post and communication, shipping, and industrial mining enterprises. In addition, the Chinese government had been implementing a healthcare scheme for senior Party officials.[16] These schemes resulted in unrestrained waste of medical and health resources.[17]

However, the peasants, who comprised the majority of the Chinese population, had no such free medical provision. The structural inequity of medicine and health was not challenged until Mao's criticism of the Ministry of Health that it was "only able to serve 15 percent of the total population, and this 15 percent is made up mostly of the privileged" and he called on them to "stress rural areas in medical and health work!" Mao's statement later became known as the June 26 Directive for medicine and health work.[18] However, the structural inequity of medicine and health based on "inequality of treatment based on social distinction" was maintained intact and continued until the late 1990s.[19] Even though the governments at each level were committed to implementing the "June 26 Directive," the gap between urban and rural areas and across sociopolitical groups continued to great extent.

In the meantime, the government addressed the discrepancies between ideological and structural inequities through administrative interference, the redistribution and reutilization of medical resources, and disciplinary schemes. Administrative interference included the reduction of pharmaceutical prices

---

[13] Zhongguo weisheng nianjian bianzhuan weiyuanhui (Editorial Board of China Health Yearbook) (ed.), *Zhongguo weisheng nianjian 1985 (China Health Yearbook 1985)* (Beijing: Renmin weisheng chubanshe, 1986), 59.

[14] Qian, "Woguo weisheng shiye shengli fazhan de huigu," 54; Zhongguo weisheng nianjian bianzhuan weiyuanhui (ed.), *Zhongguo weisheng nianjian 1984*, 18.

[15] Zhongguo shehui kexueyuan renkou yanjiu zhongxin (Demographic Research Centre of the China Academy of Social Sciences), *Zhongguo renkou nianjian 1985 (China Population Yearbook 1985)* (Beijing: Zhongguo shehui kexue chubanshe, 1986), 811.

[16] Gao Hua, *Lishi biji (Historical Notes)* (Hong Kong: Oxford University Press, 2019), vol. 2, 85.

[17] Huang Shuze and Lin Shixiao (eds.), *Dangdai zhongguo de weisheng shiye (Health Development in Contemporary China)* (Beijing: Zhongguo shehui kexue chubanshe, 1986), vol. 2, 53–4.

[18] Zhu Chao, *Xin zhongguo yixue jiaoyushi (The History of Medical Education in New China)* (Beijing: Beijing yike daxue, Zhongguo xiehe yike daxue lianhe chubanshe, 1990), 112–20.

[19] Fei-ling Wang, *Organizing through Division and Exclusion: China's Hukou System* (Stanford, CA: Stanford University Press, 2005).

and assigning urban mobile medical teams to rural areas. As discussed earlier, the popularization of barefoot doctors was very significant for villagers' access to pharmaceuticals. However, network, prices, and quantity were all crucial factors. For example, villagers would have to work for three years to buy a single bottle of tetracycline or Terramycin.[20] As such, the reduction of prices was crucial for villagers. By 1971, medicinal retail prices were only one-fifth of what they had been in 1949.[21] Affordable pharmaceuticals contributed to the equity of access to medical and health service when limited medical resources were otherwise unfairly distributed.

In the meantime, the Chinese government organized urban mobile medical service teams for rural areas and to train rural health workers in order to improve the rural medical situation in response to Mao's criticism of the Ministry of Health.[22] Medical graduates were assigned to rural areas and urban doctors were "sent down" to rural areas (either temporarily or permanently), following Mao's instructions.[23] Urban medical staff and graduates played important roles in training barefoot doctors and delivering medical and health services to rural areas.[24]

To address the shortage of medical resources, Chinese herbal medicine and acupuncture as low-cost methods were promoted nationwide, as reflected by the slogan, "one silver needle and a bunch of herbs."[25] The Chinese herbal medicine movement was of tremendous significance as it indicated that the state, for the first time, officially legitimated the folk medicine consumed by vast rural populations prior to the advent of biomedicine.[26] The inclusion of Chinese herbal medicine into the barefoot-doctor program also enhanced the symbolic relationship between urban doctors and rural medical practitioners in terms of political connections and the transmission of medical knowledge,[27] which justified the legitimacy of this nationwide scheme that aimed to bring social equity into the revolutionary campaign.

---

[20] Wang Wenzhi (ed.), *Fuyang xianzhi (Fuyang County Gazetteer)* (Hangzhou: Zhejiang renmin chubanshe, 1993), 218.

[21] Fang, *Barefoot Doctors*, 78.

[22] Mao Zedong, *Jianguo yilai Mao Zedong wengao (Mao Zedong Manuscript since the Founding of the People's Republic of China)* (Beijing: Zhongyang wenxian chubanshe, 1992), vol. 11, 318–19.

[23] Xiaoping Fang, "From Union Clinics to Barefoot Doctors: Village Healers, Medical Pluralism, and State Medicine in Chinese Village," *Journal of Modern Chinese History* 2, no. 2 (2008): 234–5.

[24] Miriam Gross, "Between Party, People, and Profession: The Many Faces of the 'Doctor' during the Cultural Revolution," *Medical History* 62, no. 3 (2018): 333–59.

[25] World Bank, *China: Long-Term Issues and Options in the Health Transition* (Washington, DC: World Bank, 1992), 18.

[26] Sean Hsiang-lin Lei, *Neither Donkey nor Horse: Medicine in the Struggle over China's Modernity* (Chicago, IL: The University of Chicago Press, 2012), 257.

[27] Gross, "Between Party, People, and Profession," 333.

In the meantime, the government adopted disciplinary actions to promote the barefoot-doctor program. During the Cultural Revolution, barefoot doctors were hailed as "the great revolution of the medical and health front." The government extended criticism and prohibition policies to medical practitioners belonging to "class enemies" and it also cracked down on "illegal healers" who may have continued practicing medicine by labeling them negatively as "superstitious healers." These disciplinary actions marginalized competitors of the barefoot doctors and provided them with a much bigger space in which to practice medicine and develop their professional authority in villages.

Among these efforts, pharmaceutical price reduction, the dispatch of mobile medical teams to rural areas, and the legitimization of Chinese herbal medicine all belonged to the redistribution and reutilization of medical resources without the radical changes of the extant distribution scheme. The disciplinary scheme was a politically coercive measure aimed at strengthening the restructured sociopolitical relations of health and medicine brought about by barefoot doctors. However, these efforts that addressed the discrepancies between ideological equity and structural inequity did not solve the critical issue of limited funding, which posed severe practical problems for the daily operation of the cooperative medical service. By 1973, only four years after the cooperative medical services had been implemented nationwide, the percentage of production brigades implementing them had dropped to the lowest level in the history of the program. After adjustment and improvement, the cooperative medical service reached its peak in the historical record in 1976 and then declined soon throughout China as a whole. While cooperative medical services that offered a partial waiver of medical and pharmaceuticals fees fluctuated, barefoot doctors and medical stations maintained different degrees of stability, which retained the key features of social medicine in rural China.

Notwithstanding, the end of the Cultural Revolution in 1976 and the initiation of the Reform and Opening-Up in 1978 redefined the official discourse of social medicine. In answer to the criticisms of the Cultural Revolution during the time, the Ministry of Health called for "a correct understanding of major medicine and health-work policies since 1949 that had been distorted during the Cultural Revolution." The minister criticized the practice of sending urban medical staff to rural areas. He pointed that it was wrong to believe that only a constant reduction of medical service rates and pharmaceutical prices could show the superiority of socialism.[28] In this sense, the criticism refuted the legitimacy of the redistribution of medical resources based on the restructuring of sociopolitical relations of medicine and medicine.

Following the reassessment of medicine and health strategies and policies in rural China in Mao's era, the key work of health sectors was now required

[28] Qian, "Woguo weisheng shiye shengli fazhan de huigu," 13–14.

to shift toward "medical and pharmaceutical modernization," which was different from the low-cost solution built around easily available indigenous medicine promoted during the Cultural Revolution. The new government was instructed to reform and strengthen around one third of county medicine and health networks from 1979 to 1985, such as training medical talents with modern science and technology and motivating barefoot doctors to improve their medical proficiency.[29] In October 1979, the State Council proposed holding examinations to certify the barefoot doctors.[30]

Through the new medical certification system, the state effectively changed the definition of medical legitimacy by prioritizing medical proficiency over medical equity. Simultaneously, barefoot doctors lost their core institutional context with the end of the People's Commune system in 1983. On January 24, 1985, the Ministry of Health officially announced that the term "barefoot doctor" would no longer be used in China.[31] Barefoot doctors who passed medical examinations and continued practicing medicine in villages were renamed "village doctors." Thus, the new sociopolitical and economic reforms brought about more professionalized medical practitioners and more commercialized services, which shaped the features of social medicine in rural China and impacted on the delivery of medical and health services.

Epidemiological Transition: Another Determinant of Social Medicine

From the "Newly Emerged Thing" of the Cultural Revolution in 1968 to the renaming of "village doctors" in 1985, the history of barefoot doctors shows how the Chinese Communist government defined and practiced social medicine according to political ideologies, developmental strategies, socioeconomic system, resource distribution schemes, operational procedures, and disciplinary mechanisms. But, the disease was also a determinant factor that shaped social medicine.

By 1949, rural China was still afflicted by acute and chronic infectious diseases, parasitic diseases, and endemic diseases. For example, plague, cholera, and smallpox were three major acute infectious diseases. Among chronic infectious diseases, the incidence rate of tuberculous was 4 percent, while the number of leprosy patients reached 0.5 million.[32] In terms of parasitic diseases, schistosomiasis affected an estimated 10 million patients in twelve

[29] Qian, "Woguo weisheng shiye shengli fazhan de huigu," 12–14.
[30] Fang, *Barefoot Doctors*, 166.   [31] Ibid.
[32] Huang and Lin (eds.), *Dangdai zhongguo de weisheng shiye*, vol. 1, 1–2.

provinces and 324 counties in southern China.[33] Hookworms existed in almost all provinces. In the fifteen provinces of southern China, the infection rate even reached 80–90 percent of the population.[34] Each area had its endemic diseases. Schistosomiasis and Keshan disease (an endemic cardiomyopathy) were the most typical endemic diseases of southern and northern China, respectively.[35]

From the early 1950s, prevention and treatment of acute infectious diseases, parasitic, and endemic diseases were mainly focused on two aspects.[36] First, the Chinese government launched continuous public healthcare and epidemic prevention campaigns, including the Patriotic Health Campaigns (i.e., ceremonial campaigns), ordinary schemes for eradicating endemic parasitic, and infectious diseases (i.e., regular campaigns), and emergency responses toward the pandemics like plague and cholera.[37] Second, the Chinese government committed to improving pharmaceutical and vaccine technology. By 1965, six categories of Active Pharmaceutical Ingredients (antibacterial, sulfonamide, antipyretic, vitamin, anti-tuberculosis, endemic medicine) were able to meet the demands of domestic prevention and treatment work and some medicines were exported.[38] In terms of vaccines, by the 1960s, various vaccines produced by biological product institutes guaranteed the implementation of immunization planning against major infectious diseases except epidemic meningitis and measles.[39]

During this process, the sociopolitical scheme played a crucial role in mass campaigns and technological improvements. This developmental path continued into the barefoot-doctor program in the late 1960s. The significance of the barefoot-doctor scheme lay in that it radically increased the number of healthcare workers who could actively participate in epidemic prevention in this nationwide program because the work did not require high medical proficiency.

The further progress of pharmaceuticals and vaccines, together with the epidemiological features of infectious diseases, facilitated epidemic prevention and treatment. Among them, the vaccine for measles and the epidemiological feature of epidemic meningitis were especially significant because the

[33] Qian Xinzhong, "Chengsheng qianjin, jiasu xiaomie wuda jishengchongbing" (March Forward Triumphantly, Eradicate Five Major Parasitic Diseases), *Renmin baojian* (People's Health Care) 5 (1959): 395.

[34] Zhonghua yixuehui (Chinese Medical Association), "Xinzhongguo gouchongbing diaocha yanjiu de zongshu" (Summary of the Hookworm Survey in New China), *Renmin baojian* (People's Health Care) 1 (1959): 1.

[35] Huang and Lin (eds.), *Dangdai zhongguo de weisheng shiye*, vol. 1, 1–2.

[36] Huang and Lin (eds.), *Dangdai zhongguo de weisheng shiye*, vol. 1, 6.

[37] Xiaoping Fang, *China and the Cholera Pandemic: Restructuring Society under Mao* (Pittsburgh, PA: University of Pittsburgh Press, 2021), 228–9.

[38] Huang and Lin (eds.), *Dangdai zhongguo de weisheng shiye*, vol. 1, 13.

[39] Huang and Lin (eds.), *Dangdai zhongguo de weisheng shiye*, vol. 1, 8–10.

mortality rates of measles and epidemic meningitis were the highest of all the infectious diseases affecting rural China throughout the 1950s and 1960s.[40] In China as a whole, the specific death rates from infectious disease kept dropping from 1957. By 1980, this figure for rural areas had dropped to 20 per 100,000 and was maintained at this level until 1984.[41] All in all, the epidemic control model based on mass campaigns and technological progress could effectively address the issue of the infectious diseases that afflicted the predominant majority of populations in rural China. This method guaranteed basic access to medicine and health and facilitated the implementation of social medicine when China's medical system and resource distribution suffered serious structural inequity.

However, infectious diseases were no longer the main cause of threats for rural populations by the mid 1970s. The percentage of infectious diseases of all causes of death in rural areas dropped from 3.49 percent in 1975 to 2.76 percent in 1980, though they were much higher than those of urban areas in the same year. Infectious disease ranked between eighth and ninth among causes of death from 1975 to 1983. The first five causes of death in both rural and urban areas were heart disease, malignant tumors, cerebrovascular disease, respiratory system disease, and digestive system disease.[42] That means that China had completed the epidemiological transition from infectious to chronic diseases. And there was not much difference between urban and rural areas. For barefoot doctors, their high profile was closely associated with improvement in basic indicators under the infectious disease model from the 1950s to the 1970s. However, the advent of the chronic disease model challenged the barefoot doctors' mediocre medical proficiency and the country's limited medical resources. It also subsequently impacted on social medicine in a commercialized market during the following two decades.

Barefoot Doctors, the Evolution of Community Medicine, and Social Medicine

In all, by the late 1970s and early 1980s, barefoot doctors suffered legitimacy and practical crises brought about by the renaming of village doctors and epidemiological transition. The development of community medicine, due to the changing roles of barefoot doctors, shows evolutionary features of social medicine in rural China. Up to the late 1940s, community medicine did not exist because of the individual, fragmented, and independent nature of professional

---

[40] Fang, *Barefoot Doctors*, 80.

[41] Zhongguo weisheng nianjian bianzhuan weiyuanhui (ed.), *Zhongguo weisheng nianjian 1985*, 55–6.

[42] Zhongguo weisheng nianjian bianzhuan weiyuanhui (ed.), *Zhongguo weisheng nianjian 1985*, 55–6.

medical practice and the vague distinction between medical practice and the agricultural production of medicine in rural areas. The concurrent downward extension of sociopolitical and medical systems gradually facilitated the rise of community medicine based on one specific administrative region. Because of the nationwide promotion of barefoot doctors in 1969 and 1970, a medical community, which geographically coincided with the People's Commune, formally emerged. Within a medical community, barefoot doctors provided preliminary medical and health services as discussed earlier. Outside the community, as medical staff at the lowest level of the three-tier medical system, with their counterparts at the commune and county levels, the barefoot doctors finally accomplished and enhanced the technical stratification and cooperation of the medical system through a patient referral system. As a result, villagers' encounters with doctors increased and they began to receive treatment outside their home villages and communes at county hospitals. Therefore, the emergence of community medicine embedded in an extant sociopolitical structure was significant for social medicine.

It was more significant that barefoot doctors further changed the structure of community medicine due to their dual role of healthcare workers and physicians throughout the 1970s. Particularly because they fulfilled healing roles, barefoot doctors had similar medical expertise to commune clinic doctors. Furthermore, the popularization of brigade medical stations, which had the authority to refer patients to the top of the medical hierarchy, made villagers bypass the commune clinics altogether. Barefoot doctors in practice thus further embarrassed the commune clinics, which now suffered mediocre proficiency, a shortage of the necessary equipment, supplies, and personnel to provide the medical services designated to them by the system.[43] The decline of the commune clinics made the rural medical network take on a dumbbell shape: the middle part (the commune clinics) shrank, while the top and bottom (the county hospitals and the brigade medical stations) became increasingly important. Therefore, barefoot doctors started to take over medical practices in the local community, that had previously been the domain of commune clinics. The dominance of barefoot doctors in community medicine provided villagers with timely and convenient access to basic medical services.

By the late 1970s and early 1980s, the epidemiological transition and the renaming of village doctors pushed the remaining barefoot doctors to improve their medical proficiency in response to legitimacy and practical crises. Barefoot doctors' efforts facilitated their professional development and further posed more intense challenges to township clinics (former commune clinics) because they had accumulated even more medical expertise and had grown yet more familiar with their patients in the villages than had the township clinic

---

[43] Fang, *Barefoot Doctors*, 139–44.

doctors. Therefore, the dumbbell-shaped structure has continued to characterize community medicine in rural areas since the early 1980s. However, this structure brought about a few serious problems in the new era. The most immediate problem was the overuse of Western pharmaceuticals because of village doctors' prescription preference for profit and rural residents' healthcare seeking behavior.[44] Another critical issue is that each level of the three-tier medical system was increasingly dysfunctional. The basic aim of this hierarchical structure is to divide patients among the three service points. However, as discussed above, there were no noticeable medical advantages to township clinics in comparison with the barefoot doctors' medical stations. Furthermore, barefoot doctors did not have any incentive to play the dual role of public health centers – service provider and "gatekeeper" of the whole system.

All of these features further resulted in unique healthcare-seeking behavior because there was "an elevated trust in high-level hospitals (with corresponding low trust in clinics and their staff) and the Chinese patient's high degree of autonomy."[45] When the medical market was highly commercialized in China in the 1980s and 1990s, all the costs incurred by the overuse of pharmaceuticals and hospital services were passed on to patients. Together with growing income gaps among social classes and regional differences, the full medical marketization in the late 1990s thus worsened accessibility and affordability of medicine and healthcare for rural populations. This change indicated the collapse of the traditional structure of community medicine that seriously impacted on the social equity of access to medical and health services.

Given the structural issue of community medicine in rural China in the last two decades of the twentieth century, the Chinese government conducted a readjustment – the "integrated management of rural health" – from 2008 to 2010. Each former township hospital was converted into a community health service center. Extant village clinics were abolished, while county governments established new health service stations, which were located according to the "20-minute service circle." Village doctors were incorporated into these health service stations. These health service centers and stations provided "six-in-one" services to villagers, which encompassed prevention, treatment, promotion of health and well-being, rehabilitation, health education, and family-planning advice. In all, the community health service mainly focused on public health work and minor illness treatments, which largely include medical examinations, home follow-ups, and health archives, and so on. To curb the overuse of pharmaceuticals, the Chinese government designed catalogues

[44] Liu Yuanli, "China's Public Health-Care System: Facing the Challenges," *Bulletin of the World Health Organization* 82, no. 7 (July 2004): 536.
[45] Michele Renshaw, "The Evolution of the Hospital in Twentieth-Century China," in Bridie Andrews and Mary Brown Bullock (eds.), *Medical Transitions in Twentieth-century China* (Bloomington, IN: Indiana University Press, 2014), 332.

for medical units at each level. Doctors at the community health service centers could only prescribe the pharmaceuticals listed by the catalogues. For these pharmaceuticals, the health service centers implemented zero-profit sales.

Through these measures, the government aimed to fulfil the integrated management of rural health in China in terms of medical services, public health, pharmaceuticals, personnel, and finance. Within this new structure, the role of barefoot doctors (now village doctors) was redefined and public health was re-emphasized. To some extent, the structures and function of this system were similar to those government and non-government experimental programs in the 1930s. This means that the ultimate goal of medicine and health in rural China continued across the new millennium – to provide basic medical and health services to the vast majority of the Chinese population and to guarantee accessibility and affordability of medical and health services, which has been the essence of social medicine in China's sociopolitical contexts.

Global Reception and Implications

The key features of social medicine in China represented by the barefoot-doctor program was in alignment with sociopolitical and medical systems. However, as the Chinese approach to healthcare delivery and provision from 1949, this method echoed the pursuit of accessibility, affordability, and equity of public health and medical care in both developing and developed countries. The former suffered the serious shortage of medical resources, while the latter encountered the issue of health distribution under the dominance of biomedicine. Thus, the Chinese government quickly utilized health and medicine as special international politics and diplomacy tactics in the geopolitical context of the Cold War from the 1960s.[46]

As early as 1963, China dispatched its first medical aid team to a foreign country as part of the Asian, African, and Latin American people against "colonialism, imperialism and hegemonism." After the initiation of the barefoot-doctor program, the Chinese government usually would include a model barefoot doctor in its "friendship delegations" to African countries. Together with other health collaborations, the barefoot-doctor model quickly got noticed in Asia, Africa, and Latin America.[47]

---

[46] Li Anshan, "Zhongguo yuanwai yiliaodui de lishi, guimo jiqi yingxiang" (The History, Scale, and Impact of Chinese Medical Aid Teams in Foreign Countries), *Waijiao pinglun (Foreign Affairs Review)*, 1 (2009): 25–45.

[47] Xun Zhou, "From China's 'Barefoot Doctor' to Alma Ata: The Primary Health Care Movement in the Long 1970s," in Priscilla Roberts and Odd Arne Westad (eds.), *China, Hong Kong, and the Long 1970s: Global Perspectives* (London: Palgrave Macmillan), 144–45.

The Chinese medical model based on the barefoot-doctor program also caught the World Health Organization's (WHO) attention as the Chinese approach fitted its grand goal of meeting basic health needs in developing countries. In 1976, the World Health Assembly released the "Health for All by the Year 2000" Declaration as a moral imperative and a commitment to achieving universality and equity. The declaration highlighted three key ideas – appropriate technology (criticism of the negative role of disease-oriented technology), opposition to medical elitism (disapproval of the overspecialization of health personnel in developing countries), and health as a tool for socioeconomic development.[48] In September 1978, the WHO publicized the Chinese barefoot-doctor system as a model of primary healthcare for developing countries in Alma-Ata, USSR.[49]

Though the barefoot-doctor program officially disintegrated in China in 1985, it was still influential in Asia, Africa, and Latin America. For example, as Anne-Emanuelle Birn and Raúl Necochea López noted, in Peru, barefoot doctors caught health policy-makers' attention as an inexpensive way of delivering primary care to rural areas when Chinese bilateral cooperation in health was blossoming through formal diplomatic ties and the Instituto Cultural Peruano-Chino.[50]

In the meantime, the barefoot-doctors scheme facilitated medical exchanges between China and the West and played a specific role of non-governmental diplomacy in the geopolitical context of the Cold War. The first USA medical delegation visited China in September 1971, prior to President Richard Nixon's official visit to China in February 1972.[51] From then on, many American medical delegations visited China. These American medical physicians introduced China's medical and health system to American society, including the implementation of barefoot doctors in rural areas.[52] Unlike the controversial acupuncture anesthesia, the barefoot doctors concurred in the ongoing People's Free Medical Clinics (PFMC) of the Black Panther Party due to its health

---

[48] Marcos Cueto, Theodore M. Brown, and Elizabeth Fee, *The World Health Organization: A History* (Cambridge: Cambridge University Press, 2019), 174–8.

[49] The World Health Organization and the United Nations Children's Fund, "Primary Health Care: A Joint Report by the Director-General of the World Health Organization and the Executive Director of the United Nations Children's Fund," International Conference on Primary Health Care, Alma-Ata, USSR, September 6–12, 1978.

[50] Anne-Emanuelle Birn and Raúl Necochea López, "Epilogue. A Lingering Cold (War)? Reflections for the Present and an Agenda for Further Research," in Anne-Emanuelle Birn and Raúl Necochea López (eds.), *Peripheral Nerve: Health and Medicine in Cold War Latin America* (Durham, NC: Duke University Press, 2020), 277.

[51] Victor W. Sidel and Ruth Sidel, "Barefoot in China, the Bronx, and Beyond," in Anne-Emanuelle Birn and Theodore M. Brown (eds.), *Comrades in Health: U.S. Health Internationalists, Abroad and at Home* (New Brunswick, NJ: Rutgers University Press, 2013), 121.

[52] Victor W. Sidel and Ruth Sidel, *Serve the People: Observations on Medicine in the People's Republic of China* (Boston: Beacon Press, 1973).

activism, which was an outgrowth of contemporary currents and of its own organizational evolution.[53]

The barefoot-doctor program also influenced some medical professionals and organizations. For example, in 1978, the Black Acupuncture Advisory Association of North America dispatched barefoot doctor acupuncture cadres into the South Bronx in an effort to heal and resuscitate improvised and minority neighborhoods.[54] Barefoot doctors as alternative modes of health provision alerted a few American public health and social medicine professionals to reflect on the equity of health access in American society.[55]

Conclusion

The history of barefoot doctors shows a unique developmental path of social medicine in the changing sociopolitical context of China. The state played decisive roles in defining social medicine, shaping medical and health development strategies, and establishing and reforming medical systems in Mao's era, in the post-Mao era, and in the new millennium. During this process, the crucial and challenging issue for the state was to deliver its limited medical resources to the huge rural populations according to its proclaimed political ideologies of social equity and justice. Social medicine in rural China's sociopolitical context was essentially healthcare provision within the basic units of its administrative system, such as the production brigade in the socialist era and the administrative village in the post-socialist era. In this sense, social medicine is a grand aim, while community medicine is a changing operational scheme in different sociopolitical eras.

Barefoot doctors as representative of China's social medicine involved two sets of relationships, that is traditional Chinese medicine versus modern biomedicine and administrative versus medical systems. This scheme aimed to provide low-cost healthcare to Chinese rural populations through the de-medicalization of biomedicine, de-professionalization, and localization in the institutionalization of the medical system. However, the history of barefoot doctors indicated that social medicine in China could not avoid the dominance of biomedicine, the trend of professionalization, and the emergence of de-localization, while medical institutionalization continued its momentum. This process occurred in the broader context of China's sociopolitical structural inequity from 1949, which has been further exacerbated by marketization and

---

[53] Alondra Nelson, *Body and Soul: The Black Panther Party and the Fight against Medical Discrimination* (Minneapolis, MN: University of Minnesota Press, 2011), 17.
[54] Emily Baum, "Acupuncture Anesthesia on American Bodies: Communism, Race, and the Cold War in the Making of 'Legitimate' Medical Science," *Bulletin of the History of Medicine* 95, no. 4 (2021): 521–2.
[55] Baum, "Acupuncture Anesthesia," 526; Nelson, *Body and Soul*, 8.

globalization since the early 1980s. The epidemiological transition has been another factor in shaping social medicine. As this chapter indicates, pharmaceuticals and vaccines have played crucial roles in shaping disease models and impacting on barefoot-doctor programs. Invention, production, and distribution involved both medical technological and sociopolitical factors. Among them, the latter is the most crucial determinant factor.

In the last two decades of the twentieth century, the state demonstrated both its ambivalent and crucial role in social medicine. On the one hand, the state's dereliction of duty in curbing the over-commercialization of the medical market seriously undermines equity of social medicine. On the other hand, the state has made steady progress in regulating and managing village doctors and contributing to addressing emerging issues of social medicine in rural areas. Entering the twenty-first century, the state continued to play a leading role in radical medical reform, which was intended to tackle a few thorny challenges, such as the overuse of pharmaceuticals, the dysfunctional medical system, and the proficiency of rural medical personnel.

As a Chinese approach to social medicine, the concept and practice of barefoot doctors are transhistorical and its aims and efforts continued throughout the late twentieth century into the new millennium. As a local solution to healthcare provision in China, the barefoot-doctor program echoed the transnational theme of social medicine in developing countries in Asia, Africa, and Latin America with different historical and sociopolitical settings. For example, compared with China, David Bannister's research on colonial and postcolonial Ghana in Chapter 13 in this volume shows tremendous similarities with China in terms of crucial factors at major stages of development. These include a village-dispensary program, a staff-selection scheme for Medical Field Units, the end of the Medical Field Unit program, and the establishment of community-based health planning and service programs. As an approach entangled with limited resources, huge populations, and radical politics, barefoot doctors also provided the inspiration for the development of social medicine in the Third World. In the new century, as in other parts of the world, population mobility, the radical change of sociopolitical structures, and the unbalanced economic development, brought about by urbanization and globalization, are posing new challenges for the state to address social medicine in China. The effect of the Chinese new approach is to be observed and assessed.

11 From *"Saúde Pública"* to *"Medicina Social"* to *"Saúde Coletiva"*
The Emergence of a Transepistemic Arena in Brazil

*Kenneth Rochel de Camargo**

The development of new scientific domains arises from the interaction of specific inquiry communities, the construction of research objects, and the consequent stabilization through academic associations, teaching institutions, and publishing journals. This process was described by authors with very different approaches, such as Hall's account of the development of modern science,[1] or Kuhn's seminal work on the historical development of a scientific discipline.[2] Bourdieu's description of a scientific field also sheds light on such developments,[3] showing how the social structuring of scientific communities and the consequent power relationships help shape the scientific endeavors. Knorr-Cetina's concept of transepistemic arenas as the basic sociological unit of the scientific enterprise builds upon the work of the preceding authors (especially Kuhn and Bourdieu) and provides a key support for the analysis of that development, as it proposes that "science" and "politics" are never completely apart and that the production of knowledge includes elements and interactions that extrapolate the closed walls of laboratories.[4] This is even more relevant when one considers an area with such broad interface with general human affairs, such as public health.

This chapter is an attempt to show some of the threads that were woven into an intricate tapestry over a considerable time span, involving many actors, both individuals and institutions, in order to develop a new, interdisciplinary approach to public health in specific institutional Brazilian settings,

---

* *For my dear Professor Hesio Cordeiro, in loving memory.*
[1] A. Rupert Hall, *The Revolution in Science 1500–1750* (Abingdon-on-Thames: Routledge, 2014).
[2] Thomas S. Kuhn, *The Structure of Scientific Revolutions*, 3rd ed. (Chicago, IL: University of Chicago Press, 1996).
[3] Pierre Bourdieu, "The Specificity of the Scientific Field and the Social Conditions of the Progress of Reason," *Information (International Social Science Council)* 14, no. 6 (1975): 19–47.
[4] Karin D. Knorr-Cetina, "Scientific Communities or Transepistemic Arenas of Research? A Critique of Quasi-Economic Models of Science," *Social Studies of Science* 12, no. 1 (1982): 101–30.

even under adverse social and political conditions. *Saúde coletiva* (collective health) arose from particular historical conditions, as both an intellectual enterprise that drew from traditional social medicine and part of the political resistance to a dictatorial regime, giving it a unique aspect in the global panorama of social medicine.

As Vieira-da-Silva stated in a work that provided much of the background for this text, "one can say that *saúde coletiva* was born in Bahia, Rio de Janeiro and São Paulo."[5] Here I will focus more on Rio de Janeiro, more specifically using the historical development of a particular research/teaching institution, the Instituto de Medicina Social Hesio Cordeiro (Hesio Cordeiro Institute of Social Medicine, IMS). Part of the Universidade do Estado do Rio de Janeiro (UERJ, Rio de Janeiro State University), IMS is highlighted throughout the text as a paradigmatic example of the institutional trajectories that took place in the general process. The reference to Rio de Janeiro as a state can be considered as a sort of metonymy; previously to 1975, the key institutions discussed here existed at first at the city with the same name, which was a capital of the country for a large part of its history, becoming a city/state (Guanabara State) in 1960 and later the capital of the recreated Rio de Janeiro State in 1975. Having been the country's capital, the city concentrated a number of institutions and agencies that played a major role in the development of the field, such as several federal hospitals, one of the larger and most relevant medical research institutions in the country (Fundação Oswaldo Cruz) and three different public universities, all of them with university hospitals and medical schools which provided a Foucaultian surface of emergence for the transformations in traditional public health.

This chapter relies heavily on the in-depth historical works done by colleagues, mostly Brazilian, but also on personal memories of the author as a participant observer of the latter part of the unfolding history of this arena. I opted to keep the term "*saúde coletiva*" in Portuguese throughout the text, in order to emphasize its specific Brazilian origin.

Political and Historical Background

So as to make sense of the development of *saúde coletiva* in Brazil, one has to consider the unfolding historical and political context in which it occurred. During the first decades of the twentieth century, there was an incipient organization of workers, in many ways connected to the massive immigration influx from Europe at the final decades of the previous century. This led to the

---

[5] Ligia Maria Vieira-da-Silva, "Gênese Sócio-Histórica da Saúde Coletiva No Brasil," in *Lima NT, Santana JP, Paiva CHA, Organizadores. Saúde Coletiva: A ABRASCO Em 35 Anos de História*, vol. 35 (Rio de Janeiro: Editora Fiocruz, 2015), 61.

emergence of self-funded forms of social security, initially geared toward pensions and retirement funds, but which included in varying degrees some ways of helping with medical assistance.

Workers' rights were gradually enshrined into laws, sometimes through paradoxical means. As an example, the creation of the first rudiment of a public social security system was coded into law by a representative who, in 1917, was ahead of public security in the State of São Paulo and violently repressed a general strike. A body of laws encoding several workers' protections, such as paid vacations, limited working hours, and so forth, was created during the Vargas dictatorship (1930–45), inspired by the Italian fascist *Carta del Lavoro* (Charter of Labor, 1927). Social security was granted to formally employed workers, through institutions (*Institutos de Aposentadoria e Pensão* –Institutes for Retirement and Pensions, IAPs) organized according to economic sectors (bank workers, industry workers, sales people, and so on).[6] Under pressure from their affiliates, those institutes implemented different ways to provide healthcare, ranging from creating their own hospitals and clinics to purchasing care from extant private organizations.

The Vargas dictatorship was responsible for the creation of the Ministry of Health in 1930 (originally as Ministry of Education and Public Health, being split in 1953). Healthcare outside the IAPs was provided by the public sector only for destitute people and was organized along programs geared toward specific conditions, such as tuberculosis or mental disorders. The public sector was in charge of preventive measures as well, especially vaccines.

The construction of the Volta Redonda steel mill in 1942 with US support as part of the negotiation that led to Brazil entering the Second World War on the Allied side is an important milestone in the industrialization of the country. Strategically situated halfway between the then capital, Rio de Janeiro, and São Paulo, the capital city of the homonymous state, it would play a major role in the development of industrial plants in both areas, a movement which would gain momentum in the following decade, culminating with the introduction of an economic development policy known as import substitution industrialization,[7] which would have the beginning of a Brazilian auto industry in the late 1950s as a hallmark.

With industrialization came the creation of an urban working class, in contrast with the agricultural workforce that had previously predominated and a massive migration from the fields to larger urban centers, especially the two

[6] Sonia Fleury, "Assistência Médica Previdenciária – Evolução e Crise de Uma Política Social.," *Revista Saúde Em Debate* 9 (1980): 21–36.
[7] Carlos A. Primo Braga, "Import Substitution Industrialization in Latin America: Experience and Lessons for the Future," in Hadi Salehi Esfahani, Giovanni Facchini, and Geoffrey J. D. Hewings (eds), *Economic Development in Latin America* (London: Palgrave Macmillan, 2010), 34–42.

aforementioned cities. In the span of a generation Brazil went from a majority agrarian population to an urban concentration in the late 1960s, with the consequent problems of increasing substandard housing, overcrowding, and a lack of adequate sanitation infrastructure.[8] Such conditions favored the emergence of non-communicable chronic diseases in the poor population, which still had to struggle with traditionally poverty-related infectious diseases.

The emergence of an urban working class led to a slow organization of workers and a more active political claiming of better livings conditions, with progressive, left-wing parties playing a major role. Among those, the *Partido Comunista Brasileiro* (Brazilian Communist Party, PCB), albeit being founded in 1922, was forced into clandestine operation for most of the period. Up to the 1960s, slow progress in social protections, including measures related to health in general, were then a result of workers' pressure through strikes and organization in unions and ruling elites concessions, even through the dictatorship that marked that period. During this period, a number of workers' rights were secured, such as a minimum wage, limits to working hours, paid vacancies, and maternity leave, among others.

The combination of social demands and political action created a favorable ground for the emergence of a critical approach to social theory, with a noticeable Marxist influence, which would provide one of the mainstays for the development of Brazilian social medicine. Brazilian social sciences were boosted by the creation in 1934 of the Universidade de São Paulo (São Paulo State University, USP), which hired eminent European professors, such as French scholars Claude Lévi-Strauss, an anthropologist, and Roger Bastide, a sociologist, to kickstart its courses. Some of the most relevant Brazilian intellectuals arose from that university, like Caio Prado Junior (1907–90), a trailblazing Marxist historian, or Florestan Fernandes (1920–95), a pioneering sociologist who played a major role in modernizing Brazilian sociology. This academic lineage would later intersect with the origins of *saúde coletiva*, by means of the seminal work of Maria Cecília Ferro Donnangelo, as described further on.

The democratic development of the country was halted by yet another military coup d'état that took place in 1964. Detailing all the events that led to and resulted from that coup d'état would go far beyond the scope of this chapter. Suffice to say it marked a clear rupture with the progressive gains of the working class in the previous years. Despite (arguable) economic growth, wages were depressed and the general living conditions deteriorated for the poorer population, with a consequent decline in the overall health of that segment. A hardening of the military regime took place in 1968 (described by

---

[8] Célia Regina Pierantoni, "20 Anos Do Sistema de Saúde Brasileiro: O Sistema Único de Saúde," *Physis: Revista de Saúde Coletiva* 18 (2008): 617–24.

many as a "coup within the coup"), leading to a "dirty war" against urban guerrilla groups which never represented a real threat to the dictatorship but served as an excuse for heightened repression, including torture and the "disappearing" of many individuals.[9]

The IAPs were consolidated into a single institution in 1966, the Instituto Nacional de Previdência Social (National Institute for Social Security, INPS). The different IAPs had varying models for providing healthcare for its associates, ranging from fully owned medical facilities to purchase of services provided by the private sector, which were in many cases of poor quality.[10] The model adopted by the INPS for providing healthcare was for the most part based on the latter, which was facilitated by the resulting large budget derived from worker's mandatory contributions over their wages now concentrated in one single institution. This model was rife with corruption, as denounced by one of stauncher critics of the public policies in the health sector that were then in place, Dr. Carlos Gentile de Mello (1918–82), who characterized that model as a privatization of profit and socialization of deficits.

Important population movements, such as the migration to cities, coupled with low wages, a lack of investment in infrastructure, and a wholly dysfunctional healthcare system created the perfect storm in terms of challenges to public health. Social disparities became even larger, healthcare was ineffective, expensive, and had many barriers to access.[11]

Healthcare reform became a rallying cry and a spearhead for the struggle for democracy, which resulted in the organization of the Movimento de Reforma Sanitária (Health Reform Movement, MRS), which would become a focal point for both the formulation of public policies and academic development.[12] This is one of the main axis of articulation of *saúde coletiva* as a transepistemic arena. The political (or "non-technical") aspect of the MRS had an immediate policy goal – healthcare reform – as part of a broader alliance that sought the end of the dictatorship. At the same time, the intellectual actors that were part of the movement were active academics, who proposed pertinent "technical" research programs that were at the same time drivers of and driven by the political platform, in close co-production of those aspects and multiple ramifications within the academic world and society at large.

---

[9] Comissão de Familiares, Grupo Tortura Nunca Mais-RJ, and Grupo Tortura Nunca Mais-PE, "Dossiê Dos Mortos e Desaparecidos Políticos a Partir de 1964," *CEV-PR*, n.d.

[10] Fleury, "Assistência Médica Previdenciária."

[11] Celia Iriart, Howard Waitzkin, Jaime Breilh, Alfredo Estrada, and Emerson Elías Merhy, "Medicina Social Latinoamericana: Aportes y Desafíos," *Revista Panamericana de Salud Pública* 12, no. 2 (2002): 128–36.

[12] Jairnilson Silva Paim, "A Reforma Sanitária Brasileira e o Sistema Único de Saúde: Dialogando Com Hipóteses Concorrentes," *Physis: Revista de Saúde Coletiva* 18, no. 4 (2008): 625–44.

A period of distension began in 1975, leading to a criticized amnesty in 1979 that nevertheless allowed for the return of many prominent political figures who were in exile. The cracks in the dictatorship began to widen as the economy deteriorated, especially after the Mexican default in 1982, in a scenario of economic crisis all over Latin America, which was aggravated by the so-called Structural Adjustment Programs sponsored by the World Bank and the IMF, which further impacted negatively the health of the less affluent strata of the Brazilian population.

In 1982, direct elections for state governors and representatives took place for the first time since 1965, and key opposition politicians were elected in some of the most important states, such as Rio de Janeiro, São Paulo, Minas Gerais, and Rio Grande do Sul, a political development that would become very important in the development of the healthcare sector reform that would take place later on.

The opposition to the dictatorship gained momentum at the beginning of the 1980s, with a growing popular pressure to reinstate direct elections for president. The military dictatorship created an indirect system of election, previously unheard in the country's history, in order to assure a semblance of formal democracy but with a very manipulated electoral college that basically rubberstamped whatever general was chosen by the armed forces, especially the army, to be the next president. The movement to regain the right to the full popular vote was known as *Diretas Já* (literally, "direct [elections] now"), which peaked with huge rallies in São Paulo and Rio de Janeiro, having all the main opposition leaders, including the recently elected state governors, and massive popular participation (over a million people were estimated to attend each of those events).

The manipulated election system was put in place by a revised constitution imposed by the military in 1967 and returning to the previous system required a constitutional amendment. Despite gaining a majority of votes, the proposed amendment failed to reach the necessary two-third majority and was rejected. The writing was on the wall for the dictatorship, however, and it would end in the last indirect election in the following year, 1985, which was won by a candidate of the then main opposition party, Tancredo Neves, with a running mate from a split faction of the then ruling party. The latter, José Sarney, would end up as president, after the death of Neves soon before the inauguration, in another bizarre turn of events that punctuate Brazil's story.

Despite his conservative origin, Sarney had to govern with an elected Congress that had many progressive representatives, and the new Speaker of the House was Ulysses Guimarães, one of the most prominent figures in the resistance against dictatorship, who played a major role in the *Diretas Já* movement.

A milestone in the return of democracy was the elaboration and approval of a new constitution to replace the authoritarian version imposed by the military. This task was undertaken by the newly elected Congress, led by Guimarães. The struggle for including in the new Constitution advances in social protections, including the health of the population, the important participation of the Movimento de Reforma Sanitária. This resulted in the effective adoption of many of the propositions of that movement in the final text.[13] Once again, this political achievement was heavily influenced by academic works, showing the hybrid nature of *saúde coletiva*. A document elaborated by IMS professors was at the same time the basis for a political platform that seeded those policies and the result of accumulated reflection within the academic circles.

The 1988 Constitution, Article 196, states: "Health is a right of everyone and a duty of the State, warranted through social and economic policies that aim to reduce the risks of diseases and other offenses to health and to provide universal and equal access to the actions and services for its promotion, protection, and recuperation."[14]

This provided the institutional platform for the development of the Sistema Único de Saúde (SUS), the Brazilian National Health System, as proposed by the Movimento de Reforma Sanitária. This development will be further explored.

The Development of Public Health

Traditional Brazilian Public Health has a longer history, with remote antecedents that can be traced back to the colonial period,[15] and even more so after a major historical milestone, when the Portuguese Royal Court, escaping from the Napoleonic invasion, moved to Brazil in 1808, effectively making the colony the seat of the Portuguese Empire. During that year, many key institutions were created on Brazilian soil, in particular the first medical schools, providing among its graduates the first local intellectuals who would concern themselves with the health of the population, albeit from a very conservative and racist point of view, concerned with the "Brazilian race" and the purported

---

[13] Kenneth Rochel de Camargo, "Celebrating the 20th Anniversary of Ulysses Guimarães' Rebirth of Brazilian Democracy and the Creation of Brazil's National Health Care System," *American Journal of Public Health* 99, no. 1 (2009): 30–1.

[14] Brasil, *Constituição (1988). Constituição da República Federativa do Brasil* (Brasília: Senado Federal: Centro Gráfico, 1988).

[15] Roberto Machado, "Danação da Norma: A Medicina Social e Constituição da Psiquiatria No Brasil," in Roberto Maclado, Angela Loureiro, Rogerío Luz, and Katia Muricy, *Danação da Norma: A Medicina Social e Constituição da Psiquiatria No Brasil* (Rio de Janeiro: Graal, 1978).

negative impacts of miscegenation with the large population of enslaved people of African origin.[16]

This school of thought gained even more traction after Brazil's independence in 1822. Many of the theses produced by the graduating physicians by the end of the nineteenth century were concerned with one of the key pillars of traditional public health, the hygiene of populations, conceived in a broad sense that encompassed the aforementioned racist theories and normative views on families and upbringing children, including, but not limited to, elementary school curricula and furniture.[17]

The arguments about the health of the population, especially in the (then) capital city of Rio de Janeiro had an important economic component, given that it was the most significant port, playing a key role in the economy of the young nation. The poor sanitary conditions of port cities was a cause of distress throughout the Americas and a motivating factor for the creation of the Pan-American Health Organization (PAHO),[18] which would have an important role in the development of public health in Brazil, with a long tradition of partnerships and support for various governmental and academic initiatives. A Brazilian physician, educated in modern microbiology at the Pasteur Institute in Paris, played a crucial role in the sanitization of the city: Oswaldo Cruz (1872–1917).[19] With good reason, he is considered a kind of patron saint of Brazilian public health and was the founder of one of the most prestigious Brazilian research institutions in health, the Fundação Oswaldo Cruz (Oswaldo Cruz Foundation, Fiocruz), which bears his name for obvious reasons. Cruz introduced new, science-based practices in the management of the health of population, having as one of his greatest accomplishments the eradication of yellow fever in the country's capital at the beginning of the twentieth century. This, however, was achieved with somewhat forceful means which included the forced eviction of poor people from substandard housing and the tearing down of considerable areas in the city, acting jointly with its mayor, Francisco Pereira Passos (1836–1913), a policy that became popularly known as *bota abaixo* (loosely translated, "tear it down"). This was met with resistance from the population, translated, for example, in riots against the mandatory smallpox vaccination in 1904.[20]

---

[16] Machado, "Danação da Norma"; Everardo Duarte Nunes, "Sobre a História da Saúde Pública: Idéias e Autores," *Ciência & Saúde Coletiva* 5 (2000): 251–64, at: www.planalto.gov.br/ccivil_03/leis/l6683.htm.

[17] Jurandir Freire Costa, *Ordem Médica e Maria Cecília Ferro Donnangelo Norma Familiar* (Rio de Janeiro: Graal, 1979).

[18] Marcos Cueto, *The Value of Health: A History of the Pan-American Health Organization* (Washington, DC: PAHO, 2006).

[19] Nunes, "Sobre a História da Saúde Pública."

[20] Nunes, "Sobre a História da Saúde Pública."

The early years of the twentieth century (1910s–30s) were also marked by the activities of the Rockefeller Foundation, especially in the State of São Paulo, where it helped to create what became later (1945) one of the most relevant teaching and research institutions in public health in the country, the Faculdade de Saúde Pública (Faculty of Public Health).[21]

The deterioration of health conditions for a large part of the Latin American population during the late 1960s and 1970s was the background for the development of a local critical approach, inspired by nineteenth-century social medicine and with a strong Marxist influence, the so-called Latin American social medicine.[22] Social medicine was in a sense a development following the traditional Public Health, but developed against it as well. The critique of the latter was based on its de-politicization of the health status of the population, narrow focus on the biomedical aspects of disease, and disregard for social context.[23]

A key figure in articulating people and institutions in this period was the Argentinian physician and social scientist Juan Cesar Garcia (1932–84),[24] who, working with the PAHO, was instrumental in fostering several initiatives in the continent, including the creation of the first graduate programs in Social Medicine in the early 1970s in Mexico and Brazil. The graduate programs that were created in Brazil will get more consideration further on in the chapter. Garcia "developed from 1966 to its his death in 1984 important research and analysis on of medical education, social sciences in medicine, the social class determinants in the health-disease process and the ideological bases of anti-Hispanic discrimination."[25] Garcia's role in the origin of *saúde coletiva* cannot be overestimated. At its inception, the group of intellectuals who would develop both the political and scientific aspects of the field were potential targets of the military regime, at a time where opposing the dictatorship presented serious risks for those involved. The international connections that were developed through his work, as well as the academic nature of the research program

---

[21] Lina Rodrigues de Faria, "Os Primeiros Anos da Reforma Sanitária No Brasil e a Atuação da Fundação Rockefeller (1915–1920)," *Physis: Revista de Saúde Coletiva* 5 (1995): 109–30; Lina Rodrigues de Faria, "A Fundação Rockefeller e Os Serviços de Saúde Em São Paulo (1920–30): Perspectivas Históricas," *História, Ciências, Saúde-Manguinhos* 9, no. 3 (2002): 561–90.

[22] Iriart et al., "Medicina Social Latinoamericana"; Howard Waitzkin, *The Second Sickness: Contradictions of Capitalist Health Care*, 2nd ed. (Lanham, MD: Rowman & Littlefield Publishers, 2000); Howard Waitzkin, Celia Iriart, Alfredo Estrada, and Silvia Lamadrid, "Social Medicine Then and Now: Lessons from Latin America," *American Journal of Public Health* 91, no. 10 (2001): 1592–601.

[23] Sergio Arouca, *O Dilema Preventivista: Contribuição Para a Compreensão e Crítica da Medicina Preventiva* (São Paulo: Editora Unesp, 2003).

[24] Iriart et al., "Medicina Social Latinoamericana"; Everardo Duarte Nunes, "Juan César García: A Medicina Social Como Projeto e Realização," *Ciência & Saúde Coletiva* 20 (2015): 139–44.

[25] Iriart et al., "Medicina Social Latinoamericana."

that was being nucleated at different sites in Brazil, provided some degree of protection to the field's founding figures, such as many of those named here. Once again, the intertwining of the political and the academic characterized the transepistemic nature of the emerging field.

The strong Marxist influence was, however, only part of the theoretical kaleidoscope that was forming. The cooperation between a UN organ geared toward economic development (United Nations Economic Commission for Latin America) and the PAHO resulted in a very influential health-planning program,[26] with a strong Keynesian influence and French philosophers, most notably Michel Foucault, also had a role in the development of this arena, at least in Brazil.[27]

Social medicine in Brazil had among its pioneers a handful of young physicians, among them Guilherme Rodrigues da Silva (1928–2006), Sebastião Loureiro (1938–2021), Hesio de Albuquerque Cordeiro (1942–2020), and Antonio Sergio da Silva Arouca (1941–2003), who played relevant roles both in the establishment of an academic field and the political organization of the public health sector from the early 1970s onward, taking part in the resistance to the dictatorship and subsequently in the rebuilding of democratic institutions.[28] Rodrigues da Silva created the embryo of what would later become the Instituto de Saúde Coletiva at Universidade Federal da Bahia (ISC/UFBA), and later was at the head of the department of preventive medicine at the medical school of Universidade de São Paulo (USP). Loureiro was one of the key leaderships in the creation of ISC/UFBA; and Arouca was a leader both in the theoretical development of *saúde coletiva* and in the political arena. With the exception of Arouca, the other three were at some point presidents of the main *saúde coletiva* academic association, Associação Brasileira de Pós-Graduação em Saúde Coletiva (Brazilian Association of Graduate Collective Health Programs, Abrasco).

Hesio Cordeiro (Figure 11.1), along with Moyses Szklo (who would later have a stellar career at the Johns Hopkins University) and Nina Vivina Pereira Nunes, all physicians, graduated from the medical school (Faculdade de Ciências Médicas, FCM) of the (then) Universidade do Estado da Guanabara (UEG, later Universidade do Estado do Rio de Janeiro, Rio de Janeiro State University, UERJ), under the guidance of Professor Americo Piquet Carneiro, a

[26] Lígia Giovanella, "As Origens e as Correntes Atuais Do Enfoque Estratégico Em Planejamento de Saúde Na América Latina," *Cadernos de Saúde Pública* 7, no. 1 (1991): 26–44.

[27] Nunes, "Sobre a História da Saúde Pública."

[28] Ligia Maria Vieira-da-Silva, *O Campo da Saúde Coletiva: Gênese, Transformações e Articulações Com a Reforma Sanitária Brasileira* (Rio de Janeiro and Salvador: Editora FIOCRUZ/EDUFBA, 2018); Nunes, "Sobre a História da Saúde Pública"; Moisés Goldbaum, "Guilherme Rodrigues da Silva: A Formação Do Campo da Saúde Coletiva No Brasil," *Ciência & Saúde Coletiva* 20 (2015): 2129–34.

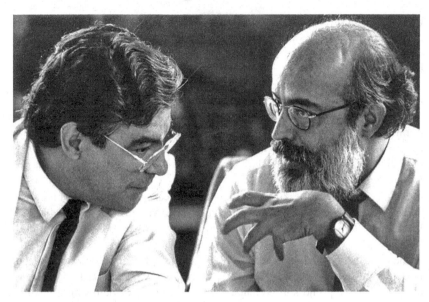

Figure 11.1 Sérgio Arouca and Hésio Cordeiro.
Source: Casa de Oswaldo Cruz/Fiocruz.

respected leadership, physician, and professor of that same school, were tasked with the reorganization of what was then the Medical Hygiene discipline at the FCM. This resulted in the creation in 1970 (approximately, there are controversies about the date) of the Instituto de Medicina Social (Social Medicine Institute, IMS, since 2021 Instituto de Medicina Social Hesio Cordeiro, again for rather obvious reasons), as an offshoot of the medical school (although it would take decades for it to acquire its full independence).

The first director of the IMS (1971–8) was a very respected traditional Public Health professor, Nelson Luiz de Araújo Moraes, who had developed a method for the quick assessment of a population's health status based on its graphic representation of proportional mortality in key age strata. During his tenure as director, Moraes also held the second position in the hierarchy of the Ministry of Health, covering the hardest period of the dictatorship. Given his national prestige, he sheltered the young progressive IMS professors – who had connections to political organizations forced into the underground, such as the Brazilian Communist Party – from the repressive regime.[29]

The pioneering IMS physicians were very critical of the traditional medical approach and were originally intent on reforming medical education and

---

[29] Reinaldo Guimarães, "Hesio Cordeiro e o Instituto de Medicina Social," *Physis: Revista de Saúde Coletiva* 31, no. 3 (2021): e310307.

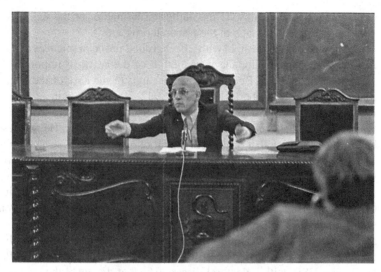

Figure 11.2 Michel Foucault lecturing at the Instituto de Medicina Social.
Source: Arquivo Nacional, Brasil. BR RJANRIO EH.0.FOT, PPU.7879.

practice. With the guidance of Juan Cesar Garcia, Cordeiro complemented his
studies in the US and returned to Brazil to continue his career. His Master's thesis as well as his doctoral dissertation were both published as books,[30] and had
a seminal role in the field. He was one of the first Brazilian authors, if not the
first, to develop the concept of the medical-industrial complex as a critical tool.

A key feature of the budding field was its intense interdisciplinary dialogue.
The aforementioned physicians started a nucleation process that aggregated
researchers from other areas, notably from the social sciences. An important pioneer was Maria Cecília Ferro Donnangelo (1940–83), a professor at
USP's Department of Preventive Medicine, whose Master's and doctoral
works explored the connections between living and working conditions and
the health–disease processes with a Marxist perspective.[31]

In the early 1970s, the first graduate programs in Public Health were created,
mostly at the Master's level, with the IMS beginning its Master's program in
Social Medicine – the second in Latin America – in 1974. The beginning of the
program was marked by a series of lectures given by none other than Foucault
himself (Figure 11.2). This program had international support (funding from
the Kellogg Foundation and the PAHO) and, paradoxically, from Brazilian

---

[30] Hésio Cordeiro, *A Indústria da Saúde No Brasil* (Rio de Janeiro: Graal/CEBES, 1981); Hésio
Cordeiro, *As Empresas Médicas: As Transformações Capitalistas da Prática Médica* (Rio de
Janeiro: Graal, 1984).
[31] Nunes, "Sobre a História da Saúde Pública."

government agencies, despite the authoritarian nature of the regime and the inherently critical approach of the research program.[32]

The newcomers to the field with a background in social sciences and humanities were responsible for the introduction of the work of important French authors, such as Pierre Bourdieu and Foucault. In the case of the IMS, a key role was played by Roberto Machado (1942–2021) a prominent philosopher who worked there from 1974 to 1978. Machado was a disciple and friend of Foucault as well as the translator of his books to Portuguese. He was responsible for the invitation that resulted in the aforementioned series of conferences. The IMS counted in its origins with other relevant intellectuals who had a founding role for the whole field, as, for instance, Maria Andrea Loyola, an anthropologist; Madel Luz, a sociologist and philosopher; and Jurandir Freire Costa, physician, psychoanalyst, and philosopher. All of them had strong ties with French-speaking institutions and were responsible for introducing those authors to the fledgling *saúde coletiva* field. Luz, in particular, after obtaining her Master's degree in Louvain, Belgium, went on to a doctorate in Political Science at USP, with a doctoral dissertation that dissected the origins of the IAPs, with a theoretical approach that connected Gramsci and Foucault. Soon after it was published as a book, it became a classic reference.[33] The infusion of diverse theoretical approaches was in general well received and integrated into the body of knowledge that was being formed.

By the late 1970s, a discomfort with the "Social Medicine" moniker became prevalent; it was perceived as excluding from the field all the other researchers who were not physicians. The name "*saúde coletiva*" (collective health) emerged and was slowly adopted in the field, with a formalization at a meeting of graduate programs that occurred in 1978.[34]

The creation of institutions that congregated researchers in the field was an important milestone of that period, with the Centro Brasileiro de Estudos de Saúde (Brazilian Center of Health Studies, CEBES) arising in 1976 and the Associação Brasileira de Pós-Graduação em Saúde Coletiva (Brazilian Association of Graduate Collective Health Programs, Abrasco, later just Associação Brasileira de Saúde Coletiva for greater inclusiveness), founded in 1978, became important focal points for the development of knowledge and political action.[35]

The role of progressive physicians in the creation of what would later be *saúde coletiva* meant that healthcare was from the start an integral component of the field, marking one important distinction from a more traditional conception

[32] Guimarães, "Hesio Cordeiro."
[33] Madel Terezinha Luz, *As Instituições Médicas No Brasil: Instituições e Estratégias de Hegemonia* (Rio de Janeiro: Graal, 1978).
[34] Everardo Duarte Nunes, "Saúde Coletiva: História de Uma Ideia e de Um Conceito," *Saúde e Sociedade* 3 (1994): 5–21; Guimarães, "Hesio Cordeiro."
[35] Nunes, "Saúde Coletiva"; Vieira-da-Silva, *O Campo da Saúde Coletiva*.

of Public Health and arguably even Social Medicine at large. The development of a network of primary care facilities in Montes Claros, a medium-sized city in the State of Minas Gerais, in 1975 is considered a milestone of the development of healthcare models that contemplated both the managerial and service delivery aspects, serving as the prototype for a countrywide program to further extend primary care to a wider share of the population.[36] This program was coordinated by Francisco de Assis Machado, yet another physician with a relevant participation in the constitution of the field. The connection with the medical profession had repercussions in the development of community and family medicine in Brazil. As an example, in the specific case of UERJ, which has had a seminal role in that area,[37] the key leaders of its development, such as Ricardo Donato Rodrigues and Maria Inez Padula Anderson, obtained their Master's and PhDs at IMS/UERJ.[38]

The implementation of graduate courses in the area that would later be termed "*saúde coletiva*" began in 1971 and until 1989, counted only with 5 programs. In 2018, however, it had been expanded to a total of 93 programs, albeit with a skewed distribution in the national territory, with a great concentration in the most affluent parts of the country.

In the early (pre-1990s) years, given the scarcity of doctoral programs in the country, many individuals sought those in other countries, especially the US and the UK, to complement their academic development, bringing diverse collaborations with other researchers from all over the world.

The overall field tended to coalesce along three main axes: Epidemiology, Social Sciences and Humanities in Health, and Health Planning and Management, with different traditions in terms of methods, priorities, and publishing patterns, sometimes threatening the integrity of the field as a joint enterprise and its interdisciplinary character.

This expansion shows the academic mainstreaming of the field, which consolidated its position as a scientific domain, although this has brought some trade-offs as well, linked to how academic hierarchies are established in Brazil.

Graduate programs in Brazil are strictly regulated by the Ministry of Education, specifically by the Comissão de Aperfeiçoamento de Pessoal de Nível Superior (Commission for the Improvement of Higher Education Personnel, CAPES), which holds regular evaluations of all the graduate programs (Master's and doctoral) in the country. The evaluation process relies heavily on numeric indicators and those related to scientific publishing have great weight in the final result. This means that those who publish more tend

---

[36] Vieira-da-Silva, "Gênese Sócio-Histórica da Saúde Coletiva No Brasil."
[37] João Werner Falk, "A Medicina de Família e Comunidade e Sua Entidade Nacional: Histórico e Perspectivas," *Revista Brasileira de Medicina de Família e Comunidade* 1, no. 1 (2004): 5–10.
[38] My own academic career began as a medical student under their supervision.

to be better evaluated and this somewhat skewed the better grades toward the epidemiologists, creating resentment among the other subdomains and further threatening the unity of the field.[39]

The greater academic emphasis may have dulled the political edge of the field as a whole, which lost some of the political capital that it held during the struggle for healthcare reform.

In the case of the IMS, the original Master's in Preventive and Social Medicine, which was for institutional reasons grouped with other Master's programs in Medicine, was replaced by a Master's in *saúde coletiva* in 1987.[40] Whereas the previous program only admitted physicians, the new one was open to all kinds of undergraduate studies, which were more in-line with the interdisciplinary nature of its faculty, which included sociologists, anthropologists, philosophers, economists, psychoanalysts, and demographers, among others. In 1991, a doctoral program in the same area was created, showing the maturity of the institution.[41] In the same year, the IMS started a regular journal, *Physis*, which is still going strong.[42]

The first generation of IMS professors was very active in the political scene; aside form Hesio Cordeiro's tenure at the helm of INAMPS (and later president of the university), Nina Pereira Nunes was subsecretary of the State Health Department in the first freely elected state government in Rio de Janeiro after the 1964 coup; José Carvalho de Noronha was secretary of the State Health Department at a later date; Reinaldo Guimarães headed a research funding agency, Financiadora de Estudos e Projetos (Funding Authority for Studies and Projects, FINEP); and Maria Andrea Loyolla was president of CAPES. As the academic aspect of the institution gained more weight though, there was a considerable reflux in the participation of its professors in the general political arena, despite some participation in several Abrasco administrations, including a recent presidency (Gulnar Azevedo e Silva, 2018–21).

The Sistema Único de Saúde – Brazilian National Health System

As stated before, throughout the military dictatorship, as the field itself self-organized and matured, *saúde coletiva* actors played a significant role in the opposition to the regime, with systematic criticism of the overall health

---

[39] Jorge Alberto Bernstein Iriart, Suely Ferreira Deslandes, Denise Martin, Kenneth Rochel de Camargo, Marilia Sá Carvalho, and Cláudia Medina Coeli, "A Avaliação da Produção Científica Nas Subáreas da Saúde Coletiva: Limites Do Atual Modelo e Contribuições Para o Debate," *Cadernos de Saúde Pública* 31 (2015): 2137–47.

[40] On a personal note, I was the last graduate of the old program.

[41] On another personal note, I was the first graduate of the new doctoral program.

[42] Full Open Access at: www.scielo.br/physis.

status of the population and the proposal of alternatives for prevention and healthcare functioning as a spearhead in the struggle for democracy. The CEBES, as previously stated, was one of the focal points of that process, publishing books by many of the relevant organic intellectuals of the movement and, since 1977, its own journal, *Saúde em Debate* (Health in Debate), which still runs today.

In 1980, a position paper, titled "A Questão Democrática na Área da Saúde" (The Democratic Issue in the Domain of Health) was published in *Saúde em Debate* in the name of the organization – its authors were not disclosed until much later: Hésio Cordeiro, José Luis Fiori, and Reinaldo Guimarães,[43] all of them IMS professors. That document consolidated the critiques and proposals of the Movimento de Refoma Sanitária and the field of *saúde coletiva* in general, becoming a kind of blueprint for many of the discussions that came afterwards. It contained a scathing – and accurate – critical assessment of the Brazilian populations' living standards: infant mortality was increasing, as were several chronic conditions, work-related accidents, and traditional endemic diseases. At the same time, public sanitation was deteriorating, environmental pollution was becoming worse, and nutritional levels were alarming, linked to what was dubbed "absolute [economic] misery." It pointed to the need to reformulate the economic model, to buttress social security, and to provide government-backed health protection and care for the whole population.

The ideas contained in that document were instrumental in shaping the discussions of the 8th National Health Conference, which took place soon after the end of the dictatorship, in 1986. The National Health Conferences (*Conferências Nacionais de Saúde*) were huge assemblies with representatives from health professionals, civillian society, and government organizations, having as their objective formulate political guidelines for the public health sector. They continued to be held during the dictatorship but mostly as political theater, with no actual consequences. The 8th Conference, however, reflected the overall drive of the previous years, with effective popular participation, having Antonio Sérgio Arouca, then president of Fundação Oswaldo Cruz, as its president and counting relevant contributions from Hesio Cordeiro, among others. With the new government, Hesio Cordeiro was installed as the president of the Instituto de Assistência Médica da Previdência Social (National Health Care Institute of the Social Security, INAMPS), the arm of the National Social Security that dealt with healthcare, at that point only for those who were formally employed. One of his first measures as president was opening the doors of the INAMPS-funded care to all Brazilians, regardless of the occupational status. This implemented in practice one of the

[43] Pierantoni, "20 Anos Do Sistema de Saúde Brasileiro."

main tenets of the Movimento de Reforma Sanitária: that access to healthcare should be universal, for all citizens. Other proposals were to have a unified system instead of complexity.[44]

The political directive for the SUS was given by the 1988 Constitution, but the actual implementation began in 1990 with the drafting and approval of laws that would provide the legal infrastructure for its operation.[45] Despite its shortcomings, mainly related to its chronic underfunding (which worsened in recent years),[46] it is the largest public healthcare system in the world, in terms of the population that it covers, and has provided in the intervening years a research and testing ground for *saúde coletiva* practitioners and researchers. It has developed one of the largest and most comprehensive immunization programs and has provided healthcare for millions of Brazilians who would otherwise be destitute. It is still plagued by problems of inequality of access, in high-cost interventions, but has enormously expanded access to care via the Family Health program since the 1990s, with demonstrable impacts on the population's health.[47]

The SUS is, arguably, the greatest achievement of Brazilian *saúde coletiva*. Despite being chronically underfunded and threatened in its basic principles by the 2019–2022 administration,[48] it has provided services for a large part of the Brazilian population that would not have otherwise access to healthcare and prevention, especially during the Covid pandemic, despite the erratic response from the federal government.[49]

What is "Saúde Coletiva," After All?

Important scholars in the field made valiant attempts to provide a formal definition of *saúde coletiva*.[50] As many philosophical problems, finding a single, definite solution has proven elusive, beginning with a key component of

[44] Cristiani Vieira Machado, "Political Struggles for a Universal Health System in Brazil: Successes and Limits in the Reduction of Inequalities," *Globalization and Health* 15, no. 1 (2019): 1–12.

[45] Guimarães, "Hesio Cordeiro"; Machado, "Political Struggles."

[46] Paim, "A Reforma Sanitária Brasileira."

[47] James Macinko, Matthew J. Harris, and D. Phil, "Brazil's Family Health Strategy – Delivering Community-Based Primary Care in a Universal Health System," *New England Journal of Medicine* 372, no. 23 (2015): 2177–81.

[48] Gulnar Azevedo e Silva, Ligia Giovanella, and Kenneth Rochel de Camargo Jr, "Brazil's National Health Care System at Risk for Losing Its Universal Character," *American Journal of Public Health*, 110, no. 6 (2020): 811–12.

[49] Francisco Ortega and Michael Orsini, "Governing COVID-19 without Government in Brazil: Ignorance, Neoliberal Authoritarianism, and the Collapse of Public Health Leadership," *Global Public Health* 15, no. 9 (2020): 1257–77.

[50] Jairnilson S. Paim and Naomar de Almeida Filho, "'Saúde Coletiva: Uma' Nova Saúde Pública 'Ou Campo Aberto a Novos Paradigmas'?," *Revista de Saúde Pública* 32, no. 4 (1998): 299–316.

the name itself – what is health, for starters? As the French philosopher of Medicine Georges Canguilhem pointed out,[51] it might not be possible to come up with a definitive conceptual definition but the process of discussing it is, in itself, an important endeavor.

Vieira-da-Silva, whose work was a key reference for this chapter,[52] took a different approach to this question, relying on a sociohistorical perspective to describe and analyze the constitution of what she defined as a field, borrowing from the conceptual framework created by Bourdieu. According to her, that field had components in academia, politics, and governmental bureaucracy, with the former having a more relevant role in its structuring, which nevertheless had relevant participation from all of those sectors – including actors who transited between them, such as Antonio Sergio Arouca and Hesio Cordeiro.

The hybrid aspect described by Vieira-da-Silva is even better characterized as a transepistemic arena, following Knorr-Cetina.[53] It encompasses the production of knowledge about the health of populations (but individuals as well), human resources training at various levels and capacities for working in the public health sector, and providing direct intervention in healthcare and prevention. It includes a wide gamut of theoretical perspectives, from epidemiological and biological analyses of the health–disease process to philosophical critiques and analyses of that same approach, and is very inclusive in terms of the professional trajectories of its participants, after an initial development nucleated by physicians pushing forward the traditional boundaries of public health and clinical medicine.

This is reflected in the structuring along the three sub-areas or subdomains previously cited, taken as a canonical organization by the majority of the actors in the arena, with some other themes, such as environmental or workers' health drawing from the three main subdomains. Whether this characterizes multi/inter/transdisciplinarity is another (quite likely endless) discussion in itself, with different views expressed by different authors. It can be said, though, that that this rich mix of theoretical and professional perspectives has over time experienced a certain degree of fragmentation and many opportunities for true interdisciplinary work have been missed as a result. The variety of theoretical approaches adopted in the area is not without its own contradictions; Marxist and Foucaultian approaches, for instance, can be at odds with each other. This essential tension (paraphrasing Kuhn), however, can be – and has been – very productive in terms of the development of critical approaches that continuously challenge established views about how to solve the health problems of diverse populations, providing innovative solutions for them.

---

[51] Georges Canguilhem, "La Santé: Concept Vulgaire et Question Philosophique," *Cahiers Du Séminaire de Philosophie* 8 (1988): 119–33.
[52] Vieira-da-Silva, *O Campo da Saúde Coletiva*.   [53] Knorr-Cetina, "Scientific Communities."

It values a critical, reflexive approach to the problems within its domain and has a strong ethical/political commitment to social justice and equity. As an academic–bureaucratic–political arena, it has provided important services for the Brazilian population, especially among those for the design and implementation, always ongoing, of the SUS, despite the numerous setbacks it has faced, especially in recent years. The connection with the provision of healthcare on the one hand, and with organized segments of the civil society (such as the Movimento de Reforma Sanitária) on the other, is arguably the major distinctive trait of *saúde coletiva* as it developed in Brazil.

The term "*saúde coletiva*" originated in Brazil, has spread to other Latin American countries, especially Argentina, where it was adopted (as "*Salud Colectiva*") in graduate programs which have professors who had part of their own studies in Brazilian institutions.

The creation of IMS in 1970 as an offshoot of the medical school of the same university, the beginning of its graduate program in 1974 and later expansion, and the participation of many of its professors in major health-related political events is singular but at the same time representative of the institutional trajectories in *saúde coletiva*.

The previous pages barely scratched the surface of a rich and complex history; many important actors were not mentioned and relevant developments related to the area, such as psychiatric reform or the national AIDS program, were not included in the narrative. Nevertheless, they provide an overview of the development of a complex network of individual and institutional actors, who have deeply impacted the country's health policies.

12 Settler Colonial Social Medicine and Community Health

Australasian Adaptations, Reinventions, and Denials

Warwick Anderson, James Dunk, and Connie Musolino[*]

Social medicine emerged during the long economic depression in 1930s Australia, nebulous and indefinite. A few socialist physicians and fellow travelers advocated structural reform of capitalism and the expansion of state medicine, while several senior public health officers, often sympathetic to European fascism, aimed to enhance vitality of "the white race" in supposedly hostile environments, whether in the burgeoning urban slums or the tropical north and harsh desert interior. Disparate in their politics, the promoters of "social medicine," an elastic category, shared a belief in social and environmental influences on disease patterns and a conviction that the state must intervene to manage population health. Some radical pioneers of settler colonial social medicine, such as Eric P. Dark, sought inspiration from British social reformers, especially the Fabians, while others, more conservative and race-minded, such as Raphael W. Cilento, learned about the impact on health of socioeconomic conditions and cultural mores from experience in Australian colonies in the Pacific and the British Empire in Asia. For the first group, social medicine proved a potent criticism of the workings of capital, while for the latter, social medicine became a portable technology of imperial settlement. For those on the left, it was a means of combatting the pathologies of global capitalism, while for those on the right, it constituted a strategy for advancing white nationalism, a mobilization of the state to promote white racial hygiene.

In this chapter, we explore the multiple meanings of social medicine as it has developed in Australia since the 1930s. Inevitably, this requires us to situate its various and sometimes amorphous manifestations in diverse settings, including progressive politics, colonial health services, and tropical medicine. As a label, "social medicine" was used sparingly. Rather, the common concern

[*] We are grateful to Anne Kveim Lie, Hans Pols, Jeremy Greene, and other participants in the Rosendal workshop for comments on earlier versions of this chapter. We also thank the interviewers and those who consented to be interviewed for the "History of Community Health in Australia" research project, led by Fran Baum. Our research has been supported by grants from the Australian Research Council (SR200200920 and DP220100624).

to recognize and manage the sociological dimensions of population health was likely to find expression through various surrogates like social work, occupational health, maternal and child health, geriatrics, non-institutional mental health services, nutrition, racial hygiene, and later Aboriginal health programs and generic "community health." Gradually, the colonial racial ties of social medicine in Australia were loosened and shed. An influx of white South African medical firebrands, such as Sidney Sax, in the 1960s and 1970s, strengthened connections with progressive politics and structural reform. A new generation of medical liberals and renegades – clustered around the medical schools of Monash, Adelaide, Queensland, and Sydney – felt comfortable talking about critical health social sciences and imagining national health schemes. Within those national imaginaries, some began to see the society implied by social medicine more ecologically. For Adelaide physician Basil Hetzel, the health of Australian society became ever more a matter of assisting individuals and communities to adapt to the distinctive Australian physical and social environments. Hetzel's student A. J. "Tony" McMichael, galvanized by the threat of nuclear catastrophe, worked to bring the entire planet into this ecological frame. He and others turned their attention to the impact on global human health of the destruction of planetary life-support systems, thereby offering to return to social medicine its neglected, almost forgotten, environmental and ecological purposes – a reinstatement still largely unacknowledged or refused.

From the late 1960s, reformist politicians and public health leaders in Australia began to support nation-wide projects in "community health," influenced by models in North America and Southern Africa, as well as endorsing strong local campaigns for women's health, sexual health, Indigenous health, and worker's health. The network of community health centers found some inspiration also in earlier settler-provided Aboriginal health services, women's health organizations, Australian colonial health services in the Pacific, and urban charitable initiatives. The goal was to "develop" communities through interdisciplinary and integrative centers (including social workers, nurses, mental health workers, and sometimes medical practitioners), embedded in and engaging with local structures and leadership. Collaboratively, they would practice a mixture of disease prevention, counselling, and conventional therapeutic intervention or primary care.

We will examine here the distinctive (and occasionally contradictory) concepts of human collectivity implied by social medicine and community health. Was "community" simply a substitute for "society"? Or did it suggest a different politics of life? What was lost and what gained through the shift from structural elements of social medicine to community health rollouts in the 1970s? Perhaps most tellingly, how did the difference in the constitution of the two – one thoroughly medical, one mostly medicine-adjacent – shape their health interventions? Due consideration of the history of Australian community health begs the question about where the "medicine" properly belongs in social medicine infrastructure. Did "community medicine" provide a means for the medical establishment to bring the problems of social medicine into its domain, on its own terms, allowing community health to rise and fall, comfortably at arm's length? Did the later decline in the 1990s of community development models, at least in some Australian states, allow a resurgence of social medicine – expressed structurally as a desire for "health equity" – or did it really mean the rise of neoliberal forms of health management? How does this history enable us to reimagine possibilities for social medicine and community health in the contemporary health field in Australia, the Pacific, and elsewhere?

Settler Colonial Dawn: Cilento and Dark

Growing up in South Australia, Raphael Cilento worried about the perceived taint of his Italian ancestry, attempting to expunge the smear through devotion to literary nationalism, boxing, and other demonstrations of manly white virtue.[1] At the end of the First World War, he served briefly as a medical officer in Rabaul, New Guinea, which Australia had acquired from Germany under a League of Nations' mandate, becoming enthralled by opportunities in tropical medicine. In the 1920s, he took over as director of the Australian Institute of Tropical Medicine in Townsville, Queensland, while seconded long-term as the director of public health in colonial Papua and New Guinea.[2] (In 1926, on the island of New Britain, momentarily abandoning public health responsibilities, he proudly reported turning a machine gun on some rebellious Nakanai people, who had threatened local whites, killing several of the "savages."[3]) Shaped by colonial experience, Cilento dedicated his career to the surveillance and regulation of potentially degenerate white bodies in the tropics and the urban slums, seeking to fashion for them a corporeal white armature. Dispelling older fears of the insalubrious tropical climate, he believed that the Australian state should intervene to protect the health of pure white

---

[1] Although we focus on Cilento, attention should be given to an earlier generation of advocates of state medicine and national health insurance – especially J. H. L. Cumpston and J. C. "Jack" Elkington – who were also votaries of a purely white Australia. See Warwick Anderson, *The Cultivation of Whiteness: Science, Health and Racial Destiny in Australia* (Durham, NC: Duke University Press, 2006); and Milton J. Lewis, *The People's Health: Public Health in Australia, 1788–1950* (Westport, CT: Praeger, 2003).

[2] Fedora Gould Fisher, *Raphael Cilento: A Biography* (St Lucia: University of Queensland Press, 1994); A. T. Yarwood, "Sir Raphael Cilento and The White Man in the Tropics," in Roy M. MacLeod and Donald Denoon (eds.), *Health and Healing in Tropical Australia and New Guinea* (Townsville: James Cook University, 1991), 47–63; Anderson, *The Cultivation of Whiteness*; and Alexander Cameron-Smith, *A Doctor across Borders: Raphael Cilento and Public Health from Empire to the United Nations* (Canberra: ANU Press, 2019).

[3] R. W. Cilento, "Story of a Massacre," *Sydney Morning Herald*, December 30, 1928.

settlers especially vulnerable to "disease-ridden natives," unhygienic Asians, dirty Jews, and dubious swarthy immigrants.[4] Once any "native reservoir" of disease was removed or any "foreign pool" of disease contained, whites might flourish anywhere, with proper conduct and care of the body. Cilento therefore fervently demanded improvements in nutrition, housing, clothing, exercise, and behavior. Indeed, productive male labor became for him the main index of success in implanting the white race in harsh and stressful Australian conditions.[5]

As director-general of health and medical services in Queensland from 1934, Cilento expressly began to couple social medicine to his white nationalist aspirations. The goal was still to impower the state to intervene to prevent white decadence and degeneration – only now social medicine seemed to offer a fresh rationale and new methods to do so, thereby arresting white population deterioration. Cilento's earlier work in New Guinea and the Pacific had taught him that racial purity and social homogeneity conferred public health benefits; it divulged to him the risks supposedly attendant on contact with other races; and it imparted the value of surveillance and prevention, organized by the state and focusing on hygiene, nutrition, and housing. Since populating the continent was imperative, he resisted any negative eugenic measures such as sterilization of the "unfit" – in exigent circumstances, no white body could be regarded as irredeemably unfit, all must be salvaged for the nation. More and more, Cilento supplemented his colonial know-how with close reading of social medicine tracts by Alfred Grotjahn, René Sand, and Arthur Newsholme – along with growing enthusiasm for fascist techniques of governance in Italy and Germany, which nearly led to his incarceration during the Second World War.[6] An honorary professor of Social and Tropical Medicine at the University of Queensland from 1937, Cilento agreed with Sand that, "almost every medical question ends in a social question."[7] In his *Blueprint for the Health of the Nation* (1944), the Queensland health officer defined social medicine as "an attempt to determine the principles by which circumstances can be scientifically influenced in the interests of the

---

[4] R. W. Cilento, *The White Man in the Tropics, with Especial Reference to Australia and Its Dependencies*, Department of Health Service Publication No. 7 (Melbourne: Government Printer, *c*.1925).

[5] Warwick Anderson, "Coolie Therapeutics: Labor, Race, and Medical Science in the Australian Tropics," *International Labor and Working-Class History* 91 (2017): 46–58.

[6] Alfred Grotjahn, *Soziale Pathologie*, 3rd ed. (Berlin: Springer, 1923); René Sand, "The Rise of Social Medicine," *Modern Medicine* 1 (1919): 189–91; and Arthur Newsholme, *Health Problems in Organised Society: Studies in the Social Aspects of Public Health* (London: P.K. King and Sons, 1927). On Cilento's adoration of Benito Mussolini, see Fisher, *Raphael Cilento*.

[7] Sand, "Rise of Social Medicine," 190. See Patrick Zylberman, "Fewer Parallels than Antitheses: René Sand and Andrija Stampar on Social Medicine, 1919–1955," *Social History of Medicine* 17 (2004): 77–92.

individual and of the race." He adhered to the "ideal that a health service is intended to provide positive health, preventive care and medical aid at need, to every member of the community" – by which he meant the fortified *white* community.[8]

Cilento's advocacy of group practices with salaried medical staff irritated his professional colleagues after the war. The Australian branch of the British Medical Association denounced his proposals along with the plans of the Labor federal government for a national health service.[9] Social medicine thus was first associated with eugenic ideas and then, in time, elided by "socialized medicine," falling into disfavor in those flat post-war years. Cilento departed for ravaged Europe, becoming director of the British zone of occupied Germany for the United Nations Relief and Rehabilitation Agency, trying to suppress infectious diseases among refugees and displaced persons. Later, as director of disaster relief in Palestine, his fierce antisemitism alienated incoming Jewish settlers. Returning to Australia, Cilento struggled to find a position in the health bureaucracies or medical schools and failed as a parliamentary candidate for various far-right groups. Increasingly bitter and disillusioned, he ended up ever more stridently denouncing inferior races and imagining Jewish conspiracies everywhere.

As a communist fellow traveler, Eric Dark grounded his ideal of social medicine in very different political terrain. He agreed with Cilento, however, that in the 1930s a choice had to be made between fascism and socialism – but he, unlike the two-fisted Queenslander, would join the "rising tide of socialism." He thus uttered a "plea for socialism as the only alternative to a recoil into a darker age."[10] But regardless of which pole they drifted toward, both Cilento and Dark came to understand social medicine in relation to the augmented role of the nation-state in everyday life. A medical graduate of the University of Sydney, Dark distinguished himself in the army medical corps on the Western Front in the First World War, before taking up general practice and rock-climbing in the Blue Mountains outside Sydney. War had radicalized him, so unlike most of his class he joined the Australian Labor Party, while cautiously skirting the margins of communism. His wife Eleanor Dark, from a raffish literary family, became a celebrated novelist, known especially for *Prelude to Christopher* (1934), an exploration of mental illness and eugenics, and *The Timeless Land* (1941), a critical narrative of the European invasion of Australia. In a series of articles in the *Medical Journal of Australia*,

---

[8] R. W. Cilento, *Blueprint for the Health of the Nation* (Sydney: Scotow Press, 1944), 91, 48.

[9] National Health and Medical Research Council, "An Outline of a Possible Scheme for a Salaried Medical Service," *Medical J. of Australia* ii (1941); 710–25. See James Gillespie, *The Price of Health: Australian Governments and Medical Politics, 1910–1960* (Cambridge: Cambridge University Press, 1991).

[10] E. P. Dark, *Medicine and the Social Order* (Sydney: F.H. Booth and Son, 1943), 116, 6.

published in the late 1930s, Eric Dark explained how "health is bound up with the political and economic structure of society."[11] The Great Depression had revealed the impact of the workings of capital on the health of the people. Dark perceived the urgent need to improve labor practices, nutrition, and housing – which would imply nothing less than the overthrow of the existing social order. Reading the encomiums of Henry Sigerist, Arthur Newsholme, and radical Melbourne psychoanalyst Reg Ellery, left Dark enamored of Soviet experiments in social medicine.[12] Medicine in the Soviet Union is "PREVENTIVE medicine," he joyfully announced. As living conditions and diet were ameliorated, and medicine reformed, morbidity and mortality rates plunged. "Nothing like them could have been achieved," Dark enthused, "except by a socialized medical service, backed by all the resources of the community."[13] But as the campaigning general practitioner learned after the war, the time was not ripe for avocations of socialized medicine. There was some support for Dark's approach from his colleagues – one correspondent described the sociologists as prophetic figures, "like those crying in the wilderness" – but most others, like University of Sydney-trained physician Harry Herbert Lee, expressed aggressive opposition to the national health insurance legislation then being drafted and to any peers supporting it.[14] A long period of conservative government in Australia, compounded by the encroaching Cold War, soon saw support for social medicine dry up and wither, tainted as it was both by communism and eugenics. In Australia, at least, the fortunes of social medicine followed the global contours of ideological conflict.

The 1960s and 1970s: The Revival of Social Medicine

In the late 1960s, medical reformers began infiltrating state and federal health bureaucracies, concerned about persisting limitations to medical care and pervasive inequality in population health outcomes. Sidney Sax, an émigré medical doctor from South Africa, was one of the more prominent of these advocates of social medicine and the establishment of a national health service. Sax's training at Witwatersrand in the 1940s and subsequent experiences

---

[11] Dark, *Medicine and the Social Order*, 7. Dark was particularly indebted to Beatrice and Sidney Webb, Harold Laski, and René Sand for his analysis. See E. P. Dark, "The Inductotherm," *Medical Journal of Australia* (September 19, 1936): 397–99; "Some Recent Advances in Physical Therapy," *Medical Journal of Australia* (August 1, 1938): 243–44, and "Property and Health," *Medical Journal of Australia* (March 4, 1939): 345–52.

[12] Henry E. Sigerist, *Socialized Medicine in the Soviet Union* (New York, NY: W. W. Norton, 1937); Arthur Newsholme and John Adams Kingsbury, *Red Medicine: Socialized Health in Soviet Russia* (Garden City, NY: Doubleday, Doran, 1933); and Reg S. Ellery, *Health in the Soviet Union* (Melbourne: Rawson's Bookshop, 1942).

[13] Dark, Medicine and the Social Order, 107, 114.

[14] Harry H. Lee, "National Health Insurance," *Medical Journal of Australia* (March 4, 1939): 369.

working in African communities had sensitized him to how socioeconomic disadvantage and racial discrimination under settler colonialism determined patterns of illness and immiseration.[15] Appalled by the rigid system of apartheid, he immigrated to Australia in 1960, where he soon became director of geriatric services in New South Wales, a field of clinical endeavor he regarded as a proxy for social medicine. He developed aged care assessment teams and promoted community healthcare delivery across the state. During this period, momentum for change within the Labor Party culminated in a meeting on June 6, 1967 convened by Moss Cass, the founding medical director of the Trade Union Clinic in Melbourne, to discuss the merits of an alternative health insurance program.[16] Attendees included influential Labor politicians, key figures in the healthcare services, and University of Melbourne health economists John Deeble and Richard Scotton.

After the election of the reforming federal Labor government in 1972, Sax was appointed to lead a new Hospitals and Health Services Commission – a body that would bridge the administrative gap between hospital and community. For a decade, the Commission directed the vast expansion of national responsibilities in disease prevention, clinical care, and medical funding, developing policies for the effective allocation and distribution of new federal health programs. Together with Scotton and Deeble, Sax helped to devise Medibank, Australia's first national health insurance scheme, which aimed to provide universal free access to medical care.[17] When a conservative government in the late 1970s abolished the Commission and closed Medibank, Sax became chair of the national Social Welfare Policy Secretariat. Like other health reformers in this period, he was dedicated to increasing state action to improve the living conditions and health outcomes of citizens, regardless of race.[18] Influenced by his reading of Sigerist and Thomas McKeown, Sax hoped "social and economic progress [would enable] people to live in an environment from which present health hazards had been removed." But, he lamented, "as the pursuit of technology became a dominant feature of our healthcare system, concepts of health maintenance and social well-being were relegated to positions of low priority."[19]

---

[15] Sidney Sax, "The Introduction of Syphilis into the Bantu Peoples of South Africa," *South African Medical Journal* ii (1952): 1037–9.

[16] Jennifer DeVoe, "A Policy Transformed by Politics: The Case of the 1973 Australian Community Health Program," *Journal of Health Politics, Policy and Law* 28, no. 1 (2003): 77–108.

[17] Richard B. Scotton, "Medibank: From Conception to Delivery and Beyond," *Medical Journal of Australia*, 173 (2000): 9–11.

[18] Sidney Sax, *Medical Care and the Melting Pot: An Australian Review* (Sydney: Angus and Robertson, 1972).

[19] Sidney Sax, "Are Health and Medicine in Conflict?" *Medical Journal of Australia* i (1977): 357–62, at 357, 358. Sax refers to Henry Sigerist, *Medicine and Welfare* (New Haven, CT:

Sax worked instead through the federal government to improve health education and promotion, while ensuring wider access to reliable medical, nursing, and supportive services, focusing on the health of the whole person rather than the failing of specific organs.

The bureaucratic or governmental matrix for social medicine was thus enriched in the 1970s, in parallel with the proliferation of medical school teaching and research in the subject. Over the course of the decade, it became increasingly likely that medical students would learn a little about social aspects of healthcare. A few departments of social and preventive medicine opened, offering research pathways in connecting medicine with critical social sciences and somewhat more rarely, with political economies of health. These advances were not unprecedented. Fleeing grim post-war England, Eric Saint had earlier found opportunities to develop or augment programs in social medicine in Western Australia and Queensland. His medical training had revealed to him the health effects of poverty in Tyneside, Newcastle, an "unpropitious and conscience-awakening milieu." There he felt the influence of James Spence, the leader of social pediatrics, who studied nutritional deficiencies in poor families and taught students "to look beyond the individual problem, to the ecology of disease."[20]

Arriving in Australia in the early 1950s, Saint worked initially in the asbestos-mining town of Wittenoom, trying futilely to alert authorities to an impending industrial health disaster, the emergence of the world's largest cluster of asbestosis. He also spent time in Aboriginal communities, where he sought to eliminate yaws and leprosy. By the time he took up clinical research at the Perth Hospital, and then the new chair of medicine at the University of Western Australia, Saint was all too familiar with disease as "a social problem requiring administrative action." He became a leading advocate for social medicine, by which he meant "an attitude of mind which views the pattern of disease in a population as a reflection of the cultural structure of society and the occupational pursuits of its members."[21] Sometimes he wondered if the name bore "a rather dreary connotation with sanitary inspectors and water closets"; perhaps "human ecology" was a more appealing description, signaling as it did the "total environment," internal and external to the human body. In any case, as dean of the medical school at the University of Queensland in the 1970s, Saint continued to explore "the no-man's land which lies between medicine and sociology and social anthropology," urging curriculum reform and

Yale University Press, 1941); Thomas McKeown and C.R. Lowe, *An Introduction to Social Medicine* (Oxford: Blackwell, 1966); and Thomas McKeown, *The Role of Medicine: Dream, Mirage, or Nemesis?* (London: Nuffield Provincial Hospitals Trust, 1976).

[20] Eric Saint, "On Men and Institutions," *Medical Journal of Australia* ii (1971): 67–71, at 67.
[21] Eric Saint, "Social Perspectives in Medicine," *Medical Journal of Australia* i (1955): 161–5, at 162, 161.

stronger medical engagement with social science research.[22] "The reminder that medicine has a sociological and humanitarian content," he wrote, "is important in an era when a visitor from another planet might think that its practice was either a technology or a business." It was evident to Saint that the typical Australian medical professional:

should listen with patience and understanding to what the psychologist and social scientist have to tell him [sic] about cultural patterns and human behaviour in relation to the origins and consequences of disease, and that he should learn to work in close and friendly collaboration with a new generation of social workers, hospital administrators, industrial personnel officers, rehabilitation officers, child guidance workers, infant health nurses, all of whom have accepted and share responsibility for the prevention of mental and physical ill health.[23]

As Saint repeatedly observed, "the good doctor develops an awareness of his place in a complex network of social interrelations."[24]

An expert in human nutrition, Basil Hetzel had been attracted to social medicine in the 1940s through the Student Christian Movement at the Adelaide medical school. The social gospel convinced him "of the importance to health of social and community life and the social environment."[25] He became engrossed in medical research in colonial Papua New Guinea (PNG) – but with motives and inferences quite distinct from Cilento's. Hetzel's experiences of the health aspects of "native administration" underscored the medical significance of nutrition and living conditions, as well as accenting the psychosocial dimensions of well-being. On the remote Huon Peninsula of PNG, he determined that iodine deficiency was causing endemic goiter and cretinism and he showed that dietary supplements might remedy it.[26] Through the Iodine Global Network, he campaigned tirelessly for dietary iodine supplementation, attempting to eliminate iodine-deficiency disorders worldwide. Associating his nutritional studies with the "holistic" approaches of social medicine, Hetzel founded in 1968 the Department of Social and Preventive Medicine at Monash University, in Melbourne, based on an ecological model of health, which included human biology, environmental health, health services analysis, and social and behavioral sciences.[27] "Social medicine," he wrote, "is concerned with the importance of social factors in prevention,

---

[22] Saint, "Social Perspectives in Medicine," 162, 163.
[23] Saint, "Social Perspectives in Medicine," 164.
[24] Eric Saint, "On Good Doctoring," *Medical Journal of Australia* ii (1972): 121–6, at 124.
[25] Basil S. Hetzel, *Chance and Commitment: Memoirs of a Medical Scientist* (Adelaide: Wakefield Press, 2005), 108.
[26] Mandy Brener, "Infectious Personalities: The Public Health Legacy of Three Australian Doctors in Papua New Guinea," *Health and History* 17 (2015): 73–96.
[27] Basil S. Hetzel, *Health and Australian Society* (Melbourne: Penguin, 1974). See also Basil S. Hetzel, *Life and Health in Australia: The Boyer Lectures* (Sydney: Australian Broadcasting Commission, 1971).

cause, and treatment of illness."[28] According to Hetzel, "the ultimate goal that confronts us in social medicine is the provision and delivery of medical care, including the benefits of medical science and technology, to the whole community."[29] Increasingly, he concentrated on problems in urban health, particularly the social environment of new suburbs, on Aboriginal health, and on the need more generally to bolster teamwork in community medicine – but in most of this, eschewing interest in more fundamental questions of structural accountability.[30]

The new program in social medicine at Monash – like those developing at the medical schools of Sydney and Newcastle universities, among others[31] – became a nidus for training and research in the health social sciences and in preventive medicine. Social medicine gradually shifted from the singular expression of isolated charismatic men to an institutionalized orientation toward the relations of health and social structure, a more democratic and diffuse point of view shared among teachers, and sometimes students, of medicine and public health. Never a popular movement, social medicine in the 1970s eventually came to appear a didactic necessity in major schools of medicine and public health, even if marginalized and discounted, rendered anodyne and abbreviated, in most curricula. Reference to socioeconomic determinants of health generally was muted. As John Powles, briefly a leading figure in the Monash department, put it, there was simply a widespread, if grudging, admission that teaching the technics of medical diagnosis and treatment –

---

[28] Basil Hetzel, Report on Special Leave, 1968, Monash University, in Basil Hetzel collection, University of South Australia archives, series 1, box 15.

[29] Basil S. Hetzel, "The Role of the Behavioural Sciences in Medicine: Social Medicine," *Medical Journal of Australia* ii (1969): 47–51, at 51. Hetzel referred to the sociological studies of Robert K. Merton, Elliot Freidson, Howard Becker, and David Mechanic.

[30] See Basil S. Hetzel, "Health for Aborigines: A New Approach?," *Medical Journal of Australia* ii (1972): 693; Basil S. Hetzel and H. J. Frith (eds.), *The Nutrition of Aborigines in Relation to the Ecosystem of Central Australia* (Melbourne: CSIRO (Commonwealth Scientific and Industrial Research Organisation), 1978); Basil S. Hetzel, "The Impact of a Changing Society on Community Health Programmes," *Medical Journal of Australia* ii (1971): 881; and comments on Glenn McBride, "Social Adaptation to Crowding in Animals and Man," in Stephen V. Boyden (eds.), *The Impact of Civilisation on the Biology of Man* (Canberra: ANU Press, 1970), 154–8. Hetzel returned to Adelaide as the director of the CSIRO's Division of Animal Nutrition.

[31] The program at Sydney, and the activities of Charles Kerr, John Last, and Michael Marmot (as a medical student), should also receive attention. The University of Melbourne's medical school, in contrast, proved especially resistant, aside from tolerating a few figures such as Ross Webster, David Christie, and Hedley Peach in what was fundamentally a department of general practice, though sometimes called "community medicine." When Warwick Anderson, fresh from the Department of Social Medicine at Harvard, set up the Centre for the Study of Health and Society (now the Centre for Health Equity) in 1997, he was advised (perhaps facetiously) not to mention "social medicine" at Melbourne as it sounded too much like socialized medicine. In 2000, the Centre, focusing on social sciences and medicine, was merged into the new School of Population Health, separate from the medical school.

medicine as an "engineering strategy" – was no longer sufficient. According to Powles, medicine now had to abandon its "technological 'overreach'" and instead address "the wider crisis in industrial man's [*sic*] relationship to his environment," coming to grips with the diseases of "civilization" consequent on social maladaptation.[32] Having inserted the "social" into the medical curriculum, Powles wanted to find further space for ecological perspectives. Thinking about social medicine became for him "an urgent precondition for the articulation of an alternative 'ecological' strategy for the improvement of health."[33] But he soon found there were limits to the medical school's embrace of social medicine and disease ecology, both at Monash and later at Cambridge University. Medical deans might gesture favorably, if vaguely, toward things social or ecological, but laboratory research and individualized clinical care would always take precedence.

At least one Monash graduate student, Tony McMichael, heeded the teaching of Hetzel and Powles. As a radical medical student and antinuclear activist at Adelaide in the 1960s, McMichael had been inspired by Hetzel's commitment to social medicine and engagement with the politics of healthcare. He followed his mentor to Monash to undertake graduate studies, where he conducted research in the health consequences of lead pollution, UV radiation, solvent exposure, alcohol consumption, and passive smoking. McMichael then spent a few years in the 1970s in public health at the University of North Carolina, Chapel Hill, at the suggestion of the planetary-minded disease ecologist René Dubos, before returning to Adelaide as professor of Occupational and Environmental Health, his concerns becoming ever more ecological and less sociological.[34] At Chapel Hill, McMichael encountered an epidemiology

---

[32] John W. Powles, "On the Limitations of Modern Medicine," *Science, Medicine and Man* 1 (1973): 1–30, at 13, 1. As a medical student at the University of Sydney, Powles had taken leading roles in the local campaign for nuclear disarmament and in Student Action for Aborigines, participating in the 1965 Freedom Ride across outback New South Wales. Influenced by René Dubos, McKeown, and Stephen V. Boyden, Powles was in the Science Policy Research Unit at Sussex University between 1970 and 1975, when he moved to Monash to join Hetzel; from 1991 he lectured in public health at Cambridge University.

[33] Powles, "On the Limitations of Modern Medicine," 23.

[34] A. J. McMichael, "Global Warming, Ecological Disruption and Human Health: The Penny Drops," *Medical Journal of Australia* 154 (1991): 499–501; and A. J. McMichael, *Planetary Overload: Global Environmental Change and the Health of the Human Species* (Cambridge: Cambridge University Press, 1993). See Colin Butler, Jane Dixon, and Tony Capon (eds.), *Health of People, Places and Planet: Reflections Based on Tony McMichael's Four Decades of Contributions to Epidemiology Understanding* (Canberra: ANU Press, 2015); Howard Frumkin, "The Sage of Canberra: Tony McMichael on Climate, History, and Health," *EcoHealth* 14 (2017): 425–47; James Dunk and Warwick Anderson, "Assembling Planetary Health: Histories of the Future," in Samuel S. Myers and Howard Frumkin (eds.), *Planetary Health: Protecting Nature to Protect Ourselves* (Washington, DC: Island Press, 2020), 17–35; and Warwick Anderson and James Dunk, "Planetary Health Histories: Toward New Ecologies of Epidemiology?" *Isis* 113, no. 4 (2022): 767–88, doi.org/10.1086/722308.

department in the act of establishing an interdisciplinary "social epidemiology," shaped by the experience of John Cassel and Sidney Kark at the Pholela Community Health Centre in South Africa.[35] That experience in rural, multidisciplinary health work embedded both in social and ecological systems proved formative for epidemiology's pivot to the social causes underlying patterns of health and illness – though ecological interest at the time was typically limited to the neighborhood environment, filled with occupational and industrial work threats, the products of social injustice.[36]

The ravaging of the environment and the dire consequences for animal life and human health, were always front of mind in a settler colonial society, in an ecologically transformative polity like Australia, especially in a sensitized desert city like Adelaide, McMichael's early habitat.[37] In the 1990s, as Professor of Epidemiology at the London School of Hygiene and Tropical Medicine, McMichael continued to sound a tocsin to the world to address the human health impacts of degradation of the earth's life-support systems, principally through the effects of anthropogenic global heating. By the turn of the century, he demanded that epidemiologists try to "understand the determinants of population health beyond proximate, individual-level risk factors."[38] "Modern epidemiology's search for specific proximate causes has deflected us from social-contextual models of disease causation," McMichael wrote. "We epidemiologists must broaden our causal models and recognize the important ecologic dimensions of social-environmental influences on health and disease."[39] Against simplistic assumptions of contamination and pollution, McMichael posed more complex and biologically realistic epidemiological models that drew on social science and systems ecology. But he no longer called this social medicine. That mode of inquiry had long ago, in Cilento's time, jettisoned its connections to medical geography and environmental reckoning on a large scale, so it seemed inadequate to his task. Moreover, the bonds of social medicine with the declining nation-state still seemed too adherent to permit the earth-system vision and global action that was required. Eventually, then, McMichael's proposals to address the health

---

[35] Judith Winkler and Victor J. Schoenbach, *The UNC Department of Epidemiology: Our First 40 Years, 1936–1976* (Chapel Hill, NC: The UNC Gillings School of Global Public Health, 2018), 11–12.

[36] Ana V. Diez Roux, "Social Epidemiology: Past, Present, and Future," *Annual Review of Public Health* 43, no. 1 (2022): 79–98.

[37] Anderson, *Cultivation of Whiteness*, chapter 7; and Libby Robin, "Ecology: A Science of Empire?," in Tom Griffiths and Libby Robin (eds.), *Ecology and Empire: Environmental History of Settler Societies* (Melbourne: Melbourne University Press, 1997), 215–28.

[38] A. J. McMichael, "Prisoners of the Proximate: Loosening the Constraints on Epidemiology in an Age of Change," *American Journal of Epidemiology* 149 (1999): 887–97, at 887. See Warwick Anderson, "The History in Epidemiology," *International Journal of Epidemiology* 48 (2018): 672–4, doi.10.1093/ije/dyy247.

[39] McMichael, "Prisoners of the Proximate," 895–6.

impacts of global heating would acquire another name, planetary health.[40] Few discerned its origins in settler colonial social medicine.

The Rise of Community Health: Substitute or Elaboration?

"I was always quite cynical about medical dominance, always looking for it," Fran Baum, Professor of Health Equity at the University of Adelaide, reflected in 2021. "And I guess for me, social medicine might have been a turn off ... It's a claiming of space by medicine that shouldn't have been defined by medicine."[41] As an insurgent health social scientist, Baum was more attuned to community health programs, dependent on multidisciplinary teamwork, as they were developing in Australia and elsewhere during the 1970s. Social medicine also seemed too biomedical to Denise Fry, a leader of the community health movement in Sydney: "I think [social medicine] was a way for medicine to expand its view, and address social issues, and social concepts. It did privilege doctors of course, but that's how things were at the time." Certainly, for non-medical activists like her, it was not a usable framework.[42] "You see, the medicine word was used as an exclusion," Chloe Mason told James Dunk.[43] Jim Birch, the manager of a South Australian community health center, recalled social medicine was "very much associated with trying to move the medical model into social settings or situations beyond the traditional structures and hierarchies that they formerly existed in, or still exist in, but it's not a term I use very much."[44] Some saw a neat progression which displaced medical dominance from what some fashioned – provocatively, perhaps – as "social health."[45] "Social and preventive medicine was the forerunner of community health and epidemiology," recalled Howard Gwynne.[46] Other community health campaigners were more dismissive. "That's something the British invented," Tony Adams insisted. "It doesn't mean anything, it's too waffly."[47]

---

[40] Dunk and Anderson, "Assembling Planetary Health"; and Anderson and Dunk, "Planetary Health Histories." After 2001, McMichael became director of the National Centre for Epidemiology and Population Health at the ANU.

[41] Fran Baum, interviewed by Connie Musolino, June 22, 2021. The term "medical dominance" was popularized in Australia by Evan Willis, *Medical Dominance: The Division of Labour in Australian Health Care* (Sydney: George Allen & Unwin, 1983).

[42] Denise Fry, interviewed by Connie Musolino, June 24, 2021.

[43] Chloe Mason, interviewed by James Dunk, November 24, 2021.

[44] Jim Birch, interviewed by Paul Laris, July 22, 2021.

[45] Peter Ruzyla, interviewed by Virginia Lewis, February 26, 2022. Rusyla, a psychologist who directed Maroondah Social Health Centre, recalls that at an earlier chair, Clarrie Armstrong, had been influenced by social health movements in Scandinavia when the center was founded in 1974.

[46] Howard Gwynne, interviewed by Connie Musolino, May 4, 2022.

[47] Tony Adams, interviewed by James Dunk, November 11, 2021.

Like social medicine, community health was a global movement – but neither simply diffused from some "central" northern site to the remainder of the world. To be sure, in Australia, models of social medicine derived mostly from European and colonial endeavors, while the community health movement in the 1970s often found its exemplars in North American experiments. But the aspirations and practices of both social medicine and community health would be adapted and transformed in local usages, giving rise to fresh visions and unanticipated actions, and taking on vernacular forms. Though ostensibly different – even, for some, incommensurable – social medicine and community health in Australia corresponded at several points. There was common advocacy of disease prevention, attention to the "person" more than the specific pathogen, recognition of the importance of the socioeconomic matrix, and an emphasis on multidisciplinary approaches, sometimes including teamwork. Several community health leaders who were familiar with the language of social medicine (typically those who had trained in medicine), saw the two as members of the same family. "Community health is an attempt at social medicine," reflected Ben Bartlett, a medical doctor who worked in women's health and workers' health centers and in Aboriginal health. "I don't really see a fundamental difference."[48] Other medicos saw a divergence in emphasis, with community health a sort of parochial enterprise preoccupied with primary care and social medicine standing above with a wider vision. "Community health is much more related to primary healthcare delivery at the community level," stated one medical doctor. "Social medicine probably encompasses that but places more emphasis on what we now call the social determinants of health, looking at health within the broader social context, not just the local community context."[49]

From the 1970s, many advocates for social medicine pragmatically reframed their arguments in terms of community health or community medicine. As Hetzel observed in 1971: "I believe that new thinking in healthcare should be going outside the traditional medical viewpoint of health into a much wider context of society and the individuals in it to health in the community."[50] Accordingly, Sidney Sax laid out the "community" agenda in *A Community Health Program for Australia* (1973), a report of National Hospitals and Health Services Commission. His ambitious recommendations focused on primary healthcare and whole-of-life care in a community setting, conscious of interdependent "medical and social aspects" of health and illness, including family breakdown, poverty, school truancy, alcoholism, and child abuse.

[48] Ben Bartlett, interviewed by Connie Musolino, September 20, 2021.
[49] Anonymous doctor, South Australia, interviewed by Fran Baum, December 8, 2021.
[50] R. McEwin, Opening Address, Community Health Action Seminar, North Ryde Staff Development Centre, August 6–8, 1975 (Health Commission of New South Wales), 3–4.

Better individual understanding of disease and disability conditions, for the sake of prevention and effective care, would be promoted in community settings. Led by a reforming Labor prime minister, Gough Whitlam, the federal government at the time was eager to invest in such new modes of disease prevention and healthcare delivery, conventionally domains of the states.[51] The new community health services were explicitly modelled on women's health centers and the clinics established by the union movement, along with the Aboriginal urban medical services, which had been inspired by Black Panther initiatives in the United States.[52] Although activists could look to some isolated exemplars in Britain, including the Peckham Experiment, it was clear that community health work was more advanced in North America, frequently in association with US medical schools.[53] The international institutional shift, at the WHO especially, toward expanding access to primary healthcare, culminating in the 1978 Alma-Ata Declaration, also shaped and encouraged local campaigns.[54] In Australia, nurses, social workers, and local representatives tended to dominate the ramifying network of community health centers, often in tension with medical doctors who were either incorporated in the agency or competing in the surrounding neighborhood. The emphasis was on disease prevention and health education and integrated, multidisciplinary care – not routine medical consultations. Although most community health workers recognized the socioeconomic determinants of health, they rarely had the time and resources to address them critically and structurally. Nonetheless, community health managed to improve the lives of the poor and disadvantaged in Australia in ways that formal social medicine, despite its lofty goals, never did – though it could still be contended that community health actually was a practical, if partial, instantiation of the concept, despite the protestations of its participants.

At least initially, community health was imagined as constructing networks of care, clusters of multidisciplinary local health centers, from the ground

---

[51] Parliament of the Commonwealth of Australia, *A Community Health Program for Australia: Report of the Interim Committee of the National Hospitals and Health Services Commission* (Canberra: Government Printer of Australia, 1973); and Gough Whitlam, "1974 Election Policy Speech," delivered at the Blacktown Civic Centre, April 29, 1974, at: https://whitlamdismissal .com/1974/04/29/whitlam-1974-election-policy-speech.html.

[52] Kathy Lothian, "Seizing the Time: Australian Aborigines and the Influence of the Black Panther Party, 1969–1972," *Journal of Black Studies* 35, 4 (2005): 179–200.

[53] W. R. Willard, "Report of the National Commission on Community Health Services: Next Steps," *American Journal of Public Health* 56 (1966): 1828–36. A notable UK center was the Pioneer Health Centre, in southeast London, home to the Peckham Experiment, in which physicians looked to diet, exercise, and community itself to build health (rather than treat illness). See Philip Conford, "'Smashed by the National Health'? A Closer Look at the Demise of the Pioneer Health Centre, Peckham," *Medical History*, 60, no. 2 (2016): 250–69, doi.org/10.1017/ mdh.2016.6.

[54] As did the 1986 Ottawa Charter for Health Promotion, also sponsored by the WHO.

up, generated or supported by local groups, rather than a function of medical dominance in the interests of the nation-state.[55] Certainly the Aboriginal and women's health centers which were co-opted into the community health movement by the lure of federal funding had emerged from the periphery of power, and from specific communities, writing their own mandates to care for those who were overlooked by existing, centralized systems.[56] From 1973, the Community Health Program sought to enfold those centers and services into a model of centralized health provision. Although community health might be imagined from the ground up and invested, at least theoretically, in the idea of community involvement, it turned out to be largely driven in Australia by a concern to rationalize and economize health delivery, both across regions and states and between levels of government and health specializations.

It proved hard to ward off creeping medical dominance, often under the rubric of *community medicine*, not community health. Boundaries blurred between social medicine, community medicine, and community health during the 1970s, in part because rapidly expanding medical schools saw professional opportunities in their erasure. The slippage from social medicine to community medicine, often evading community-grounded *health*, became commonplace in the medical profession.[57] Thus B. A. Smythurst, a reader in Social and Preventive Medicine at the University of Queensland, could write, eliding any distinction: "Social or community medicine is that branch of medicine which deals with populations or groups rather than with individual patients."[58] Other medicos also were prone to amalgamate social and community medicine while hedging on community *health*. "Community has to do with aggregates of people, and medicine has to do with alleviation of suffering which presents as sickness and disability," Ian W. Webster, a leading medical reformer, explained in 1984, "community medicine is about societal analyses and prescriptions, and about individual therapeutic action in the community."[59] He

---

[55] Health Commission of New South Wales, *Community Health Book No 1: General Concepts* (Sydney: Health Commission of New South Wales, 1977), front matter.

[56] The original Aboriginal health center, in Redfern, Sydney, emerged in response to a rapid influx of Aboriginal people from rural NSW after the 1967 referendum precipitated the repeal of mission and reserve legislation. The Aboriginal Legal Service – the first of the "community-controlled, community-survival programmes" – helped protect those arriving from prejudicial enforcement and sentencing, and the need for a community *health* center grew from the intertwined legal, social, and medical concerns of this "community of refugees." See Gary Foley, *Redfern Aboriginal Medical Service 1971–1991: Twenty Years of Community Service* (Sydney: Aboriginal Medical Service Cooperative, c.1991), 5.

[57] Raymond G. Brown and Henry M. Whyte, *Medical Practice and the Community* (Canberra: Australian National University Press, 1970).

[58] B. A. Smythurst, *Fundamentals of Social and Preventive Medicine* (St Lucia: University of Queensland Press, 1976), 1.

[59] Ian W. Webster, "Where Healing Starts," in Rex Walpole (ed.), *Community Health in Australia*, 2nd ed. (Ringwood, Vic: Penguin, 1984), 37–52, at 37.

spoke for many advocates of social medicine and community medicine when he observed: "Illness takes place at the point of intersection between biology, emotional experience, and the physical and social environment, and a prior decision to deal with one and not the others cannot be justified." He wondered whether the biomedical sciences had anything more than marginal relevance to community health. "The greatest need for the future," Webster concluded, "is a conjunction across the boundaries of the biological and social worlds because herein lies the greatest opportunity for our society to benefit human health and set people free from suffering." Accordingly, "social policy and health policy need to be developed simultaneously – and in this process social justice and health justice are the overriding principles."[60]

The Australian Universities Commission's Committee on Medical Schools reported in July 1973 that virtually all universities were looking to give community medicine more weight in medical training, which had until then included at best gestural treatments of the subject. Those universities looking to create new medical schools – like Newcastle and Wollongong – saw a special need to "fit the doctor better for community practice."[61] The Committee described a "mutually" beneficial relationship for community health centers and the medical schools, with centers offering necessary training in primary healthcare for medical students as well as employing medical staff. The Whitlam government was rarely accused of moving slowly and later that year it awarded the Royal Australian College of General Practitioners a large grant to establish a Family Medicine Programme.[62] What would later develop into a specific program of "general practice" or family medicine training was initially channeled into support for new hires or even departments in community and social medicine. Announcing the funding, Whitlam linked the new community practice schools and courses with community health centers, including extra funding to accommodate teaching within the centers themselves.[63] Sidney Sax noted, with satisfaction, that in the ten years from December 1973, departments of "community practice" had been created in every medical school in the country. The medical graduates partly shaped by such departments, which generally offered some social medicine teaching,

---

[60] Webster, "Where Healing Starts," 43, 51.

[61] Expansion of Medical Education: Report of the Committee on Medical Schools to the Australian Universities Commission, July 1973, Parliamentary Paper No. 110, ordered to be printed 11 September 1973 (Canberra: Commonwealth of Australia, 1973), 84.

[62] Stephen C. Trumble, "The Evolution of General Practice Training in Australia," *Medical Journal of Australia* 194, no. 11 (2011): S59–62, doi.org/10.5694/j.1326-5377.2011.tb03129.x.

[63] The Federal Government offered $35,000 funding in the first year and $75,000 in subsequent years, with an added $50,000 to facilitate teaching in community health centers associated with university departments. Prime Minister's Press Conference, Parliament House, Canberra, December 4, 1973, at: https://pmtranscripts.pmc.gov.au/sites/default/files/original/00003093.pdf.

entered uneasy relations with community health services, with some health centers employing general practitioners and others not – whichever way the prejudice ran – and with frequent tense debates about fee-for-service and salaried employment.

In the 1980s, the community health movement in Australia entered the doldrums. "Then, of course," said Kathy Eagar, a community health leader in New South Wales, "the Commonwealth turned the tap off and froze everybody where they were."[64] Some states were more advanced than others, having done more "community development" earlier and more effectively – but even so, their health centers felt the strain. Throughout the process, it had never been clear what "community" was signifying, or how a community might announce itself, or be fashioned into a functional entity. As Chris Scarf told us, "I'm struggling, I guess I didn't know what the community was, you know?"[65] Lou Opit, Hetzel's successor in Social and Preventive Medicine at Monash, tried to explain what it might mean. "Community health," he wrote, "expresses a desirable social state believed to be attainable without recourse to the orthodox medical approach to health care." And yet, the "community" in community health – like "health," too, of course – was an ambiguous concept, perhaps generatively so. It could imply "a collection of persons who share some attribute, and the property which is shared defines the nature of the community." But Opit still had to admit, "if community health has a useful unambiguous meaning, we cannot find it within the existing logic of language."[66] What had the discursive shift in the 1970s from "society" to "community" represented functionally? How had these different collective worlds shaped the configurations of medicine and healthcare? When, in the early years of the twenty-first century, health equity became ascendant, eclipsing or overshadowing community development, did this augur a return to social medicine, with its critique of the structural violence of capitalism and the nation-state? Or was it, yet again, just another means of mitigation and extenuation, of tinkering at the edges?

Conclusion

In reflecting on his career in social medicine in 1976, Douglas Gordon, Professor of Social and Preventive Medicine at the University of Queensland, observed that the postwar enthusiasm for biochemistry, pharmacology, and

[64] Kathy Eager interviewed by James Dunk and Warwick Anderson, October 13, 2021.
[65] Chris Scarf interviewed by James Dunk and Warwick Anderson, August 5, 2021.
[66] L. J. Opit, "Community Health," in Rex Walpole (ed.), *Community Health in Australia*, 2nd ed. (Ringwood, Vic: Penguin, 1984), 84–90 , at 84, 85. Another Adelaide medical school graduate, Opit, taught social medicine at Birmingham (1970–6) before taking up the Monash position (1976–85), after which he returned to Britain as Professor of Community Medicine at the University of Kent (1985–98).

genetics, medical attention had shifted in the late 1960s toward the impact of social disadvantage and environmental degradation on health. This decentering of molecular and cellular pathologies showed "balance being restored" in understandings of disease processes.[67] Influenced professionally, though not politically, by Cilento, Gordon regarded the increasing concern for the social, economic, and political dimensions of population health as a manifestation of social medicine. For him, it was an expansive category. "Social medicine," Gordon declared, "is the study of the collective health of groups of people, of the collective efforts which such a group takes to prevent disease and promote health, and of the manner in which the group organizes care for those suffering ill health."[68] Social medicine began, he argued, with epidemiology and demography, veered into "human ecology" (understood as studies of the interaction of physical environment and human health) and, in the interrogation of social determinants of health and disease, strayed even into sociology, anthropology, and history to plumb "the philosophies and essential mysteries of human behaviour insofar as these affect health."[69] These overlapping contexts and terms had led to "an unholy confusion" of fields, particularly since "departments of community medicine or community practice or community care are springing up like the flowers of the fields," especially in North America, where the phrase "social medicine" had never been "acceptable due to its probable confusion with socialized medicine."[70] Indeed, Gordon wondered if community medicine might be a convenient shorthand both for social medicine and preventive medicine since it avoided the inscrutability of the former ("since only the experts know what 'social' implies in this context") and the "mouthful" of using both terms. "Perhaps community health might be a more fitting designation," he ventured, apparently oblivious to his own assumptions of medical dominance.[71]

Gordon's concluding remarks on social medicine, a field he helped to reestablish in Australia, display an unstable mixture of assertion and vulnerability. Like so many others in Australia in the 1970s, he was acutely aware of the social and political dimensions of health and disease, especially at a large scale, at population level. He embraced the need for interdisciplinary collaborations, particularly with social scientists and epidemiologists – sometimes even with human ecologists. He understood that health professionals were inevitably part

---

[67] Douglas Gordon, *Health, Sickness, and Society: Theoretical Concepts in Social and Preventive Medicine* (St Lucia: University of Queensland Press, 1976), 11. Gordon was appointed to the position in 1957.

[68] Gordon, *Health, Sickness, and Society*, 3–4.   [69] Gordon, *Health, Sickness, and Society*, 5–6.

[70] Gordon, *Health, Sickness, and Society*, 11. David Pennington, a dean of medicine at Melbourne, recalled that hospital clinicians tended to view social medicine and even community health as "wicked socialist medical activity" (interviewed by Tim Walsh and Bill Newton, May 25, 2016).

[71] Gordon, *Health, Sickness, and Society*, 11. See Willis, *Medical Dominance*.

of the political process, as advocates for their patients against health inequities. At the same time, he clearly had a sense that something else was happening in the 1970s, something he could never quite formulate. It sometimes seemed as if both the "social" and the "medicine" of social medicine were under erasure or at least subject to challenge. The rise of community health was shifting the ground on which judgments about health equity could be made – and by whom they could be made. Conceits and evasions such as "community medicine" neither revived the political agenda of social medicine nor shored up physician authority. Community medicine tended to dwindle into a medical teaching and training stratagem – while never quite restoring medical dominance in community health. As neoliberalism became entrenched in health arenas during the 1990s, neither the older statist social medicine nor the newer activist community health would thrive. Yet within a few decades, both timeworn social medicine and cognate community health now appear together again to offer potential blueprints for addressing health inequity and environmental injustice in Australia and elsewhere.

13 Social Medicine beyond Colonial Rule
The Medical Field Units of Ghana, 1930–2000

David Bannister

In the interwar 1930s, in an outlying district of the British Gold Coast colony (now Ghana), itself on Britain's imperial periphery, a group of activist officials and African traditional elites created a self-sustaining community-based health network. The region was the Northern Territories Protectorate, a third of the colony's total area and home to almost a third of its people, but enduringly marginalized within the colonial and postcolonial states. During the indirect-rule austerity which followed the Great Depression from 1929, a system of village clinic-dispensaries was built by "Native Authority" (NA) chiefs and the communities whom they represented with varying degrees of legitimacy. Staffed by locally trained health workers and sustained by communities themselves with little central support, the new dispensaries were an immediate success. They provided treatment and medical advice to thousands of outpatients, often at higher rates than better resourced facilities in the colony's wealthier south. The program was explicitly intended to address what local officials and community leaders understood as a central underlying determinant of widespread poor health in the north: that the region and its peoples were seen as a low-cost migrant labor reserve by central governments in Accra, and were therefore accorded little political importance in the colony's healthcare plans or allocations of central funds.

Despite its success, the north's rural dispensary program was dismantled in the late 1930s. After 1945, a new service was created, also attempting to circumvent the political and economic exclusion which increased health problems in the north. The Medical Field Units (or MFUs) grew into a far-reaching mobile community health service, staffed by local employees with little formal education, serving extensive rural areas that lay beyond the reach of both the colonial and early post-independence states. With reduced dependence on funds from the central government, and a training program which passed relatively complex knowledge of clinical and public health methods directly from one fieldworker to another, the MFUs were to some extent self-sustaining, independent from the fixed facilities and patronage networks of the national health system. Their successes were recognized by the first government of independent Ghana and after independence in 1957, the MFU program was expanded countrywide. This ad hoc service, created in response to the political neglect and limited funds that underpin poor healthcare at the margins, had become a national healthcare institution.

Over the decades of instability which affected many African countries in the 1970s and 1980s, shaped by the Cold War, global oil shocks and structural adjustment, Ghana's Medical Field Units became central to the continued provision of basic health services, under conditions of collapse in other parts of the national health system. But adjustment brought ideologies of reduced welfare and severe austerity and the program was closed down in the early 1990s, after a half-century of success which is evident in state documents, World Health Organization (WHO) archives, and community oral histories across Ghana.

This chapter examines northern Ghana's Native Authority dispensaries and the Medical Field Units as programs which embodied many ideas and practices of social medicine over the twentieth century, although the term was rarely used by the actors themselves. The evolving terminology and central historical figures of "Social Medicine" were largely absent, but these Ghanaian programs were produced by similar ideas and practices (regarding underlying determinants of poor health, community health needs, and just distributions of care) as many contemporary, self-identified social medicine movements elsewhere. In this chapter, "social medicine" is used as an analytical category, comprising these fundamental ideas and practices. The chapter relates the evolution of the MFU program to social histories of individual advocacy, healthcare reforms from colonialism to independence, and shifts in internationally circulating economic beliefs regarding the role of welfare and the state.[1] African countries have often been represented as places in need of social medicine, suggesting a diffusion of ideas from somewhere else. This chapter discusses locally inflected African social medicine programs which endured for decades, complicated by their origins in the administration of the colonial periphery. Their development calls the notionally monolithic character of colonial medicine into question. This was the case for northern Ghana, where a lack of attention from central colonial governments, who saw the region as unprofitable, meant that there was sometimes more scope for alternative institutional ethics, notions of solidarity, and understandings of the determinants of poor health.

This analysis is based on sources from Ghanaian and WHO archives, and community oral history interviews carried out in Ghana during 2015–22. I also use interviews with current and former Ghanaian health officials and national planners and retired health workers who held positions from c.1960 to the

[1] See J. Manton and M. Gorsky, "Health Planning in 1960s Africa: International Health Organisations and the Post-colonial State," *Medical History* 62, no. 4 (2018): 425–48; Giovanni Carbone, "Democratic Demands and Social Policies: The Politics of Health Reform in Ghana," *Journal of Modern African Studies* 49, no. 3 (2011): 381–408.

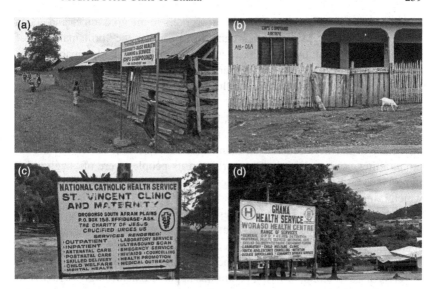

Figures 13.1 (a)–(d) Community health facilities in rural Ghana, 2018. Many of these frontline health facilities in Ghana have grown on the same sites as the Local Authority health system of the 1930s, having changed hands with national- or mission-based ownership. They embody many of the same aspirations, at the necessary convergence of social and community medicine. Photo: David Bannister.

present, notably in community medicine and rural public health. From these sources, some key observations emerge: about the role of the political and economic margins as an enduring test-bed for social medicine's ideas and about the cyclical creation, decline, and recreation of similar social medicine and community health programs on these margins, in places like northern Ghana (see Figures 13.1(a)–(d)).

Native Authorities and Community Health, 1930–9

It is important to understand the north's relationship to Ghana's centers of political and economic power, comparable with circumstances that have fostered the emergence of social medicine advocacy elsewhere. Separated from the coast by the West African forest belt, the north's weather, ecologies, and agricultural potentials were (and are) substantially different to the rest of the country. Unlike southern Ghana, the north has no cocoa production, the crop most valued and supported by colonial and postcolonial governments. When attempts to force cultivation of alternative export crops like cotton were unsuccessful, the colonial government designated the north as a migrant labor reserve from the early 1900s, supplying low-cost workers to the gold mines and cocoa farms of the south.[2] Migrant labor came to be seen as the "principal asset of the dependency" and by the 1920s, many of the region's work-capable adults migrated annually as low-cost laborers.[3] Colonial-era neglect also stemmed from the north's lack of political influence. With little access to the central government at Accra, which imposed policies to restrict the development of northern education and infrastructure, the region was kept at a political arm's length over the colonial period.[4] There were few opportunities for African advocates or northern officials to counter the perception of the colony's governing elites, who argued that the north and its peoples were of "negligible" importance and that the region "imposes a burden upon the Gold Coast for which it makes no adequate return."[5]

These problems persist into the present. The north has been a periphery of both the colonial and postcolonial state: in terms of administrative attention and spending from central government, access to education and economic opportunities, and relative political influence.[6] Following its annexation in 1903, poverty, disease, and poor living conditions appeared increasingly regularly in descriptions of northern communities, contributing to an enduring public discourse which has represented northerners as unhealthy, second-class citizens. By the mid 1920s, orientalist official reports of "the wild tribes" who "leapt out with twanging bows and bloodcurdling yells, in apparent ecstasies of joy," had been replaced by "the immigrant labourer from the North, who generally reaches the cocoa areas in poor physical condition and is often diseased."[7]

These were the structural conditions faced by northern societies under colonial rule and since. Beyond economic privation and resulting poor health, however, the north's peripheral situation shaped healthcare in less expected ways. Necessity was often the mother of invention, when long-term underfunding compelled local officials to find novel answers to problems of health provision.

[2] See 1924–1925 Northern Territories Annual Report (hereafter, NTAR), 3.
[3] See 1928–1929 NTAR, 12; and Roger Thomas, "Forced Labour in British West Africa: Northern Territories of the Gold Coast 1906–1927," *Journal of African History* 14:1 (1973), 79; Meyer Fortes, "Culture Contact as Dynamic Process: An Investigation in the Northern Territories of the Gold Coast," *Africa* 9 (1936), 37.
[4] Roger Thomas, "Education in Northern Ghana, 1906–1940: A Study in Colonial Paradox," *International Journal of African Historical Studies* 7, no. 3 (1974): 427–67.
[5] 1918 NTAR, 2–3.
[6] For example, Yakubu Saaka, "North–South Relations and the Colonial Enterprise in Ghana," in Saaka (ed.), *Regionalism and Public Policy* (Lausanne: Peter Lang, 2001), chapter 7; Rhoda Howard, *Colonialism and Underdevelopment in Ghana* (London: Croom Helm, 1978); Inez Sutton, "Colonial Agricultural Policy: The Non-development of the Northern Territories of the Gold Coast," *International Journal of African Historical Studies* 22, no. 4 (1989), 637–69; Thomas, "Education," 427–67; Alexander Moradi, "Colonial Legacies: Lessons from Human Development in Ghana and Kenya, 1880–2000," *Journal of International Development* 20, no. 8 (2008): 1115.
[7] 1910 NTAR, 12; 1923–1924 NTAR, 21.

These innovations included Native Authority community healthcare from the 1930s; the Medical Field Units, which operated for decades before and after independence; and the later co-optation of vertical donor-funded campaigns (notably the Carter Centre's guinea-worm program in the 1980s–90s) to serve broader public health needs. Neglect and underdevelopment created the moral basis for sustained healthcare advocacy by northern communities and officials, while allowing new local health initiatives to proceed with little central oversight.

This was evident in the creation of the Native Authority clinic-dispensaries scheme in the 1930s. The role of "Native Authorities" and indirect rule in colonial Africa has been a focus of critique, concerned with the illegitimacy of the institutions created when Britain began governing via its preferred "traditional" elites.[8] But there were other aspects to this transition. In the colonial north, Native Authorities became relatively effective activists and managers of health services, prepared to allocate resources to areas which been neglected under centralized British rule. The NAs were not dependent on the Accra government's largesse. They had their own treasuries, were able to raise and spend revenues locally, and were staffed by northerners, who were more responsive to health problems affecting their communities. Following their establishment during 1930–4, health became an immediate priority of the Native Authorities. Their central achievements were the rapid creation of a rural sanitation program to improve water quality and a network of village dispensaries and treatment centers were set up providing health surveillance and education, drugs, and outpatient treatments for common diseases.

These involved significant investment in local infrastructure by northern communities and from 1930–5, NA spending on new health infrastructure greatly exceeded the north's total annual medical budgetary allocations from the central government at Accra, which preferred to allocate funds for short-lived campaigns against diseases that threatened the southern labor supply (notably sleeping sickness).[9] By 1938, there were 16 large dispensaries, many smaller treatment centers, and a training program for local health workers. The north's native authorities contributed to schemes for training "village overseers," in charge of preventive rural sanitation, and the construction of a much larger School of Sanitation.[10] They also developed

---

[8] Mahmood Mamdani, *Citizen and Subject: Contemporary Africa and the Legacy of Late Colonialism* (Princeton, NJ: Princeton University Press, 1996), chapter 2.

[9] 1936–1937 NTAR, 16, 86; and David Bannister, "Wilful Blindness: Sleeping Sickness and Onchocerciasis in Colonial Northern Ghana, 1909–1957," *Social History of Medicine* 35, no. 2 (May 2022): 635–60.

[10] 1937–1938 NTAR, 77; 1940 MDAR, 16; and see NRG/8/7/9 (1949–1951), Enclosure 13, p. 28, "Notes on a Meeting with the Director of Medical Services," Undated 1949; and Enc. 15: Letter from T. A. Mead to Asst. Director Medical Services, Tamale, October 3, 1951.

a course for NA "dressers" in the regional capital, Tamale. After eighteen months of training, the dressers' work included treating yaws, sleeping sickness, round worm, scabies and ulcers, basic wound dressings, sterilization techniques, and home nursing or referrals to colonial medical officers. NA "dispensers" ran larger facilities. They were trained in similar techniques and in the provision of an expanded range of drugs, including subsidized quinine tablets and the use of new sulfonamide antimicrobials during regional meningitis epidemics.[11]

Supported by activist officials in the north's colonial administration, the NAs began to address other problems of underdevelopment related to health, including expansion of clean water supplies. These British officials, many of whom remain anonymous in colonial files, were public in their criticism of the Accra government's "belated realization" that clean water was a requirement for improved northern health, at a time when activism from colonial officials was relatively uncommon. They pointed out that in 1937, the north's Dagomba and Mamprusi Native Authorities had jointly spent £600 to employ a private engineer to develop proposals for clean water provision in their districts.[12] The north's various Native Authorities allocated £9,355 that year toward expenditures on preventive "health" initiatives for village sanitation. This far exceeded comparable funding from the government at Accra, which had allocated only £664 for village sanitation across the entire Northern Territories that year.[13]

The Native Authority health system was an immediate success from its creation in the early 1930s. With community-funded preventive sanitation, and clinical facilities staffed by northerners, its services were intended to compensate for the region's marginalization within the state and NA healthcare was soon recognized as an effective model by medical officers around the colony. This public success emboldened the region's medical and political officers in voicing direct criticisms of the central government. The protectorate's chief commissioner, W. J. A. Jones, wrote that:

The Northern Territories have seen the greatest advance in administration so far recorded in the history of the Gold Coast. Between the years 1902 and 1932 there was little or no alteration in the legislation affecting the lives of the people of the Northern Territories. This fact discloses the attitude of Government towards the people of the Protectorate. They were regarded as ... fit only to be hewers of wood and drawers of water for their brothers in the [southern] Colony.[14]

Other officials noted the "tremendous increase in the provision of facilities for medical treatment, improvement in village sanitation, and water supplies"

---

[11] 1937–1938 NTAR, 69, 77; 1936–1937 NTAR, 16; 1934–1935 NTAR, 86.
[12] 1936–1937 NTAR, 30–8.   [13] 1936–1937 NTAR, 59.   [14] 1937–1938 NTAR, 2–3.

as a result of NA initiatives, and attributed a significant fall in the colony's total number of out-patients to the work of the northern dispensaries.[15]

In the region's annual report for 1935, a district commissioner observed that, "The progress made by the Native Authorities has enabled them to obtain benefits which they would probably never have received if they had waited on Government generosity."[16] This foundational aspect of social medicine – an engagement with structural factors determining local health outcomes – is evident in many sources on health in the colonial north. The north's NA system was not simply a facade for the continued exercise of direct rule by British officials. Nor did it devolve into the "decentralised despotisms" assumed by some critiques of indirect rule.[17] From its creation, the NA health system was co-produced by northern communities, traditional leaders, and a small number of British officials in the region and almost entirely funded by the communities themselves.[18]

Medical Field Units and Ideas of Health and Development, c.1945–57

The colonial north's NA health system operated for only twenty years, despite its clear successes in improving community health and circumventing distributional inequities between the region and the wealthy south. In 1934, the north's chief commissioner had written, "it is to be hoped that these endeavors of the people to help themselves will be rewarded by the grant of generous assistance, by the central government or from the Colonial Development Fund." But no additional health funds were allocated to the region during the 1930s, perhaps because of the success of community-led NA healthcare. There was political resistance by the late 1930s, with efforts to restrict NA health services because they were seen as having expanded beyond supervision by the Accra government. Despite heated advocacy from communities and officials, northern Ghana's NA health system was shut down in the early 1950s, when the first independent government sought to centralize control of national healthcare and standardize training, considered more important than sustaining independent services in the north. Reflecting on colonial government resistance to northern community health, an activist official in the Northern Territories observed with apparent irony: "Perhaps it is a matter for congratulation, that we have

---

[15] 1936–1937 MDAR, 39; 1936–1937 NTAR 71–3; 1937–1938 MDAR, 69.
[16] 1935–1936 NTAR, 30.   [17] For example, Mamdani, *Citizen and Subject.*
[18] Among others, NRG/8/13/9 (1947–57), Enc. 35: Letter from Nandom *Na* to Ministry of Health, September 1956 and *passim*; "Native Administration," NTARs 1933–1938; David Bannister, "Public Health and Its Contexts in Northern Ghana, 1900–2015," PhD, School of Oriental and African Studies, London, 2017, doi.org/10.25501/SOAS.00026656, chapters 1 and 3, and see 86–7.

prevented them from running the risk of having a fall by trying to walk, before they can creep properly," with "creep" connoting obeisance to Accra.[19]

This would be repeated several times over the twentieth century: a northern community health initiative, designed under conditions of privation, would become a blueprint for services across Ghana, and risk becoming a victim of its own success in the interests of maintaining centralized control. The awareness of distributional inequities informed several subsequent northern health initiatives, which also embodied the ideas and practices of social medicine and were closed down in their turn. In 1938, a British official noted that health innovation of this kind was necessary for the region precisely because of persistent economic neglect: "an isolation which is inevitable, so long as the [north] is separated from the seat of Government by so valuable a crop as cocoa."[20]

With the decline of NA healthcare from the late 1930s, northerners requiring treatments beyond traditional herbalism were compelled to travel long distances to a handful of minimally funded government hospitals. Colonial medical budgets for the region in this period were allocated almost entirely to sleeping sickness control, seen as an economically important disease affecting the southern migrant labor supply.[21] Distributions of health infrastructure remained evidently unjust, driving continued advocacy on the part of northern communities and local officials. After 1945, local advocacy led to the creation of a new mobile medical service, intended to address the same problems. The Medical Field Units became one of Ghana's most enduring healthcare institutions, providing rural services across the country. It operated into the early 1980s and its northern fieldworkers became a crucial ark of local health knowledge across the independence divide. The MFUs were created in what some have seen as the "developmental" phase of colonial rule, in which Britain invested in headline infrastructure projects partly intended to improve its public support in the colonies, while privately also seeking to reduce overseas expenditure in the context of post-war austerity. With decolonization increasingly imminent, in 1948 the Gold Coast Medical Department published the *10-Year Development Plan*, which proposed that: "the future shape of medical services in the Gold Coast depends on a choice that must be made at this stage, between the rival claims of preventive and curative work. To aim at providing services satisfactory in both respects, for the entire country, is out of the question."[22] Relatively little had been done to develop preventive medical capacity under colonial rule in the Gold Coast, and the transition from colonial to independent rule (*c*.1948–57) brought an increased focus on building hospitals and urban

---

[19] 1938–1939 NTAR, 57.   [20] 1937–1938 NTAR, 38.

[21] See Bannister. "The Sorcerer's Apprentice: Sleeping Sickness, Onchocerciasis, and Unintended Consequences in Ghana, 1930–60," *Journal of African History* 62, no. 1 (2021): 29–57; Bannister, "Wilful Blindness," 635–60.

[22] NRG/8/7/9 (1949–1951), Enc. 1: Draft Ten Year Plan & Comments 1948, 2.

clinics, because curative medicine was believed to generate more immediate political support than longer-term prevention.[23]

With little central funding for preventive medicine in the north, the MFUs were created in the late 1940s with ad hoc resources available on the ground, by fusing remnant personnel from older northern treatment campaigns (against yaws and sleeping sickness) into a service designed to provide wider health services to rural communities. The MFUs did much of the same disease surveillance and treatment that characterized other mobile medical services in Africa, including the General Mobile Service of French West Africa, the Belgian FOREAMI, and the related MFUs of Nigeria.[24] Beyond this general remit, however, the foundational planning of northern Ghana's MFUs was focused explicitly on social and economic inequities which gave rise to malnutrition and endemic disease. The MFUs were founded by an Australian medical officer, B. B. Waddy, who argued that increased disease and economic decline were produced by insufficient government support for northern communities during the planting season, when stored food supplies were lowest, disease rates were high and many migrant laborers were absent. He proposed that:

the welfare of people in much of the Gold Coast turns on this vital period annually … even slight exaggerations of the difficulties may cause eventual famine, while amelioration may result in better harvests and a consequent progressive improvement in health and nutrition. With food to sell, the standard of living rises quite obviously … To achieve such a result with the limited resources available, the attack must be made first on those conditions.[25]

Waddy emphasized that this welfarist approach was central to the creation of the MFUs, concerned with precedent conditions that give rise to increased burdens of local disease.[26]

As with NA healthcare in the 1930s, the preventive, structurally aware approach to healthcare that Waddy described would seem to embody some key tenets of social medicine, whether he understood himself to be working in its traditions or not. Both programs aimed to alleviate or circumvent aspects of political and economic neglect unrelated to the immediate disease environment, in circumstances where there was little capacity to effect political

---

[23] See Bannister "Public Health," see chapters 3 and 6.
[24] 1954.GB-0809-RossInstitute.03.43, J. L. McLetchie, "Medical Field Units in Nigeria"; B; 1949.GB-0809-RossInstitute.03.23.v27, P. A. T. Sneath, "Rural Medical Services" (Tanganyika; 1951.GB-0809-RossInstitute.03.43, R. Mouchet, "The FOREAMI"; and see F. X. Mbopi-Keou, L. Bélec, J.-M. Milleliri, and C.-G. Teo, "The Legacies of Eugène Jamot and La Jamotique," *PLoS Negl Trop Dis.* 8, no. 4 (2014), doi.org/10.1371/journal.pntd.0002635.
[25] 1956.GB-0809-RossInstitute.03.43.v54; B. B. Waddy, "Organization and Work of the Medical Field Units of the Gold Coast Medical Field Units," *Transactions of the Royal Society of Tropical Medicine* 50, no. 4 (1956), 333–4.
[26] Waddy, "Organization and Work," 333–4.

change from the center. In this sense, both are comparable with the Pholela Community Health Centre in 1940s South Africa.[27] The northern Ghana health initiatives discussed above are similarly problematized by their origins on the colonial periphery, as programs co-created with colonial officers at the edges of an exploitative imperial system. It can also be argued that in many places at the rural periphery, with little state infrastructure, economic opportunity and political access, there is a necessary confluence between politically "Social" and practically "Community" Medicine, to the extent that the two are practically coterminous. At these rural margins, beyond advocacy and critique and in the relative absence of integration with the kind of social worlds which international advocates of social medicine might have conceived of (linking people through shared experiences of the state and wage labor), in these contexts "Community Medicine" often comprised all of the practicable interventions which Social Medicine practitioners could bring to bear.

Other forms of "social medicine" were understood by central British administrations in late colonial Africa. For example, in a 10-year Development Plan for Gold Coast health services, published in 1948 but never implemented, "Social Medicine" was proposed as one division of a reformed colonial health service, along with curative medicine, preventive medicine, nutrition, and laboratory services. A Social Medicine division would deal with "maternity and child welfare, school medicine, and dentistry" and planned to use women health visitors as a way of gaining community trust for increased preventive services over time.[28] Coming from the administrative center, these developments in the pre-Cold War 1940s may have been shaped by the diffusion of ideas from the 1937 Bandung Conference on Rural Hygiene, the rural health programs of the Rockefeller Foundation (which funded concurrent yellow fever research in West Africa), and perhaps by the work of Andrija Štampar and Henry Sigerist. Contemporaneous developments in social medicine may well have been known by those involved in the creation of the NA and MFU programs in the colonial north, although none are referenced in the available sources. From the 1940s "developmental" phase of colonial rule, there were other resources beyond the literature on health – related to broader discussions around labor and social welfare – which could be used to make arguments about the underlying determinants of poor health in colonial northern Ghana. Britain's 1929–45 Colonial Welfare and Development Acts offered a rhetorical resource for criticizing the colonial state using its own terms.[29] The idiom

---

[27] Abigail Neely, *Reimagining Social Medicine from the South* (Durham, NC: Duke University Press, 2021).

[28] NRG/8/7/9 (1949–1951), Enc. 2: 10-Year Plan for Hospital, Health and Nutrition Services: Social Medicine, 2–14.

[29] E. R. Wicker, "Colonial Development and Welfare, 1929–1957," *Social and Economic Studies* 7, no. 4 (1958): 172–5.

of development, and the moral language the Acts contained, were influential in shaping advocacy for health programs which aimed beyond the "great campaigns" and curative preferences of most colonial medicine.[30]

Independent Ghana: Socialized, Community, and Primary Health

At his inaugural Christmas address in 1957, independent Ghana's first president, Kwame Nkrumah, said:

> My first objective is to abolish from Ghana poverty, ignorance and disease. We shall measure our progress by the improvement in the health of our people; by the number of children in school and the quality of their education; by the availability of water and electricity in our towns and villages ... The welfare of our people is our chief pride, and it is by this that my Government will ask to be judged.[31]

Nkrumah's Convention People's Party (CPP) welfare policies set out to create a socialized health service on the British model, funded by general taxation. Fees for drugs and outpatient services were ended and government health workers were prohibited from charging for treatments away from state facilities.[32] New clinical and training infrastructure expanded across the country and there were attempts to integrate traditional healers into Ghana's health system.[33] From 1964, there was a policy shift toward the new paradigm of "community health" promoted internationally by the WHO, emphasizing basic rural healthcare and preventive medicine.[34] Ghana endorsed this model relatively early, as part of a global movement focused on community needs and primary care, aspects of social medicine which would culminate in the call for "a new global economic order" of the 1978 Alma-Ata Declaration. Nkrumah's government ran various programs oriented toward broader societal health, including national health education initiatives and a family support

[30] For example, Colonial Reports, Series 1919, on the "Economic and Social Progress of the People of the Gold Coast," The National Archives of the United Kingdom, London.

[31] Nkrumah, in Gilford Ashitey, *An Epidemiology of Disease Control in Ghana* (Accra: University of Ghana Press, 1994), 30.

[32] See Bannister "Public Health," chapters 3 and 5; Carbone, "Democratic Demands," 387–94; Daniel Arhinful, "Health Care in Ghana and How It Was Paid for: An Historical Perspective (1850–2001)," in D. Arhinful, *The Solidarity of Self-Interest: Social Feasibility of Rural Health Insurance in Ghana* (Leiden: African Studies Centre, 2003), chapter 1.

[33] See WHO/S10/372/2/GHA/6 (1965), UNSF Establishment of a Community Health Project, WHO Geneva, Enc. 1: "Report on Ghana under EPTA program," 10–20; S. Agyei-Mensah de-Graft and A. Aikins, "Epidemiological Transition and the Double Burden of Disease in Accra, Ghana," *Journal of Urban Health* 87, no. 5 (2010): 886; Arhinful, *Solidarity*, 48–9.

[34] WHO/S10/372/2/GHA/6 (1965), Enc.1: "WHO Consultant Report under EPTA," 10–20; WHO/AFR/EXT/16 (1967) Report on a Visit to Ghana, Dr. J. Vysohild, March 31, 1967, WHO Geneva, 30–50; Carbone, "Democratic Demands," 387–9.

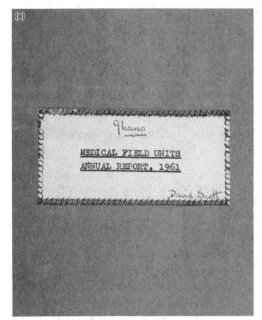
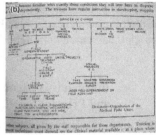
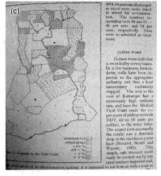

Figures 13.2(a)–(c) Internal documents, organizational structures, and reports of the Medical Field Units in 1952 and 1961 across Ghana's transition to independence. Created to address feedback loop between social conditions, nutrition, and poor health, the Units persisted from the 1940s into the 1980s as the first line of rural healthcare and disease prevention in Ghana.
Source: B. B. Waddy, "Organization and Work of the Medical Field Units of the Gold Coast," 1952–1956. GB-0809-RossInstitute.03.43.v54, (13.5 and 13.7); D. Scott, Annual Report on the Medical Field Units, 1961. PRAAD, Accra.[Uncatalogued typed report] (13.6).

program which reprised late-colonial social medicine plans for the country, sending hundreds of women health visitors to rural districts to monitor community nutrition (Figures 13.2(a)–(c) are examples of health documents produced during this transition).[35]

However, these independence-era programs were short-lived. Decolonization had relocated Ghana from the imperial to the global economic periphery, in the context of Cold War clientalism. As the world's leading exporter of cocoa in the 1950s and 1960s, there were significant foreign reserves to fund the expansion of socialized health and welfare services. But the situation deteriorated

[35] See NRG/8/13/40 (1959–65) Health Education; NRG/8/13/18 (1951–1964) "Nutrition Assistants"; NRG/8/13/26 (1953–1960), "Local Authority Health Services," all PRAAD-Tamale.

from the early 1960s. As Nkrumah's government joined the Non-Aligned Movement and partnered with several socialist states, Western cocoa buyers increasingly moved their purchasing to neighboring Côte d'Ivoire under the French-aligned government of Félix Houphouët-Boigny, during a period of global cocoa overproduction. These changes eroded the economic foundation of Ghana's independence-era health reforms, while restrictions on private enterprise generated resistance from Ghanaian elites (notably doctors who had been restricted from private practice). In 1966, Nkrumah was overthrown by West-aligned military officers who governed as the National Liberation Council. This began a twenty-year period of rapid, unstable political transition, often by military coup, which stalled plans to expand health infrastructure, and resulted in a gradual accretion of authority by transnational health organizations and NGOs, particularly in the management of rural care.

The period 1957–66 was Ghana's only experiment with extensively socialized healthcare. But the Medical Field Units persisted during Nkrumah's time and beyond. In the early 1950s, the number of mobile teams was doubled and MFU personnel were tasked with monitoring, preventing, or treating practically all of the north's principal rural health problems, including village sanitation, health education, general injuries, and obstetrics (to the extent that these were unaddressed by traditional medicine), as well as endemic and epidemic diseases including meningitis, onchocerciasis, guinea worm, tuberculosis, yaws, leprosy, malaria, smallpox, bilharzia, hookworm and other helminths, and malnutrition. At independence in 1957, Ghana's new Director of Medical Services observed that the north's MFUs were "of greater service to the community than any hospital, however large."[36] Recognizing the value of a mobile, community-oriented medical service for reaching peoples who had received little colonial-era care, the CPP government expanded the service across the country, preserving its remit but greatly increasing the national scope of MFU activities.[37] Although technically based within the Ministry of Health in Accra, the headquarters and training school remained in Kintampo, a small town on the northern edge of Ghana's rainforest belt, where MFU candidates, "accustomed to working in primitive surroundings and familiar with local languages," gathered for courses in field medicine. There are comparisons to be made with the later "barefoot-doctors" movement in 1960s China. Most learning took place by direct instruction between successive cohorts of MFU members, as opposed to book-led instruction from medical professionals, and MFU members were recruited for their local knowledge, community relations, and physical endurance, rather than formal education; many were illiterate or had a basic primary school education. With this adaptive

---

[36] NRG/8/13/11 (1949–57), Enc. 7: Cheverton, "Observations on the Medical Department," 48–9.
[37] See Ashitey, *Disease Control*, 11–12.

approach, however, the MFUs were able to sustain and transmit the knowledge necessary to perform relatively complex clinical and diagnostic tasks, including field microscopy and forms of surgery, in places beyond the road network and bureaucratic reach of the state.[38]

Beyond frontline care and prevention, Ghana's MFUs also functioned as a crucial ark of health knowledge and community relations across the independence divide and during the instability which followed the overthrow of Nkrumah. Much institutional knowledge of rural health problems was lost when British health workers left the Gold Coast en masse in the 1950s, having resisted the training of African personnel who might replace them, and problems persisted after independence when southern Ghanaian medics refused to take up vacant posts in the rural north.[39] Dr. Sam Bugri, who became the north's Regional Director of Health in 1984, recalled that for decades after independence, district physicians relied on the formally untrained staff of the MFUs as a repository of medical knowledge. Among other things, MFU personnel trained new hospital physicians in the relatively high-risk technique for lumbar puncture, used by MFUs to test for meningococcal meningitis in the field:

We had a team they called the Medical Field Units – they started way back in the colonial times … At first they focused on the North, and they were well trained. I learned how to do lumbar puncture from them, not from medical school. They could screen a village within a short period for any diseases that you want. We had a feeling that there were very few doctors who are comfortable with doing lumbar puncture. So we insisted that all doctors in the field would see this. And these MFU people were not highly educated. But they taught them how to do it safely, and very accurately – they did it with ease.[40]

Over five decades, through economic downturn and successive political upheavals, the widely remembered work of the MFUs stands as a testament to the role played by a group of "uneducated" northerners, operating in difficult environments beyond the reach of the state, in shaping independent Ghana's public health.[41] Across overthrows of successive Ghanaian governments during 1966–82 and the severe economic shortfalls experienced by most African states in the 1970s as global oil shocks destabilized poorer countries at the

[38] GB/0809/v54.6 (1957). Waddy, "Cerebro-spinal Meningitis," 11; Waddy, "Organization and Work," 313–36.

[39] Dr. Sam Adjei, Interview, Accra, June 26, 2016; Dr. Sam Bugri, Interview, Tamale, June 30, 2015.

[40] Dr. Sam Bugri, Interview, Tamale, June 30, 2015; and see PD/65/v2 Box 27/02/02735 (1972–1981), Enc. 9: "Rural Health Training Centre, Kintampo," March 7, 1969; and Enc. 10: "Development of Basic Health Services, Second Edition 1972."

[41] See among others, Thomas Bowden, "The Development of Public Health in Underdeveloped Areas," *Journal of the Royal Institute of Public Health and Hygiene* 27, no. 5 (1964), 131–9.

global periphery,[42] the MFUs played an increasingly central role in the maintenance of community-oriented health services and the preservation of medical knowledge. These disruptions diminished Ghana's record-keeping capacity and relatively few government documents were archived for these years, including on national health. Community oral histories suggest that in poorer rural districts, the MFUs were often the only persistent state health service from the 1940s to the early 1980s, offering locally adapted healthcare and screening and participating in transnational campaigns against smallpox and onchocerciasis. Reports from the WHO Smallpox campaign in the 1970s reveal the extent to which eradication in Ghana depended on the MFU network.[43] As other divisions of the national health service contracted or ceased operations, the Medical Field Units became "the pride of the Ministry of Health."[44] WHO consultants posted in Ghana consistently remarked on the importance of the MFUs under the economic conditions of the 1970s, observing that they offered the best way of "providing as much coverage to the population as is possible within the limitations of available staff and resources."[45]

National Planning and International Health

Under the unstable conditions previously discussed, it is surprising that the Medical Field Units remained in place and relatively unchanged from the colonial 1950s to the mid 1980s. Beside their practical successes, the MFUs were also sustained by the health planning orientations of the Ghanaian state, produced by Ghana's situation in the world of international health and particularly its relationship with the WHO.

The history of pre-Adjustment national health planning in Africa is an emerging area of research, discussing the interplay between domestic visions for health reform and ideas circulating internationally.[46] After independence, Ghana drew on a heterodox range of influences in the formulation of national health policy.

---

[42] Bruce Fetter, "Healthcare in Twentieth-Century Africa: Statistics, Theories, and Policies," *Africa Today* 40, no. 3 (1993): 9; Frederick Cooper, "Possibility and Constraint: African Independence in Historical Perspective," *Journal of African History* 49, no. 2 (2008): 167–96.

[43] See, for example, WHO SE/WP/75.12 (1975), Smallpox Eradication, WHO, Geneva.

[44] Ashitey, *Disease Control*, 11.

[45] WHO/P9/445/8/GHA (1973–1975), Enc. 251: Report of Duty Travel to Ghana by Drs. J. Holm and J. Stromberg, Division for Strengthening of Health Services, WHO, April–May 1974.

[46] For example, Manton and Gorsky, "Health Planning"; Martin Gorsky and Christopher Sirrs, "From 'Planning' to 'Systems Analysis': Health Services Strengthening at the World Health Organisation, 1952–1975," *Dynamis* 39, no. 1 (2019): 205–33; Carbone, "Democratic Demands"; Bannister, "Public Health," chapter 5; see also Ruth Prince and Rebecca Marsland (eds.), *Making and Unmaking Public Health in Africa* (Athens: Oxford University Press, 2014); Jean-Paul Gaudillière, Claire Beaudevin, Christoph Gradmann, Anne M. Lovell, and Laurent Pordié (eds.), *Global Health and the New World Order* (Manchester: Manchester University Press, 2014).

Early influences included Britain's late-colonial "10-year plans" and the 1953 Maude Commission *Report on the Health Needs of Ghana*.[47] Nkrumah's first independent health plan was drafted with advisors from the Israeli labor movement and, from the early 1960s, his government turned increasingly toward the socialist world as a partner and source of planning advice. After the coup d'état in 1966, the military National Liberation Council set out to "divest the state from the socialist programs pursued under Nkrumah."[48] When a second coup brought the left-leaning National Redemption Council to power from 1972, it conversely expanded state welfare and health subsidies and restored relations with the socialist world, developing bilateral relationships for trading medical goods which persisted into the late 1980s.[49]

With stasis or collapse in many areas of Ghanaian healthcare from the 1960s–80s, what sustained the Medical Field Units across these political shifts? They endured in part because the underlying inequities which the MFUs were created to address had remained constant or increased: the economic marginalization and resulting disease burden of rural communities, out of reach of state health infrastructure. But the MFU program was also sustained by the persistence of social medicine as an idea in international health. A strong Ghana–WHO relationship, across different governments, acted as a conduit for new terminologies that rested on the same fundamental orientations. From the 1950s to late 1970s, Ghana's medium-term national health plans comprised successive proposals for expanding what were variously called "Social," "Community," "Basic," and "Primary" health services, often drafted in collaboration with the staff of the WHO's Division for Strengthening Health Services.[50] While the terminology changed, social medicine's enduring currency in international health thinking and support for its ideas within the Ghana–WHO relationship may have helped to sustain the MFU program across different political regimes.

Adjustment and the End of the MFUs

The Medical Field Units were created to provide healthcare under conditions of economic and political marginality, many years before the 1978 Alma-Ata

---

[47] NRG/8/13/18 (1951–1964) "Health Needs Of Ghana," PRAAD-Tamale, Enc. 2: Circular from Minister of Labour & Health, 1951.

[48] Arhinful, *Solidarity*, 51.

[49] See Bannister, "Public Health," chapter 5; and, for example, PD/230 Box 18/02/02726 (1983–89), Enc. 6: "Negotiation of Bilateral Agreement between Ghana and G.D.R," July 21, 1986.

[50] For example, WHO/P9/445/8/GHA (1973–1975), Enc. 59: Duty Travel Report, Ghana, November 23, 1973, 127–66; PD/65/v2 Box 27/02/02735 (1972–1981), Enc. 9: "Basic Health Services"; WHO/P9/445/8/GHA (1973–1975), Study on Community Involvement in Solving Local Health Problems, Ghana, WHO, Geneva; and see also Enc. 191: Dr. M. A. Baddoo, Director of Medical Services, Accra, to Division of Strengthening of Health Services, WHO, August 31, 1973 and Enc. 251: "Duty Travel to Ghana, April to May 1974."

Declaration. They were first designed to secure community health during the vulnerable northern planting season when food stocks were low, migrant labor was absent and there was no state support, with the aim of increasing harvests, productivity and health in the longer term. Although it is unclear whether the MFUs were influenced by the development of social medicine elsewhere, the program was likely sustained by the internationally conducive climate for social medicine discussed above, adapted by health planners in Ghana.

All this changed soon after 1978, a historical high-water mark for the primary care and social medicine movements. From the early 1980s, the community-oriented mobile health services of the MFUs were undermined by centralizing budgetary micromanagement under Structural Adjustment and by competing NGOs, Christian Health organizations, and other external actors that adjustment had brought to the country. In 1983, Ghana became the first African state to accept World Bank-/IMF-mandated restructuring as a condition of development loans, after debt crises reduced national healthcare spending by almost 80 percent during 1976–80.[51] In some analyses, Ghana's adjustment program has been seen as an outstanding success. Gareth Austin suggests that the country was "one of the two most successful cases of structural adjustment in Africa."[52] Arguments of this kind are often based on aggregate growth, without regard to distributional effects, although adjustment in Ghana arguably also failed on its own macroeconomic terms.[53] Foreign debt more than doubled between 1983 and 1987 and costs of structural adjustment austerity were consistently passed to peripheral regions and the rural poor, whom the IMF and World Bank had cast as its principal beneficiaries.[54] Rising poverty resulted from trade liberalization and currency devaluation after 1983 and severe cuts to spending on health and education drove many destitute rural communities to migrate to informal settlements around southern cities.[55]

In healthcare, World Bank purchasing restrictions meant that the country completely ran out of essential medicines at several points in the 1980s, including all tuberculosis treatments and antibiotics like penicillin and ampicillin.[56]

---

[51] Carolyn Baylies, "The Meaning of Health in Africa," *Review of African Political Economy* 13, no. 36 (1986): 71.

[52] Gareth Austin, "African Economic Development and Colonial Legacies," *International Development Policy* 1 (2010): 3.

[53] See Bannister, "Public Health," chapter 2.

[54] Roger Gocking, *The History of Ghana* (Westport, CT: Greenwood Press, 2005), chapter 10; Jon Kraus, "The Struggle over Structural Adjustment in Ghana," *Africa Today* 38, no. 4 (1991): 20.

[55] Agyei-Mensah and Aikins, "Epidemiological Transition," 887; Gocking, *History*, 199.

[56] For example, PD/224 Box 1802/02726 (1986–89) World Bank Health Fund (Facility for Drugs), PRAAD-Accra, Enc. 1: Dr Moses Adibo, PNDC Secretary for Health, to UNICEF Procurement, July 14, 1986; PD/85 Box 27/02/02735 (1994) Medical Stores, General Correspondence, PRAAD-Accra, Enc. 3: "Current Drug Situation at the Department of Chest Diseases, Korle Bu," Letter from Staff Doctors to PNDC Secretary for Health, MoH Accra, March 27, 1992.

Cost-recovery measures were imposed at government health facilities, requiring full advance payment before treatments or drugs were supplied.[57] This led to a situation in which an estimated 69 percent of Ghanaians were unable to afford state care, with many people turning to traditional herbalism or forms of faith healing.[58]

Under these conditions, there might seem to have been a clear need for a low-cost, scalable model for maintaining basic health services. But Adjustment-era centralization of health authority was antithetical to a service like the MFUs, which was inherently decentralized and unpredictable by design, intended to address shifting rural health needs away from state infrastructure. The MFU program may also have been affected by changes in health accounting practices which took place concurrently with adjustment from the early 1980s, given the difficulty of calculating a neat return-on-investment for a self-organizing service operating in deep rural areas beyond regular inspection.[59] The MFU program ended in the mid 1980s and it was intended to be replaced with fewer, formally trained "technical officers" at fixed district health posts. Under Adjustment-era poverty in rural Ghana, however, it was clear that some form of mobile services were still needed to reach poorer communities, then in retreat from state health facilities and advance user fees. The new solutions to this problem reinvented the wheel. A wave of foreign-funded religious and NGO-led health services moved into rural areas and the MFUs which had served Ghana from c.1948–88 were recreated privately as "Mission Mobile Clinics" and "NGO Service Expansions," funded by external donors.[60]

Conclusion

In contemporary Ghana, there are echoes of the older social medicine initiatives discussed in this chapter. There are mission- and NGO-led mobile health services which replaced the MFUs and in the country's current frontline healthcare, an initiative which hearkens back to the 1930s. Since 1999, Ghana's

---

[57] PD/44 Box 15/02/2723 (1990–1992), Enc. 1: "Cash and Carry Design Workshop, Memorandum from Dr. Issaka-Tinorgah, Project Director for PNDC Secretary for Health," October 5, 1992; and Enc. 2: "Implementation of Cash and Carry Drug Scheme," Bombardier Matthias Cudjoe, PNDC Co-ordinator to PNDC Health Secretary, January 10, 1992; also Carbone, "Democratic Demands," 388–401.

[58] An estimate from former Director-General of the Ghana Health Service Badu Akosa, quoted in Arhinful, "Health Care in Ghana," 54.

[59] See C. Sirrs, "The Health of Nations," in Axel C. Hunetelman and Oliver Falk (eds.), *Accounting for Health: Calculation, Paperwork, and Medicine, 1500–2000* (Manchester: Manchester University Press, 2021), 359–85.

[60] See WHO/JCP, Vols. 5–6 (1980–5), pp. 9–12, Section 6: NORRIP Health Program; and Dr. Bugri, Interview, June 30, 2015.

Community-Based Health Planning and Services (CHPS) program has become the most extensive primary healthcare network in the country's history. Small CHPS compounds now cover most communities in Ghana, housing one to three health workers who serve one or two villages. CHPS was another northern innovation adopted nationally, having been proven under conditions of long-term rural poverty in a politically marginal region. For better and worse, the political and economic margins have always been social medicine's "living laboratory." If a mode of healthcare provision works where people can afford little and where little infrastructure has been provided, then it is likely to flourish (and save some money) in better resourced districts elsewhere.

This role of the margins is one central observation of the chapter. Marginalized communities are often the sites of cyclical innovation, decline (through persisting political marginality), and then recreation of similar social medicine programs. Ghana's current CHPS system was developed from a 1990s community-health study called the "Navrongo Experiment," conducted by the northern Navrongo Health Research Centre with funds from the Rockefeller Foundation and USAID. This was a large-scale demographic surveillance study of approximately 171,000 people in northeastern Ghana, designed to test new community-health interventions in comparison with existing (or non-existing) rural health services at the end of structural adjustment.[61] Offering community-based services with family planning and maternity care, the trial's clear success led to its national implementation in the early 2000s and in areas where CHPS operated, childhood mortality was halved within years of its inauguration.[62] CHPS has been hailed as a landmark in the extension of primary healthcare in Ghana and cited as an exemplar for effective community-based medicine worldwide.[63]

It is interesting to note the extent to which the CHPS system resembles a much earlier success. The 1930s Native Authority healthcare system placed trained health workers directly into rural communities, working closely with traditional leaders and their networks. Its approach to health provision was decided collaboratively, through consultation between NA health workers and the communities they served, who provided labor and funding for activities like disease surveillance, maintenance of facilities, and rural sanitation. The NA system was also recognized as an outstanding success by officials and the

---

[61] Fred Binka, Alex Nazzar, and James F. Phillips, "The Navrongo Community Health and Family Planning Project," *Studies in Family Planning* 26, no. 3 (1995): 126; Professor Fred Binka, Interview, Ho, June 21, 2016.

[62] Binka, Nazzar, and Phillips, "Navrongo Community Health," 163.

[63] Dr. K. Awoonor-Williams, Interview, Navrongo, July 2, 2016; Dr. Moses Adibo, Interview, Accra, June 17, 2016; and J. K. Awoonor-Williams, Ellie S. Feinglass, Rachel Tobbey et al., "Bridging the Gap between Evidence-Based Innovation and National Health-Sector Reform in Ghana," *Studies in Family Planning* 35, no. 3 (2004): 161–77.

northern public, who resisted its closure in the 1950s.[64] Seemingly without knowing of this earlier initiative, the 1990s "Navrongo Experiment" again proposed that successful primary healthcare in Ghana should base trained health workers in rural communities, "to mobilize the previously untapped cultural resources of chieftaincy, social networks, and village gatherings in order to promote community accountability, volunteerism, and investment in health services."[65] Beyond its testing in a large-scale trial, and differences in the availability of modern drugs and communications, the CHPS and NA models are closely comparable, based around the same collaborative, community-oriented framework that had been recognized as a success in the 1930s.

This chapter has examined two Ghanaian health programs which embodied many ideas and practices of social medicine. Both the NA system and the Medical Field Units were created in the period 1930–50, both from a foundational concern with the structural determinants of poor health, arising from the long-term political and economic marginalization of northern Ghana – a region which has been the site of multiple successful healthcare "experiments" of this kind. Both programs were responsive to community needs and operated in sequence for almost seventy years: from 1930s colonial rule, across Ghana's independence transition, and into the late twentieth century. The MFUs demonstrate a practical application of social medicine ideas outside of its main traditions – born from colonial-era advocacy and sustained by African proponents and permissive international contexts for social medicine until the 1980s. The story of these initiatives is in some ways emblematic of broader histories of social and community medicine in Africa from the 1940s. Short-term practical responses to unjust distributions of health resources have endured for much longer than their designers – imagining futures in which such programs would no longer be needed – might have hoped. In the course of group oral histories in 2015 and 2019, many rural communities across different regions of Ghana remembered the Medical Field Units kindly. Older people would sometimes laugh at questions about the availability of government doctors or fixed health facilities from the 1950s–70s. "Government – was there even government?" was one relatively typical reply. "We only had the MFUs."[66]

As a concluding thought, for these long-past health initiatives and those which succeeded them at the economic and geographical margins of the state, it is worth asking how much was achieved in advancing social medicine's aims? Initiatives like those discussed above, past and present, were envisioned as creating a virtuous cycle in which improved local healthcare and nutrition

---

[64] NRG/8/13/9 (1947–57), Enc. 35: Letter from Nandom *Na* to Ministry of Health, September 26, 1956; and see Bannister, "Public Health," 144–50.
[65] Awoonor-Williams et al., "Bridging," 162.
[66] Group 03: Sherigu Village (Guruni), Interview, July 28, 2019.

might strengthen a community's economic prospects, relative to other, better resourced places and groups within a state, ameliorating some of the precedent causes of poor health. Community health and social medicine have located many interventions in the gaps of economic opportunity and healthcare distribution which persist at the rural margins. Where did this succeed and why, in the sense of achieving some of social medicine's aims either locally and practically or as part of a broader political project in the worlds of national and global health?

In addition to research in Ghana, over the past decade this author has intermittently lived and worked near the Pholela Community Healthcare Project, discussed elsewhere in this volume – one of the earliest and most cited exemplars of social medicine in practice, located on South Africa's rural periphery. The project has been embraced by the post-Apartheid state, celebrated on national health administration websites and new community healthcare facilities and community nutrition projects have been developed as satellites to the main center. Despite the expansion of health facilities, it is hard to say whether political recognition and economic opportunities – as foundational determinants of health – have changed much for people living in these places. By tracing these and other cases over time and into the present, there is more research to be done on how success and its limits should be understood in the historiography and history of applied social medicine.

14 Changing Avatars of Social Medicine in the Indian Subcontinent

Rama V. Baru

Much of scholarly writing on the concept of social medicine traces its roots to Western Europe of the early twentieth century.[1] The core concerns that underpinned this concept were social and health inequalities, normative concerns of social justice, and equity. In order to realize these objectives, centrality was given to the role of the state to ensure access to health services and address the social determinants of health. The South Asian region, consisting of India, Pakistan, Bangladesh, Nepal, and Sri Lanka, share a common history of British colonial rule and so a common approach to several policy issues. Most of these countries gained independence during the 1940s and faced similar challenges of nation building as postcolonial states. With respect to health service development, Western European ideas of social medicine found considerable resonance. However, through the process of anti-colonial struggle there were a plurality of ideas on the relationship between society, medicine, and health. These included the world view of practitioners of indigenous systems of medicine; sections of the leadership of the nationalist movement; the communist movement that drew inspiration from the Soviet Union and later China; and radical elements within the medical community and society at large. I call this diversity of approaches as the many "avatars" of social medicine.[2]

The leadership of the social medicine movement during this period was among several physicians from Western Europe and the United States. Prominent among them were Henry Siegrist, John Ryle, John Grant, Andrew Russell, George Newman, and John Gunn, to name a few, who formed an epistemic community of doctors who advocated the idea and practice of social medicine. They were associated with institutions that included the

---

[1] George Rosen, *A History of Public Health* (Baltimore: Johns Hopkins University Press, 1993).

[2] I use the metaphor of Avatar which means descent in Hindu philosophy to denote the different ideas of social medicine that were in circulation in pre and post independent India. The term social medicine has been informed by varied ideological positions and its practice and therefore the metaphor "avatar" tries to capture the many strands of the same. The term avatar has evolved from a religious connotation to a broader idea of transformation or embodiment of ideas. In this chapter we use avatar in social medicine to elaborate on the transformation and embodiment within a historical context in south Asia.

International Health Division of the Rockefeller Foundation, Johns Hopkins University, Harvard School of Public Health, and others who were engaging with China, India, and several countries in Latin America. They contributed significantly to the debates on how to structure and organize health services in developed and developing countries. As Milton I. Roemer observes, there were debates around the importance of the integration between preventive and curative medicine by setting up health centers as the primary level of care.[3] Circulation of the ideas of social medicine had a far-reaching influence on postcolonial societies both from the West and the Soviet model of social medicine. Several postcolonial countries, including India, were founders of the Non-Aligned Movement (NAM) and thereby did not align fully with the United States or the Soviet Union. The former tried to wield their influence through economic, scientific, technological, and cultural domains, while the latter left an imprint on planned approach to the economy and health development in post-independent India.

British Colonial Rule and Social Medicine

European and American ideas of social medicine in circulation in the early twentieth century influenced health service development in India during the pre-independence period. Western concepts spread through allopathic medical institutions set up from the early eighteenth century. These institutions initially treated Europeans in India but later were opened to native population. The institutionalization of hospitals, dispensaries, and medical colleges during the colonial period was continued by the leadership of the national movement after independence. Colonial health policies were dominated by curative medicine, laboratory science, control of infectious disease, and sanitary measures. The idea of European social medicine did not find a place in the overall strategy of health services development during the colonial period since the policies were more focused on disease control and sanitary policies.[4]

Health Service Development for Independent India

The Joseph Bhore Committee on Health Survey and Development, set up in 1943 by Government of India, provided the blueprint for health services

---

[3] R. Roemer, "Milton I. Roemer, 1916–2001," *Bulletin of the World Health Organization* 79 no. 5 (2001): 481, World Health Organization, at: https://iris.who.int/handle/10665/268338.
[4] Muhammad Umair Mushtaq, "Public Health in British India: A Brief Account of the History of Medical Services and Disease Prevention in Colonial India," *Indian Journal of Community Medicine: Official Publication of Indian Association of Preventive & Social Medicine* 34, no. 1 (January 2009): 6–14, Doi: 10.4103/0970-0218.45369.

development in independent India. The influence of social medicine was visible with the representation of international experts who were its strong advocates. These included John Ryle, Henry Siegrist, and John Grant, who played an important role in contributing to the deliberations of the committee. One would argue that the influence of European social medicine was an important avatar in shaping policy for the development of health services in independent India. Sunil Amrith elaborates on the liberal and left positions that were present in the Bhore Committee that advocated strong ideas of social medicine in its deliberations.[5] The Bhore Committee advocated for a three-tier structure with a well-worked-out referral system. The design of the health services was similar to Yugoslavia and China during the 1930s. However, the investments required for a strong state-supported healthcare were inadequate and the emphasis was on curative hospital-based care. While curative medicine was dominant, several preventive programs had elements of the idea of social medicine through state-supported disease control and population -control programs. Several civil-society organizations also furthered ideas of social medicine by partnering with the government for national health programs.

Plurality of the Ideas of Social Medicine in the Indian Subcontinent

The nationalist movement was a coalition of differing ideological persuasions. Certain sections of the nationalist movement were supportive of heavy industrialization, while others presented alternate visions of development. There were four documents that represented the differing ideological positions on the future of India's development. These were the Bombay Plan representing big business; the Congress Plan that was elaborated in the National Planning Committee Report; the People's Plan representing socialist ideas; and the Gandhian Plan that was for small-scale industrialization with a focus on the needs of village India. One would argue that the very idea of development was represented by different ideological avatars. Despite the differences, there was a consensus among the various actors to bring an end to colonial rule.

The National Planning Committee that was set up in 1938 elaborated on the importance of addressing inequality, poverty, and unemployment. The vision was for a state-led development in the economy and for health, it emphasized how:

Planning must aim at liquidating illiteracy, eliminating epidemics, expanding health facilities and raising the average life span. A rational population policy would have to be framed to enable economic growth to improve the standard of living of an average

[5] Sunil Amrith, Rockefeller Foundation and Postwar Public Health in India, 2009, Rockefeller Archive Center, at: www.issuelab.org/resources/27992/27992.pdf.

Indian. Labour must be assured better and hygienic conditions of work and protection from sickness and accidents. Unemployment insurance and minimum wages must be provided statutorily.[6]

The Bombay Plan, authored by leading Indian industrialists, pro-actively sought state intervention for capitalist development.[7] Their vision included a central role for the state in the economy and social sectors. The acceptance of allopathy as rational and scientific resonated with the Nehruvian emphasis on industrial development and promotion of a scientific temper. On the other hand, the People's Plan, which was drafted by M. N. Roy, a communist leader, gave primacy to agriculture and advocated for the nationalization of agriculture and all production activities. Unlike the advocates of the Bombay Plan and members of the National Planning Committee, Gandhi was skeptical of Western ideas of development and modernity. The Gandhian Plan articulated a decentralized economic structure for India, with self-contained villages. Unlike the National Planning Committee and the Bombay Plan, the Gandhian Plan emphasized agriculture and stressed cottage and village industries.

In the case of health, Gandhi drew upon local traditions, indigenous systems, and naturopathy that had a sophisticated understanding of the relationship between the environment, society, and the individual body. This holistic understanding engaged in the complexity of the physical, social, economic, and psychological aspects of health and well-being. Gandhi was critical of the reductionism of biomedicine and emphasized the cultural rootedness of understanding health. In many of the indigenous systems, there was a great deal of emphasis on the relationship between food and health; detailed knowledge of flora for enhancing well-being and also curing illness; and individual and societal interrelationships was also given importance as determinants of health. It is interesting to note that while Gandhi engaged in folk and indigenous systems of healing, Nehru was skeptical about their value. Given the dominance of allopathy, indigenous systems were given a secondary position within the health services. Apart from the socialist influence, ideas of Gandhi's Swaraj also played an important role in shaping ideas of social medicine where the role of the state was critiqued for its inadequacy and local self-government and engagement with indigenous knowledge systems gained ground.

Babasaheb Ambedkar who was the author of the Indian Constitution and a key intellectual on the question of caste and inequality in Hinduism, was

---

[6] Girish Mishra, "Nehru and Planning in India," *Mainstream Weekly* 52, no. 47 (November 15, 2014), at: www.mainstreamweekly.net/article5320.html.

[7] Sanjaya Baru and Meghnad Desai, *The Bombay Plan: Blueprint for Economic Resurgence* (New Delhi: Rupa Publications, 2018).

an important influence for development and its implication for health.[8] His views on health are critical because he questioned and rejected the Hindu caste system, which he saw as the cause of persisting social inequalities. Keeping inequalities at its core, Ambedkar recognized how it mirrored unequal life chances, access to basic needs, health inequalities, and access to health services. Some of his ideas resonated with the ideas of Western social medicine but went beyond the importance of the state's role in public health. There was emphasis on the structural determinants of health and therefore went beyond health services or advocating particular medical interventions against diseases. Babasaheb Ambedkar argued that the state's role was to improve the social determinants of health, such as ensuring access to nutritious food, a stable income, and access to clean drinking water, the lack of which caused ill-health. In addition, Babasaheb Ambedkar argued that the removal of caste and class inequalities in access, not only to medical institutions, but to the determinants of health, was an essential responsibility of the state. Health required not just medicines and hospitals, but a grappling with India's grossly unequal social reality. As Mahanand observes:

Babasaheb's ideas on social security and public health sought to address these social realities through state efforts that could help bridge the inequalities that are deeply embedded in Indian society. His idea of a democracy emphasised a state that would intervene to break down structural divisions. His conception of public goods – such as health and education – were inclusive and equitable, seeking an equal distribution of and access to public health and social security, in order to ensure the overall well-being of the masses.[9]

Geopolitical Order and Postcolonial Societies in Twentieth-Century Asia

From the early part of the twentieth century, the rise of the Soviet Union resulted in a bipolar world. Most postcolonial societies asserted their independence by largely taking a position of non-alignment and asserting self-reliant development. This essentially meant that they were in a position to articulate and resist pressures from both the capitalist and socialist blocks. There was diversity in the politics of the Indian subcontinent during the 1940s. A stark

---

[8] Dr. Babasaheb Bhimrao Ambedkar is one of the architects of the Indian Constitution. Dr. Ambedkar fought for the rights of Dalits and other mistreated classes and to eradicate untouchability perpetuated by the upper castes in India). The caste system is a hierarchical system of socioeconomic order that is determined by birth. The Brahmins occupy the uppermost rung and the lowest rung is occupied by the Dalits. Ambedkar, B. R. (Bhimrao Ramji, 1891–1956), *Annihilation of Caste: An Undelivered Speech* (New Delhi: Arnold Publishers, 1990).

[9] Jadumani Mahanand, "India's Pandemic Response Needed Ambedkar's Vision of Social Security and Public Health," *The Caravan*, August 24, 2020, at: https://caravanmagazine.in/policy/indias-pandemic-response-needed-ambedkars-vision-of-social-security-and-public-health.

contrast in approaches to socioeconomic development was seen between India and Sri Lanka during the 1940s and 1950s.

While the leadership of the Indian nationalist movement was informed by a democratic and socialist ideology, Sri Lanka's leadership in the early years was influenced more by communism. Differences in political ideology influenced public policies both in the economic and social sectors. As observed by Rosenburg et al., "By the time Sri Lanka gained independence in 1948, government policy required health facilities to accept any patient who sought admission. In 1951, the government abolished all user fees. The idea was 'welfare first, then growth.'" Welfare, in addition to health, included investment in food subsidies, free education, and subsidized transportation. Public sector services were offered without consideration for the income or other status of beneficiaries.[10]

The approach to building welfare was shaped by differential ideologies in India and Sri Lanka. India was essentially an interventionist state, while the latter guaranteed employment, food security, health, and education. Thus, the extent of state support for welfarism varied in the South Asian region. The weakness of an interventionist welfare state in India was reflected in the underfunding of the public sector that had consequences for inequities in access to services across regions, caste, class, and gender.[11] The inadequacies of the public sector in India gave rise to diverse approaches to ensure equitable access to health services and addressing the social determinants of health by civil society groups. Another important fallout of a weak public sector was the expansion for markets in healthcare from the late 1970s.[12]

Social Medicine and the Role of Civil Society during the 1960s and 1970s

By the 1960s, social medicine acquired many avatars. American influence came through partnerships with the Rockefeller Foundation and with public health experts from the Harvard School of Public Health and Johns Hopkins University, who collaborated with the Christian Medical College in Ludhiana,

---

[10] Julie Rosenberg, Tristan Dreisbach, Claire Donovan, and Rebecca Weintraub, "Positive Outlier: Sri Lanka's Health Outcomes over Time," Harvard Business Publishing, 2018, Global Health Delivery Project, at: www.globalhealthdelivery.org/publications/positive-outlier-sri-lanka%E2%80%99s-health-outcomes-over-time-0.

[11] Niraja Gopa Jayal, "The Gentle Leviathan: Welfare and the Indian State," in Mohan Rao (ed.), *Disinvesting in Health: The World Bank's Prescriptions for Health* (New Delhi: Sage Publications,1999), 39–48; Rama Baru, Arnab Acharya, Sanghmitra Acharya, A. K. Shiva Kumar, and K. Nagaraj, "Inequities in Access to Health Services in India: Caste, Class and Region," *Economic and Political Weekly* 45, no.38 (September 18–24, 2010): 49–58.

[12] Rama V. Baru, *Private Health Care in India: Social Characteristics and Trends* (New Delhi: Sage Publications, 1998).

Punjab. The two projects, Khanna and Narangwal, were partnerships between the Rockefeller Foundation, Harvard School of Public Health, and Johns Hopkins. Rebecca Williams has documented the American influence through the Khanna and Narangwal studies in the Punjab that focused on primary healthcare and population control. The International Health Division of the Rockefeller Foundation had close links with the Harvard School of Public Health that was engaged in human ecology and population problems in developing countries. She argues that:

Gordon had been working alongside two of his MPH students, medical missionaries Carl Taylor and John Wyon, on plans for a population study as part of a broader series of epidemiological studies in the Ludhiana district of Punjab. The geographical setting was chosen for the practical reason that Taylor was set to take up a position as head of the newly-formed Department of Preventive Medicine at the Ludhiana Christian Medical College. Taylor, a medical missionary with the American Presbyterian mission, was already well known to the RF. He had been in a class of doctors that had been trained by the RF on behalf of the U.S. Army during the Second World War. In 1950 the RF awarded him a fellowship which allowed him to study at the HSPH, and in March 1952, they offered Taylor a position as head of the Department of Preventive Medicine at the RF-funded Vellore Christian Medical College in South India. Taylor declined the proposal on the basis that he was morally and mentally committed "to returning to Ludhiana. Taylor was born in North India to medical missionary parents, already spoke Hindi and Urdu fluently and was familiar with Punjab village life," and therefore wanted to work in the region.[13]

In 1961, the Narangwal study, which was similar to the Khanna Study of the 1950s, was initiated in Ludhiana under the aegis of the Christian Medical Colleges. As Chakrabarti states:

The Narangwal and the Khanna rural health-care projects, which attracted global attention, show that population control often operated as part of rural primary health-care initiatives that had started in India in the post-independence period. The Narangwal Rural Health Research Centre in three community development blocks of the Ludhiana district in the Punjab was established in 1961 and had similarities with the Khanna project of 1952 and rural health projects in other countries during the mid-20th century, such as in Danfa, Ghana, and Lampang, Thailand. Narangwal was a complex operation that established some of the basic modes of community participation in rural primary healthcare in India. The centre had its primary health clinics run by the Christian Medical College of Ludhiana.

Chakraborti describes the focus of these surveys as:

The medical team and the resident social scientists also undertook surveys on diet, nutrition, and child and maternal health. Crucially, the project also trained and

[13] Rebecca Williams, Rockefeller Foundation Support to the Khanna Study: Population Policy and the Construction of Demographic Knowledge, 1945–1953, Rockefeller Archive Centre Collection Home (January 1, 2011), at: www.issuelab.org/resources/28011/28011.pdf, p. 16.

employed nurses, midwives, and other community health workers. The family health workers, who were mostly women, had previous training as auxiliary nurse midwives and catered for various primary health concerns of the villages, including assisting in childbirth.[14]

This avatar of social medicine influenced the preventive and social medicine departments in medical colleges in India during this period. The circulation of the Americanized version of social medicine influenced the shaping of departments of preventive and social medicine in the medical colleges from the mid 1950s to the 1960s. One could argue that this version of preventive and social medicine departments in medical colleges privileged allopathic interventions and "desocialized" social medicine.

Another important avatar was that of critical social medicine from China, Latin America, and Africa that influenced several community health projects in India. Critical social medicine was heavily influenced by Marxian ideology and praxis that gave more importance to the structural factors that shape health outcomes and highlighted the limits to medicine. Several civil society movements in India in the late 1960s and 1970s were inspired by these country experiences. Social deficits in India energized non-partisan social movements around sociopolitical, living, working, and environmental conditions, with a demand to recognize that, "the struggle for liberation (was) not just from alien rule but also from internal decay."[15] These movements stimulated grassroots community health projects across different Indian states that connected health with larger social concerns and with a claim for social justice and local democratic control. These ideas, with those from other regions, had some influence in the comprehensive framing of Alma-Ata Declaration.

In the 1970s, social movements challenged the state in addressing inequality and poverty and implemented innovations at grassroots level, including community health projects. They reflected Gandhian, Christian, Marxist, and feminist ideas, most often a hybrid of the three. The Chinese idea of barefoot doctors changed the idea about a "health worker" and resonated with the Gandhian idea of "Arogya Swaraj,"[16] or "peoples' health in people's hands," a popular slogan that influenced many community health organizations that focused on social determinants of health and health systems. These social movements were of the view that only an equitable, sustainable, and just society can ensure

---

[14] Pratik Chakrabarti, "Health as Activism: Rethinking Social Medicine in India," *The Lancet* 399, no. 10341 (June 2022): 2096–7, Doi: 10.1016/S0140-6736(22)00979-5. P.2097.

[15] Rajni Kothari, "Party and State in our Times: The Rise of Non-party Political Formations," *Alternatives* 9, no. 4 (October 1984): 541–64, doi.org/10.1177/030437548400900404.

[16] Arogya Swaraj is inspired by Gandhi's ideals and it includes understanding of oneself, including one's mind, body, conscience, and conduct. It includes the idea that an individual must reduce dependency on doctors and drug manufacturers. Therefore it translates to the idea of People's Health in People's Hands.

health for all. Health action was seen to call for a struggle against harms such as pollution, poor living, dietary and psychosocial conditions, and for the promotion of an alternative, healthier pattern of development. While many actions for this lie outside the healthcare system, they saw the health system as the most visible determinant of health, calling for a public system that would be responsive to people's needs and be socially accountable. They rejected blame placed on poor people, women, and other marginalized groups for their own ill-health, seeing this as a consequence of elite dominance in decision-making, in and beyond the health sector.

These ideas resonated with (and contributed to) the principles and design of comprehensive Primary Health Care (PHC) in the 1978 Alma Ata-Declaration. While they were implemented in limited local settings, alliances were formed on specific issues in the 1980s and 1990s that gave them stronger policy visibility and influence. Diverse networks, women's and consumer movements, doctors, and social activists converged on issues such as the promotion of essential medicines, breastfeeding, local traditional farming and food security, and on the protection of medicinal plants and traditional therapies. As examples, the Medico Friends Circle (MFC) formed in 1974 by a group of doctors and social activists who broadly subscribed to Gandhian and socialist ideologies to critique technology-determined disease-control programs.[17] One of the civil society coalitions in western India led a campaign on the "right to food" through school-feeding programs, universal preschool childcare, employment, and food security for vulnerable social groups. The women's movement engaged in a diverse set of health issues like hazardous contraceptives such as EP drugs, Net En, Norplant, Depo-Provera, sex-selective abortions, and coercive state population-control policies, as well as domestic and state-sponsored violence against women.

Comprehensive PHC and rights-based approaches to health were further advanced by social movements, especially by the Indian Peoples' Health Movement (PHM), termed Jan Swasthya Abhiyan (JSA), which was formed in 2000. JSA is a coalition of about twenty national networks and more than a thousand local organizations across India working on health, science, women's issues, and development. It has opposed commercialization of medical care and argued for pro-people changes in the health sector. It has taken up research, advocacy, legal action, and alliances on the right to health and social determinants of health. It has highlighted inequities in health outcomes and access to health services, pointing also to a social gradient that has led some parts of the middle class to equally experience declining health outcomes.

---

[17] N. B. Sarojini et al., *Women's Right to Health, National Human Rights Commission* (New Delhi: National Human Rights Commission, 2006), at: http://dev.ecoguineafoundation.com/uploads/5/4/1/5/5415260/womens-health_rights.pdf.

Following the 2008 World Health Organization (WHO) Commission on Social Determinants on Health Report, JSA energized PHM branches in Asia to form a South–South alliance in order to draw attention to the inadequacy of state policies on social determinants, with different networks covering issues such as equitable social development, migrant health, pesticide safety, and the determinants of HIV.

Several of the health NGO initiatives were led by doctors and allied professionals who provided leadership to these projects, drawing from diverse ideological moorings – Marxist, feminist, populist – that broadly subscribed to the critiques of capitalist development. During this period, several resistance movements led by organized and unorganized working class, women, Dalits, Tribal, and religious minorities also had ideas of social medicine as a part of their understanding. Several of these movements highlighted social inequalities and the limits of allopathy in addressing well-being and health. This in essence formed the rubric of the radical ideology that included the organized left, Gandhian and Ambedkarites, feminist, Catholic and Christian health networks. The diverse ideological positions focused on inequality, poverty, and the unmet needs of marginalized groups. They were critical of the bureaucratic and top down approaches of the public sector and emphasized the importance of a people-centered health services, recognition and legitimization of folk practices and indigenous systems of medicine, and going beyond to address the social determinants of health.

Thus, the idea and practice of social medicine in its various avatars remained vibrant among social movements and civil society organizations in the Indian subcontinent. The influence of these various avatars remained largely outside the purview of state-sponsored medicine. However, there have been certain periods when some of the practices in community health projects were translated into mainstream health policy.

Community Health Projects

There were several community health projects that experimented with training community health workers for basic care, demystified medicine and engaged in traditional medicine in its various forms. A few of these were initiated by missionaries in remote parts of the country, where they engaged in women's health, empowerment, and education. Others were inspired by Gandhian ideology to demystify Western medicine. As Iyengar observes:

Gandhi was critical of biomedical approaches, but also and saw limitations in traditional healing systems. He saw hospitals as a "symptom of decay," and called for more focus on prevention of diseases and on mental, physical and spiritual health. Rather than the top-down application of technological approaches, he perceived that achieving health depended on living healthy lives, starting at the village level, as a form of a social determinants approach. He advocated for community health workers, or *Arogya Samrakshan Samiti* and for primary health centers that promote healthy lifestyles and family care, advise on diets and production of healthy foods, promote safe water and sanitation and apply herbal therapies based on the available biodiversity.[18]

This approach made the community and primary level of care as two important pillars for health services and healthy societies. The Gandhian paradigm was taken up by many grassroots groups and movements in the 1980s and 1990s. This led to the rise of several coalitions around specific issues of human rights, responsible development, health, and social rights. The constituents of these coalitions consisted of political parties, leftist trade unions, Gandhian, Dalit, Adivasi, and feminist groups.

It is interesting to note that elements of the American ideas of community medicine were adapted by a generation of doctors who founded a few health projects in rural India. Furthermore, the leadership of several of these community health projects were in the hands of doctors who had done their Masters in Public Health at Johns Hopkins. There was much variety in ideology, praxis, and innovations in the practice of social medicine through the 1970s and 1980s among such doctors who chose to return to India. One could argue that these projects combined the diverse avatars of social medicine in their praxis. There was uptake of these diverse experiences of community health projects that was translated into national health policy with the introduction of the Community Health Workers (CHWs) scheme in 1977. The government scheme drew inspiration from the barefoot doctor scheme in China and several community health projects in India that resonated with the Gandhian ideas of strengthening people's health in people's hands.

There are some well-known examples of community health projects that had introduced health workers and also tried to address some aspect of social determinants of health. These projects were primarily located in rural areas.[19] Several of the community health projects were initiated by clinicians. Prominent among these are the Comprehensive Rural Health (CRPH) project and Society for Education, Action and Research in Community Health (SEARCH) in Maharashtra. The former was founded by Drs. Raj and Mabelle

---

[18] Sudarshan Iyengar, "Health Care: The Gandhian Way," 13th HM Patel Memorial Lecture, Karamsad, Anand, Gujarat, 2017, at: www.charutarhealth.org/sites/default/files/13thhm_patel_memorial_lecture_text_new_0.pdf.

[19] Saroj Pachauri, *Reaching India's Poor: Non-governmental Approaches to Community Health* (New Delhi: Sage Publications, 1994). The Community Health Workers of Jamkhed; the village health workers of the Indo Dutch Project; the lay first aiders of VHS-Adyar; the link workers on the tea gardens in South India; the Family care volunteers and Health Aides of RUHSA; the MCH workers of CINI-Calcutta; the Swasthya Mithras of Banaras Hindu University-Varanasi; the Sanyojaks of Banwasi Seva Ashram, Uttar Pradesh; CHW course of St. John's Medical College – Bangalore; the Rehbar-e-sehat scheme of Kashmir government; the CHVs of Sewa Rural and the Community Health Guides of many other projects.

Arole and the latter by Drs. Abhay and Rani Bang. Both the couples had their medical education in India and later gained their Masters in Public Health from Johns Hopkins University. The Aroles set up their project in the 1970s, with a vision of providing primary healthcare services using appropriate technology. Health services were integrated within a multisectoral approach to address social inequalities and ill-health, poverty, poor women's status, and the caste system. An important contribution toward upscaling the project was their training programs for community health workers in Non-Government Organizations (NGOs) from different parts of the country. SEARCH was established in a tribal area, Gadchiroli, that had one of the poorest health indicators. The Schedule Tribe communities in India are among the most marginalized and in some cases their socioeconomic and health status is even worse than Dalits. The focus of their work was on maternal and child health in the tribal areas that did not have functional health services.

An overview of these CHWs in the non-government sector showed that frontline workers were predominantly women volunteers belonging to the lower socioeconomic groups. They were trained to use strategies to empower and represent marginalized communities across different states in India. Some of the community initiatives by NGOs were translated and upscaled into state-supported programs. An example of these are the Women's Development program in Rajasthan and the Mahila Samakhya program in 1988 by the Central government. Both of these were government-led programs in partnership with NGOs. There were specific initiatives within this program to address women's education, empowerment, health, and specifically reproductive health.

Alliances for Promotion of Social Medicine from the South Asian Region

The Non-Aligned Movement of the postcolonial societies and leadership of clinicians, public health, and civil society organizations formed alliances for the promotion of social medicine. Drawing inspiration from the Bandung Conference on Rural Hygiene in August 1937, the importance of state-funded health services and addressing intersectoral action for health was foregrounded. The ideas of the Bandung Conference were instrumental in shaping the Primary Healthcare approach in 1978.[20] The Conference drew attention to the relationship between high levels of poverty and ill-health across developed and developing countries. This was much higher in the rural as compared to urban populations. The poor bore the burden of

---

[20] Imrana Qadeer and Rama Baru, "Shrinking Spaces for the 'Public' in Contemporary Public Health," *Development and Change* 47, no. 4 (June 6, 2016): 760–81, at: https:/10.1111/dech.12246.

morbidity and mortality of communicable diseases with limited access to food, work, housing, and medical care.

The idea of social medicine was kept alive by several prominent physicians and practitioners in public health in the South Asian region. Deeply committed to the principles of equity and rational care, many formed alliances across the south to question Western dominance. Broadly, the NAM engaged in self-reliance and the need to push back on the dominance of multinationals in the economy and social sectors. Many of the ideas on rural hygiene that were discussed at the Bandung Conference in 1937 strengthened the practice of social medicine through the next few decades and many of these ideas were resurrected in the Alma-Ata Declaration for Primary Health Care in 1978.

There were discussions on how to organize health services at a population level and examples were drawn upon from Eastern Europe and later John Grant's attempts to apply the same principles in rural China. The emphasis on state intervention for comprehensive health services with a well-worked-out referral system was accepted and practiced by the advocates of social medicine.

The 1970s saw the coming together of leadership from the south of professionals within a political climate of heightened radicalism. The leadership for radical reform in an important subsystem of the health service system, namely pharmaceuticals, came from Sri Lanka during the early 1970s. It was the dominance of Left politics that provided spaces for nationalization of the pharmaceutical industry and curbing multinational corporations. Dr. Seneka Bibilie, who was a clinician and supporter of the Left parties, envisioned the Sri Lankan National Drug policy. As Perera observes:

Professor Bibile's principle of developing a rational pharmaceutical policy intended to ensure that people would get reasonable drugs at an affordable price, was based on ensuring that doctors prescribe the minimum required drugs to treat the patient's illness. This policy was used with enormous benefit to Third World countries as a model for expansion of policies based on rational pharmaceutical use in other countries as well by the WHO, the United Nations Conference on Trade and Development (UNCTAD) and NAM. Due to the far reaching effects of his proposals and policies, he has been called the "greatest medical benefactor of humanity that Sri Lanka has hitherto produced." UNCTAD, in fact scrutinized the Sri Lankan practice, concluding that an examination of the Sri Lankan model could give other third-world countries an insight into ways of devising, developing and executing integrated national medicinal drugs policies.[21]

The Sri Lankan experience found global resonance that gave rise to a number of networks in India and later Bangladesh. Dr. K. Balasubramaniam, who was Bibilie's student and protégé, became part of Health Action International (HAI).

---

[21] K. K. S. Perera, "Dr. Senaka Bibile's 'Drug Price Policy' Was Feared by Transnational Pharmaceutical Industry Known as 'Big Pharma,'" Posted by Administrator on November 26, 2016, 1:21 a.m., at: https://dbsjeyaraj.com/dbsj/archives/49865.

HAI was formed with clinicians and public health persons from both the developed and developing countries, who strongly advocated for a rational drug policy as an important aspect of social medicine. Dr. Zafarullah Chowdhury from the Gonashasthya Kendra in Bangladesh and the All India Drug Action Network (AIDAN) in India are examples of South Asian partnerships with HAI for accountability on pharmaceutical products, rational drug policies, and essential drugs. In addition, several of these movements focused on banning pesticides, banned and restricted products, and hazardous waste exports.

Institutionalization and Practice of the Many Avatars of Social Medicine

The many avatars of social medicine and its practice is seen in several community health projects and also addressed by health movements across India. In this section, I present vignettes of efforts to institutionalize the idea of critical social medicine in a university and of a network of medical practitioners, social scientists, and activists who had diverse institutional affiliations called the Medico Friends Circle.

A unique effort to institutionalize the theory and practice of social medicine as an academic discipline was the establishment of the Centre of Social Medicine and Community Health in the Jawaharlal Nehru University, New Delhi, during the 1970s. In a radical departure, the Centre was located in the School of Social Sciences in the university and not attached to a medical college. The committee that endorsed this saw the need to go beyond curative medicine and engage with the relationship between society and health. The committee was critical of the curriculum of the Preventive and Social Medicine or Community Medicine departments in medical colleges and sought to expand the scope to include the social determination of health. There was a view that innovation in approaches, curriculum, and pedagogy would be possible only outside the confines of the medical college with greater interaction with social sciences.

The Centre was founded by a public health clinician, Dr. D. Banerji,[22] who had worked in community health projects and had engaged in a study of the National Tuberculosis Institute that informed the Indian TB program. Instead of a vertically driven program, this study advocated for strengthening the general health services to address the felt needs of people suffering from TB in a community. This collaborative study of Indian scientists with the WHO was a departure from the vertical programing for controlling communicable diseases globally in the 1960s. Subsequently, Dr. Imrana Qadeer, a pediatrician by training and deeply engaged in the Medico Friends Circle and several community

---

[22] Debabar Banerji, *Health and Family Planning Services in India* (New Delhi: Lok Paksh, 1985), 174–252.

health projects, joined the Centre. Over the years, the composition of the faculty drawn from medical and social sciences for interdisciplinary approach engaged with students from diverse disciplinary backgrounds. The curriculum for the master's and doctoral programs have an interdisciplinary approach to Indian health problems. The core concerns addressed were inequality, poverty, and an intersectoral approach for health and well-being. This Centre is one of its kind in South Asia because the concerns are derived from an understanding of the relationship between society and health.

Medico Friends Circle

Many health activists from the 1970s to the 1990s were either involved in or closely followed the discussions of the MFC *Bulletin*. The exchange of mail between two young barefoot doctors, coping with the difficulties of providing rural healthcare is often credited with the formation of MFC. The first meetings of MFC in the early 1970s was a discussion group of ten to twenty persons who were keen to discuss and debate rural work and health services, rather than to institutionalize their work into more formal organizations. The group refused any external funding. This emerged as a platform for academics, practicing doctors, and civil society organizations who engaged in ideas of social medicine by emphasizing politics of health, giving priority to the health of the poor, and concerns regarding social inequalities. The membership of MFC intersected with AIDAN, HAI, and several networks of Christian and Catholic medical missions. This was a period of growth of civil society groups setting up community health projects taking an anti-state stance but campaigning, advocating, and practicing social medicine in local contexts. Several of these actors later came together to form the peoples' health movement globally and the Indian Jan Swasthya Abhiyan.

In addition to publishing the journal and carrying out studies, activists in the movement helped to create alternative hospitals whose particularity was to be co-managed by several stakeholders. These health centers could, for instance, be run by unions, workers, and civil society groups, the most famous being the Shaheed Hospital, built in 1983 in Madhya Pradesh, with the support of Dr. Binayak Sen. In doing so, they chose to bridge the cultural and epistemic boundaries between the expert doctor and the impoverished patient: all of them had to be involved on an equal footing in the construction and organization of work in health centers.

Neoliberalism, Commercialization, and Social Medicine

With the introduction of liberalization policies in the 1990s, the spaces for critical social medicine started shrinking in the Indian subcontinent. The erstwhile radical politics that informed civil society discourse were marginalized with the introduction of the Structural Adjustment Program (SAP) of the World Bank that privileges privatization. The neoliberal agenda was antithetical to social medicine perspectives and the Alma-Ata Declaration that emphasized the important role of the state to ensure redistributive justice, health as a right, and going beyond health services to address the structural determinants. On the other hand, neoliberal health reforms believes that the private sector is more efficient than the public sector. The clear demarcation in roles of the public and private sector undermined the comprehensiveness of health services as espoused by the principles of social medicine and primary healthcare approach. The private sector is responsible for the provisioning of curative services in order to ensure cost efficiency of delivery of services, freedom of consumer choice, and the promotion of competition among private entities. While the "for-profit" sector was privileged, the "non-profit" sector was seen as an important player in public–private partnerships for preventive and promotive services. This was seen in several externally funded disease-control programs for tuberculosis, HIV, malaria and blindness control.[23] Apart from existing NGOs and external funding from multilateral organizations like the World Bank in partnership with bilateral organizations, several new NGOs emerged in the health sector. These newer organizations were influenced by market models of service delivery. As a result, complex partnerships involving public, non-profit, and for-profit entities emerged.[24]

Alliances of some civil society actors against the SAP continued to pressure the state by providing evidence on rising inequities in access to health services, weaknesses of public provisioning, and the pitfalls of rampant commercialization of services. In 2004, when the United Progressive Alliance consisting of a coalition of the Congress and left-wing parties was voted to power, there was once again an opportunity for civil society to engage in policy. In health, the National Rural Health Mission (NRHM) provided a limited opportunity to restructure rural health services. Many ideas of community health volunteers as a link worker between the community and formal health services, communitization, decentralization to local levels, and so on became part of the design of the NRHM. Several civil society actors were engaged in the planning,

---

[23] Rama V. Baru and Madhurima Nundy, "Blurring of Boundaries: Public–Private Partnerships in Health Services in India," *Economic and Political Weekly* 43, no.4 (January 2008): 62–71, at: www.epw.in/journal/2008/04/special-articles/blurring-boundaries-public-private-partnerships-health-services. These complex partnerships were seen in the Reproductive and Child Health program wherein social franchising was introduced. The case of Janani in Bihar where a partnership between financing company and local actors was cited as an innovate partnership. Similar partnerships were also seen in the tuberculosis program.

[24] Rama V. Baru and Anuj Kapilashrami, "Unpackaging the Private Sector in Health Policy and Services," in Anuj Kapilashrami and Rama V. Baru (eds) and Madhurima Nundy (eds.), *Global Health Governance and Commercialisation of Public Health in India* (London: Routledge, 2018), 117–35.

training, and monitoring of innovative interventions.[25] The process of mobilization of several small and large community health projects of diverse ideological persuasions to engage with the NRHM was painstaking and commendable.
However, these initiatives could not reverse commercialization that had gained
a prominent place in the Indian health services. One could argue that commercialization had fragmented comprehensive health services broadly along the
lines of "public" and private goods. The for-profit sector dominated the health
services and reduced the role of the state to providing preventive services.

The Structural Adjustment Program of the 1990s, with its funding for select
disease control programs like HIV, malaria, tuberculosis, and blindness, promoted public–private partnerships with NGOs and "for-profit" organizations.
The external funding of the World Bank flowed to state governments and
NGOs for these select programs with the introduction of parastatal institutions. The disease-specific funding resulted in several older health NGOs shifting their priorities to attract available funds from multilateral, bilateral, and
American foundations. The funding was tied to conditionalities with the broad
agenda of privatization.

Another important area of influence of the World Bank and American
schools of public health was in education. In the 1990s, several private institutions offering Masters in Public Health were set up. Prominent among them
was the Public Health Foundation of India that was a public–private partnership with corporate funding from global and Indian companies, in partnership
with the government. Much of the curriculum was influenced by the American
schools of public health. This was broadly the trend followed by other schools
of public health across the country. The many avatars of social medicine that
were in circulation from the 1970s onward had become peripheral and there
was a tendency for homogenization and globalization of mainstream public
health curricula. This is not something that is peculiar to the Indian subcontinent and is seen in parts of Africa and Latin America, too.[26]

With the change in government in 2014 and the emergence of the right-
wing Bhartiya Janata Party, the spaces for critical engagement by civil society

[25] Kaveri Gill, "A Primary Evaluation of Service Delivery under the National Rural Health
Mission (NRHM): Findings from a Study in Andhra Pradesh, Uttar Pradesh, Bihar and
Rajasthan," Planning Commission of India, Government of India (June 2009), at: http://
environmentportal.in/files/wrkp_1_09.pdf2009.
[26] Eric D. Carter, "Social Medicine and International Expert Networks in Latin America, 1930–
1945," *Global Public Health* 14, nos. 6–7 (June–July 2019): 791–802, doi.org/10.1080/1
7441692.2017.1418902. Rene Loewenson, Eugenio Villar, Rama Baru, and Robert Marten,
"Achieving Healthy Societies – Ideas and Learning from Diverse Regions for Shared Futures,"
Training and Research Support Centre, Alliance for Health Policy and Health Systems Research
(November 2020), at: www.tarsc.org/publications/documents/Healthy%20societies%20
paper%202020%20final.pdf; Erasmus D. Prinsloo, "A Comparison between Medicine from an
African (Ubuntu) and Western Philosophy." *Curationis* 24, no. 1 (March 2001): 58–65, Doi:
10.4102/curationis.v24i1.802.

organizations started shrinking.[27] Several NGOs that were engaged in human and civil rights, health, women's issues, and aligned with social movements and political parties struggling for the marginalized, came under scrutiny. Many of them who were critical of the government were labelled as "anti-national." They had to face various forms of harassment by the government, including imprisonment of civil liberty activists. There were several efforts to curb the activities of NGOs receiving foreign funding by introducing amendments to the Foreign Contributions (Regulation) Act. Several civil society organizations that were questioning state power came under scrutiny and their sources of funding from foreign organizations were restricted. This resulted in further shrinking of spaces for strengthening ideas of social medicine.

Covid-19 and the Re-emergence of Social Medicine and Its Distortion

The Covid-19 pandemic brought back the importance of social medicine and comprehensive primary healthcare for public health. There was much debate on the need to strengthen the role of the state for health services and the social determinants of health. There was a broad agreement that public-health-strengthening was important. However, in the Indian subcontinent, this did not translate into increased public investments in health nor for addressing the economic and social disruptions for the working and middle classes. Ironically, the government advocated for greater privatization of curative services and medical education during this period. There was no effort to address the private sector that largely did not respond to the humanitarian tragedy. As Baru and Bisht observed:

The preparedness of private hospitals in dealing with the COVID-19 epidemic and the extremely variable quality of services in the poorly regulated private sector is now becoming apparent. Even internationally accredited hospitals in Mumbai and Delhi were ill-prepared to deal with the outbreak of coronavirus. A large number of health workers in these hospitals tested positive since they did not have adequate Personal Protection Equipment (PPEs) for doctors, nurses and other staff members. Once the positive cases were identified, some of these hospitals shut down.[28]

The Covid-19 pandemic has resulted in economic and political instability, especially in Sri Lanka. The rise of right-wing politics in the region has deeply

[27] Ajay Gudavarthy and G. Vijay, "Social Policy and Political Mobilization in India: Producing Hierarchical Fraternity and Polarized Differences," *Development and Change* 51, no. 2 (February 2020): 463–84.

[28] Rama V. Baru and Ramilla Bisht, "Government Must Stop Appeasing the Private Healthcare Sector," *The Wire* (April 25, 2020), at: https://thewire.in/government/coronavirus-private-hospitals.

compromised democratic spaces. These tendencies go against the ethical and moral imperatives that underline the many avatars of social medicine.

In conclusion, this chapter has tried to capture the ideological diversity that characterized the many avatars of social medicine. It elaborated on the global, national, and local avatars engaged in the idea of social medicine in the public sector and civil society organizations. It has argued that since the 1990s, neoliberal ideas and policies constituted a major setback for the idea of social medicine, both globally and in India. This led to a shrinking of the space for public health.

15   Social Medicine, *Otherwise*
Cuban Health(Care) as Political Praxis

P. Sean Brotherton

> This cancer of the mind ... consists of thinking all too sadly that certain
> things "are," while others, which well might be, "are not"
> André Breton, *Manifesto of Surrealism* ([1930] 1972)[1]

The outbreak of the highly pathogenic viral infection caused by SARS-CoV-2, popularly known as Covid-19, was declared a global pandemic by the World Health Organization (WHO) on March 11, 2020. Within days of this announcement, many countries focused exclusively on containment, treatment, and prevention among their respective populaces, quickly shuttering their national borders; implementing travel restrictions and lockdown measures; and rolling out social distancing, quarantine, and isolation guidelines. The Cuban Government implemented similar measures at home, and, confident in its strategic investments in its public healthcare system for over half a century, simultaneously embarked on another project on a global scale.

Armed with biomedical knowledge and technical expertise, on March 22, the island nation sent the Henry Reeve Medical Brigade, comprising thirty-six doctors, fifteen nurses, and additional logistics specialists, to Italy's Lombardy region. Italy had already reported 54,000 confirmed Covid cases and 4,825 related deaths. The all-too-familiar scene of arrival, a dramaturgy of Western-styled humanitarianism, captured headlines: an army of white lab coats unloading boxes of supplies, rapid deployment of medical tents, and staff poised to deliver much needed aid in a time of crisis. Under the rare glare of the global media spotlight, the Cuban humanitarian brigade of fifty-two doctors and health workers established a field hospital alongside the Crema Maggiore Hospital in Milan (see Figure 15.1). As dubbed by the media, the "army of white coats," this scene became note- and *news*worthy in no small part because of the actors involved, who inverted geopolitical, racial, and gendered hierarchies.[2]

---

[1] André Breton, *Manifesto of Surrealism*, trans. by Richard Seaver and Helen R. Lane (Ann Arbor, MI: University of Michigan Press, [1930] 1972), 187.
[2] Sarah Marsha and John Zodzi, "Cuba Punches above Weight with 'White Coat Army' During Pandemic," *Reuters*, September 14, 2020, para. 6.

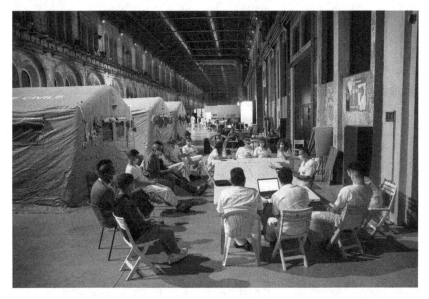

Figure 15.1 Cuban and Italian doctors meeting in Turin, Italy, to combat Covid-19. Photo: Diana Bagnoli, supported by the National Geographic Society's Emergency Fund for Journalists.

The subtext: Italy, the third wealthiest country in the European Union, struggling to manage the exponential number of coronavirus cases and a mounting death toll in the early phase of the pandemic, requests biomedical expertise from a middle-income Caribbean country. The reversal of roles of protagonists, experts, heroes, and victims that traditionally characterize Western humanitarianism and capital flows from North to South set the stage for a theater of the absurd, with a surrealist script of an illogical plot.

What makes this scene *absurd*, as the media spectacle revealed, is that the common sense of humanitarianism naturalizes certain geopolitical actors performing scripted roles of the donor (Global North) and the recipient (Global South). The illogical, or the presumed implausibility of Cuba as a principal actor in global health, disrupts the imperial gaze of humanitarianism. Such a gaze reasserts colonial legacies of empire, invoking racialized constructions of people, places, and things. Rather than analyze this as a residual artifact of history as incidental, Adia Benton stresses, this is a "foundational aspect of how humanitarianism functions."[3] Indispensable work at the intersection of global health and humanitarianism has produced a rich analytic vocabulary to

---

[3] Adia Benton, "Risky Business: Race, Nonequivalence and the Humanitarian Politics of Life," *Visual Anthropology* 29, no. 2 (2016): 187–203, at 198.

denaturalize the seemingly apolitical global health industry.[4] As a humanitarian apparatus claiming the right of intervention and interference beyond sovereign borders, global health functions as a biopolitical regime, in and through competing claims on who has duties to whom and why. Fine-tuned ethnographic studies have unraveled parts of this assemblage, including the methods, assumptions, financing, and political inner workings.[5] In so doing, these studies demonstrate how interventions, including biomedical technologies (from pharmaceuticals to health learning campaigns), are tethered to notions of standardization, economic theories of development, conditional trade agreements, and militarism.[6]

Still, what remains out of view, or to see without seeing, is the inequality built into the very design of this assemblage, coded into its DNA. Global histories of violence and subjugation, epistemic and otherwise, continually reproduce and solidify the same actors (e.g., the definition of problems, funding, and research solutions) and targets (e.g., subjects of the intervention) of this field. The assemblage moves along well-oiled paths, many long established since the beginning of European imperialist expansionism in the sixteenth century.[7] Decentering the dominant script of humanitarianism requires considering traces of other and often unacknowledged histories and political formations, experiences, and knowledge-production systems that might appear, at first, as peripheral to what has become legible as social medicine.

For example, since the Cuban Revolution of 1959, the socialist island nation, classified as a low-income country in the Global South, has invested considerable capital, labor, and infrastructure in developing a comprehensive medical program. This program includes accessible healthcare delivery integrated into an extensive, multitiered program of medical education, training, and advanced research in biotechnical innovation. Under the umbrella of medical internationalism, the country has imparted this biomedical expertise through mobile medical brigades dispatched to geographically diverse locales. Since the early 1960s, the government has sent over 400,000 medical brigades

---

[4] See, for example, Peter Redfield, *Life in Crisis: The Ethical Journey of Doctors without Borders* (Berkeley: University of California Press, 2013); Miriam Ticktin, *Casualties of Care: Immigration and the Politics of Humanitarianism in France* (Berkeley: University of California Press, 2011).

[5] Any attempt at generating a bibliography of critical global health studies would be a mammoth endeavor. A wealth of crucial interventions exists in social science journals such as *Medicine Anthropology Theory*, *Global Public Health*, and edited volumes dedicated to reimagining global health. See, for example, João Biehl and Adriana Petryna (eds.), *When People Come First: Critical Studies in Global Health* (Princeton, NJ: Princeton University Press), 2013.

[6] Didier Fassin and Mariella Pandolfi (eds.), *Contemporary States of Emergency: The Politics of Military and Humanitarian Interventions* (New York, NY, and Cambridge, MA: Zone Books, 2010).

[7] Randall M. Packard, *A History of Global Health: Interventions into the Lives of Other Peoples* (Baltimore: Johns Hopkins University Press, 2016).

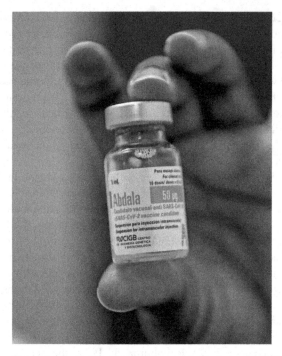

Figure 15.2 Abdala Covid-19 vaccine. Photo by Yamil Lage/AFP via Getty Images.

to provide short- and long-term healthcare in over 164 countries, more than all the G8 industrial nations combined. These brigades, engaged in "humanitarian biomedicine," address acute and chronic lack of access to primary healthcare (and, to a limited extent, secondary and tertiary care) for historically vulnerable and underserved areas and populations.[8]

Cuba has designed prize-winning primary healthcare delivery models, including tailored responses to controlling epidemics and developing innovations in vaccine production and experimental cancer therapies. In July 2021, Cuba became the first and only country in Latin America to successfully produce its Covid-19 vaccine, known as Abdala (Figure 15.2). The vaccine takes its name, Abdala, from a patriotic drama verse by José Martí, a heroic symbol of Cuba's struggle for independence from Spain. The country is also home to the world's largest medical school, the Latin American School of Medicine, which since 2005, has graduated tens of thousands of physicians from low-income

[8] I borrow the term "humanitarian biomedicine" from Andrew Lakoff, *Unprepared: Global Health in a Time of Emergency* (Oakland, CA: University of California Press, 2017).

communities in Africa, Asia, and the Americas, including the United States. Through this reshaping of economies of care, Cuba has garnered accolades for transforming the landscape and bodies in healthcare delivery in Latin America, the Caribbean, and several African countries. In scope, depth, and breadth, the magnitude of this brand of humanitarianism far outpaces the most iconic faces of the contemporary global health industry, such as Doctors Without Borders, the Red Cross, or UNICEF.[9]

Despite brandishing these evidentiary forms of success, Cuba's quest for global health equity occupies the margin or the subaltern in the global health landscape, even for a field that uncritically celebrates quantitative metrics.[10] For most observers in North America and Europe, Cuba likely occupies the rhetorical and discursive space of the singular case study or alternative, if it even makes an appearance. It is an outlier, a kind of exceptionalism marginal to mainstream discussions of global health equity; it is in the footnote or addendum of history, outside of central debates, or reduced to a compelling "theory from the South." This positionality is often glossed as minoritized or identarian and is usually significant only in unveiling moral, political, economic, and affective attachments. Ultimately, such discourses circulate in the register of singularity, a local among taken-for-granted universals.

How do we understand the absence–presence of Cuba's medical-internationalism efforts as a non-event in the contemporary global health landscape? This chapter extends and reformulates Michel-Rolph Trouillot's incisive historical analysis of how the Haitian Revolution, even as it happened, was unthinkable.[11] This event, he argues, challenged "that which one cannot conceive within the range of possible alternatives which perverts all answers because it defies the terms under which the questions are phrased."[12] As a thought experiment: what would it mean to engage seriously with Cuba's approach to social medicine – moving it from the footnote to the main text? Notes toward a speculative answer shape this chapter. I examine the foundational assertations structuring contemporary global health – the problematics, concepts, methods, and practices – that render different imaginaries of care and aid legible and thus thinkable. Many of these assertions remain unchallenged, which include world making assumptions what Trouillot terms "North Atlantic universal fictions" (e.g., progress,

[9] These numbers are reviewed in Robert Huish, "Why Does Cuba 'Care' So Much? Understanding the Epistemology of Solidarity in Global Health Outreach," *Public Health Ethics* 7, no. 3 (2014): 261–76.

[10] I borrow the phrase "avalanche of printed numbers" from Ian Hacking, "Biopower and the Avalanche of Printed Numbers," *Humanities in Society* 5 (1982): 279–95.

[11] Michel-Rolph Trouillot, *Silencing the Past: Power and the Production of History* (Boston: Beacon Press, 2015).

[12] Trouillot, *Silencing the Past*, 82.

development, modernity, nation-state, freedom, equity). More than discursive abstractions, Trouillot explains, such fictions operate as transcendental categories that "appear to refer to things as they exist, but because they are rooted in a particular history, they evoke multiple layers of sensibilities, persuasions, cultural assumptions, and ideological choices tied to that localized history."[13]

Drawing on more than two decades of extensive ethnographic research with Cuban health professionals, government officials, and everyday citizens, both in and outside of Cuba, this chapter approaches the discussion of Cuban social medicine as a form of speculative thinking, embracing possibility as an abstract noun – that is, the *what-if* – to provoke "political and ethical imagination in the present," echoing María de Puíg de la Bellacasa work. She argues that this entails drawing out the "existential domains of care as something open-ended."[14] To attend this way of seeing Otherwise requires developing an ethics of care, where ethics "cannot be about a realm of normative moral obligations but rather about thick, impure involvement in a world where the question of how to care needs to be posed."[15] Such an approach demands cultivating an analytic "toward reading and seeing otherwise; toward reading and seeing something in excess of what is caught in the frame," as argued by Christina Sharpe.[16] I commence with a snapshot of the centerpiece of Cuba's current primary healthcare system, the neighborhood clinic. Since the early 1980s, this clinic has served as a site of heated debate on the country's biopolitical project, wherein the plasticity of biomedicine, a term I unpack shortly, transforms, even distorts, the perceived rigidity of the biological and social body, and the body politic.

The Plasticity of Biomedicine

After her daily round of home visits, Dr. Ruiz,[17] flustered by the unrelenting humidity of August, was returning to her *consultorio* (clinic) in the early evening. My elderly neighbors, patients of Ruiz, introduced us in 2000. Our bustling residential block, *la Plaza*, comprising low-rise buildings and multi-level homes now converted into several apartments, was typical of this urban neighborhood a few miles west of the Havana city center. Ruiz, who lived in a small apartment adjacent to her *consultorio*, was a familiar face. She made

[13] Michel-Rolph Trouillot, "North Atlantic Universals: Analytical Fictions, 1492–1945," *South Atlantic Quarterly* 101, no. 4 (2003): 839–58, at 847.
[14] María Puig de la Bellacasa, *Matters of Care: Speculative Ethics in More than Human Worlds* (Minneapolis, MN: University of Minnesota Press, 2017), 6.
[15] Puig de la Bellacasa, *Matters of Care*, 6.
[16] Christina Sharpe, *In the Wake: On Blackness and Being* (Durham, NC: Duke University Press, 2016), 117.
[17] I have used pseudonyms to protect the identity of the individuals who participated in this research.

her daily afternoon home visits to patients who required additional monitoring and care, accompanied by one of a rotating roster of nurses. On the day we met for coffee, two cases were worrying Ruiz. A young woman had missed her prenatal checkup and an older man lived alone with chronic health problems.

"I am like an annoying family member," Ruiz joked as she discussed her patients, who were also her neighbors and friends. Most were accustomed to her cheerful nature, peppered with health promotion, education, and sometimes clinical interventions. Prenatal appointments are not optional, Ruiz asserted. The young woman's missed appointment was a reason for concern. Slightly embarrassed by the impromptu visit, the young woman assured the doctor that the appointment had just slipped her mind. Ruiz used the opportunity to discuss the additional monthly rations from the local *bodega* of food and vitamin supplements allotted for the young woman's pregnancy.

In Ruiz's interactions within the neighborhood, she always skillfully balanced admonishing and encouragement, establishing a familial rapport with many of the people of *la Plaza*. The physician, in her mid-thirties and with a family of her own, was accessible and often the person people reached out to at all hours of the day and night, asking for the cause of puzzling physical symptoms, on-the-fly blood-pressure checks, and nutritional advice. Despite the hectic, fast-paced rhythm of the dense urban block, there was also a sense of community. People, even without regular direct engagement with one another on this chaotic block, quickly recognized new faces and noted absences. For Ruiz, already embedded in multiple familial webs of care and a nodal point in diverse therapeutic itineraries of individuals and families seeking advice and treatment, this tangled involvement in people's quotidian lives was a defining feature of her medical practice.

Since 2000, I have researched the ethnographic intricacies of *consultorios* in and around the neighborhoods of Havana, scaling from individual health-related practices to the changing macroeconomic and political influences, some external to Cuba, shaping the country's healthcare system. The *consultorio* in *la Plaza* is just one among thousands (in 2020, approximately 26,173) of similar community-based clinics scattered throughout the island, serving as the bedrock of Cuba's primary healthcare system.[18] The Family Physician and Nurse Program (El Programa del Médico y Enfermera de la Familia, MEF), launched in 1984, called for physician-and-nurse teams to live and work in small clinics on the city block or the rural community they serve.

Each *consultorio* serves roughly 120 families (approximately 600–700 persons) in a designated health area. The design and structure of the MEF program

---

[18] Ministerio de Salud Pública (MINSAP), República de Cuba, "Anuario Estadístico Del Ministerio De Salud Pública, 2020," accessed September 1, 2021, at: https://salud.msp.gob.cu/portfolio/anuario-estadistico/.

are to provide greater access to healthcare services and a closer relationship between health teams and their patients. In the 1980s, Cuba's health profile underwent an epidemiological shift. This shift from so-called diseases of poverty (e.g., parasitic and infectious diseases) to "diseases of development" (e.g., heart disease and cancer). With an increase in chronic health problems and cancers linked to multicausal factors, including lifestyle (e.g., smoking, diet, and physical activity) and psychosocial and economic considerations, the success of previous curative interventions achieved through pharmaceutical prophylaxis was out of sync with the country's changing morbidity patterns. Faced with this new challenge, the Cuban Ministry of Public Health (MINSAP) overhauled the health system by training a new cohort of primary healthcare physicians. This pedagogical calibration would better equip physicians to carry out clinical and social-epidemiological vigilance of the population, promote health, and prevent disease by working with the community.

In 2023, almost forty years after its launch, the MEF program, with its mandate to train primary healthcare physicians, contributes to Cuba's reigning status of having the highest physician-to-inhabitant ratio globally. Women constitute 61.7 percent of all physicians (from primary to tertiary specialties) and 71.2 percent of healthcare workers.[19] Women also form most physicians making up the brigades on humanitarian solidarity missions. Within the past decade, these solidarity missions have tripled in size, partly owing to the domestic success of Cuba's integrated primary healthcare model, as measured by statistical indicators determined by multinational organizations. For example, the collection and circulation of nationwide vital health statistics by the WHO and World Bank form part of a complex standardization algorithm. The outcome is numerical snapshots of any country's health and social welfare (especially vulnerable populations, such as infants). As a country with scarce economic resources and modest per capita total expenditures on health, Cuba has long leveraged the political semiotics of its vital health statistics (e.g., the country's low infant mortality rate).

Physicians like Ruiz, paired with a nurse, offer a decentralized, neighborhood health(care)[20] model. As Cuba's government contends, they have a more intimate knowledge of their patients from this location, always connected to the dynamic bio-psycho-social and economic factors that shape their lives. On any given day, Ruiz and a nurse were charged with administering four priority health programs: maternal and child health, chronic non-communicable diseases, infectious diseases, and the care of older adults. Through a classification

[19] MINSAP, *Annuario*.
[20] The stylistic use of health(care) draws on Nancy J. Burke's edited volume, *Health Travels: Cuban Health(care) On and Off the Island* (San Francisco: University of California Medical Humanities Consortium, 2013).

surveillance system known as *dispensarización* or the classification and monitoring of epidemiological-risk categories, Ruiz would evaluate the overall health situation of her designated area and define the at-risk populations by a patient group – for example, hypertensive, diabetic, expectant mother, and so on. In addition to assigning a "risk group," health teams, as stipulated by the MEF methodological manual, also qualitatively assess the socioeconomic factors of each household in three categories: cultural hygiene, psychosocial characteristics, and the provision of necessities. Thus, health teams can provide immediate, continuous, and tailored forms of care.

On the surface, Ruiz's quotidian clinical practices may fit neatly within what most contemporary public experts, for example, the WHO, now defined as an attention to the structural determinants of health (SDOH), or addressing "the social, physical, and economic conditions that impact upon health." However, a fundamental difference remains, that is, the question of praxis, linking theory and action or, in the words of decolonial theorist Catherine Walsh and Walter Mignolo, constitute a "praxis of living" where theory and the action "are enacted and, at the time, rendered possible."[21] Health(care), defined through this framework, increasingly blurs the biological body as the site of medical intervention. In the twenty-first century, Cuba's primary health(care) systems, such as Ruiz's *consultorio*, which is the model that forms the basis of the solidarity humanitarian brigades, which I will discuss shortly, actively work to enact comprehensive, historically sensitive biomedical health(care). Here, SDOHs are an active component of the medical gaze, in no small part owing to the previous and ongoing transformations of social and political conditions that have radically altered the physical/biological bodies that medicine operates on and through.

More than sixty years after the Cuban Revolution, through the vagaries of radical economic setbacks, the country has remained steadfast in its commitment to address the historical reproduction of structural inequality, even if faltering at times.[22] While Cuba's socialist economy is an analytic departure point from other studies of biomedicine, my specific aim is to examine how the country's biomedical expansionism emerged in response to the structural and material conditions that gave rise to the 1959 revolution, which was an anti-imperialist movement focused on agrarian reform and ending racial and gender discrimination, predatory capitalism of economic exploitation

---

[21] Walter D. Mignolo and Catherine E. Walsh, *Decoloniality in/as Praxis* (Durham, NC: Duke University Press, 2018), 7.

[22] Numerous scholars have documented some of the failings of Cuba's domestic health(care) system. I will not rehearse those discussions. See Elise Andaya, *Conceiving Cuba: Reproduction, Women, and the State in Post-Soviet Cuba* (New Brunswick, NJ: Rutgers University Press, 2014); P. Sean Brotherton, *Revolutionary Medicine: Health and the Body in Post-Soviet Cuba* (Durham, NC: Duke University Press, 2012); Burke, *Health Travels.*

and expendability, rampant structural inequality, and widespread corruption. Cuba's variant of biomedicine is conscripted to serve as a revolutionary project and was conceived as a form of social medicine and reparative social justice.

Cuba's philosophy of social medicine as political praxis approaches health as flourishing. By extension, care *is* or *can be* "the social capacity and activity involving the nurturing of all that is necessary for the welfare and flourishing of life."[23] Through this, the practice of health(care) implodes the therapeutic boundaries of the *consultorio*, offering a generative space for reinterpreting biomedicine's transformative properties or its plasticity. Plasticity, philosopher Catherine Malabou suggests, provides an interpretive lens for exploring the creative, annihilating, and transformative meanings of organic structures and systems of thought, including ideas, discourses, or practices. She defines plasticity as the capacity to give and receive from, and as *plastique* (the French term for *explosive*), the power to annihilate form. Malabou has applied this concept to think through organic material, such as theories of the brain, to open a field of possibilities for other ways of thinking about the human condition.[24] Here, I apply plasticity to biomedicine to draw attention to its potential as a therapeutic and transformative system of social justice, wherein the corporeal, social, and political bodies are sites of historical reparations. In other words, the reparative capacity of biomedicine can be molded and transformed to alleviate the enduring material and embodied legacies of colonialism, now magnified through global capitalism. Cuba's biomedical focus on human health and, by extension, approaches to care are two sides of the same coin, configured as therapeutic and affective labor but also a political technology invested in creating the conditions for individuals, groups, and populations to flourish. As Cuba's healthcare model travels through international medical brigades, social medicine becomes enveloped in solidarity praxis, producing unexpected and expected transnational alliances and adversaries.

Solidarity Humanitarianism As Reparative Justice

Cuba's programs of solidarity humanitarianism, racially marked as the Global South, allow me to reframe the common sense of the affective and ethical bonds constituting attempts at global health equity. Here, solidarity here operates through several political valences that warrant closer examination. On the one hand, it is the provision of *care* as a response to acute suffering of humanity in post-disaster relief and, on the other, *care* as *restitution*

---

[23] Andreas Chatzidakis, Jamie Hakim, Jo Littler, Catherine Rottenberg, and Lynne Segal (The Care Collective), *The Care Manifesto: The Politics of Interdependence* (London and New York, NY: Verso, 2020), 5.

[24] Catherine Malabou, *What Should We Do with Our Brain?*, 1st ed. (New York, NY: Fordham University Press, 2008), 5–6.

to remediate what Lauren Berlant terms the quotidian "destruction of life, bodies, imaginaries, and environments by and under contemporary regimes of capital."[25]

The Henry Reeve Medical Brigade's arrival in Italy forms a much longer, complex history of Cuba's expanding approach to health(care) as political praxis. In late August 2005, Hurricane Katrina swept over southeast Louisiana and Mississippi, causing massive damage, particularly to New Orleans. The city's levee system failed, unleashing massive flood waters, and leaving tens of thousands of people, primarily Black residents, stranded without food, shelter, power, or necessities. The US federal government's response was slow and inept, exacerbating the magnitude of the disaster. Days after the storm made landfall, the Cuban government assembled 1,500 physicians with several tons of medical supplies and materials in Havana's Convention Center. Then President Fidel Castro offered to dispatch them to the devastated areas along the Gulf Coast. Addressing the brigade of physicians, Castro explained his rationale: "It was clear to us that those who faced the greatest danger [in New Orleans] were these huge numbers of poor, desperate people, many elderly citizens with health situations, pregnant women, mothers and children among them, all in urgent need of medical care." This duty to act, Castro asserted, was "writing a new page in the history of solidarity ... showing a course of peace for the suffering and imperiled human species to which we all belong."[26]

After a week of slow deliberation, the U.S. Department of State finally responded by declining the offer, citing that the United States had no diplomatic relations with Cuba. Such ties were severed in 1962 when President John F. Kennedy proclaimed an embargo on trade between the two countries, which later expanded to a comprehensive economic blockade and severe travel restrictions. Undeterred by this rebuke, the Cuban government used the opportunity to inaugurate a medical emergency response team known as the Henry Reeve International Contingent Brigade Specialized in Disasters and Serious Epidemics (HRIMB). This newly formed eponymous brigade, an army of white lab coats, honors the New York-born Brigadier General Henry Reeve, who fought in Cuba's Army of Liberation during the First Cuban War of Independence from Spain (1868–78). This act of naming transforms medicine, through the political semiotics of liberation and struggle, to Guevara's commitment to building a cadre of proletariat physicians, or "revolutionary

---

[25] Lauren Berlant, "Thinking about Feeling Historical," *Emotion, Space, and Society* 1, no. 1 (January 2008): 4–9.

[26] Fidel Castro Ruz, Meeting with the Medical Doctors Assembled to Offer Assistance to the American People in Areas Affected by Hurricane Katrin." Remarks delivered in Havana, September 4, 2005, accessed July 21, 2021, at: www.fidelcastro.cu/en/discursos/ meeting-medical-doctors-assembled-offer-assistance-american-people-areas-affected.

doctors," who now, as internationalists (*internacionalistas*), "pledge to serve wherever they are needed."[27]

A narrative history of Cuba's medical brigades through monumental events, such as their arrival in Italy or the army of physicians poised to assist after Hurricane Katrina in 2005, eclipses how emergency and disaster assistance has been a staple since the early 1960s of Cuban internationalism. For example, the first team of physicians was sent to Chile in 1960 after an earthquake. Other groups were dispatched throughout Central America and the Caribbean after hurricanes George and Mitch in 1998. In 1986, teams brought victims of the Chernobyl disaster to Cuba for treatment and rehabilitation. The HRIMB, then, is an extension of these efforts, which include the brigade's collaboration with the WHO in controlling the Ebola epidemics in West Africa in 2014; humanitarian medical teams sent to Haiti after the 2010 and 2016 earthquakes; and, more recently, sending health professionals to thirty-nine countries to assist in their battles to manage Covid-19.[28]

How, then, do these recent efforts write a new page in the history of solidarity? Since the 1960s, Cuba's approach to solidarity, within a political-epistemological context, suggests the co-emergence of interrelated forms of solidarity worth disentangling. In one instance, solidarity – invoking the writings of Simon Bolívar, Che Guevara, Jose Martí, and Karl Marx – emerges from *cooperation* rather than development assistance or aid. This shift in language highlights the non-hierarchical relations of *mutual trust and support, comradeship*, or *camaraderie*. As Robert Huish has noted, this form of solidarity contradicts normative aid frameworks or the common sense of Western humanitarianism. The latter is rooted in charity, altruism, and a moral incentive to act.[29] Cuban solidarity brigades in a post-disaster context are a form of cooperation without political conditionality or material self-interest and do not retrain the conventional power imbalances implicit in the geopolitics of donor–recipient relations. Yet this history of solidarity as cooperation also intersects with the country's humanitarian imperative through an explicitly political framework of social justice, rationalized as part and parcel of a form of ethics rooted in subaltern politics. This form of international solidarity resonates with the decolonization debates of the Bandung Conference of 1955, a meeting of twenty-nine African and Asian countries to discuss the global reconfiguration of power taking shape post-Second World War. As European

---

[27] *MEDICC*, "Cuba's Henry Reeve International Medical Brigade Receives WHO Dr. Lee Jong-Wook Memorial Prize for Public Health," May 26, 2017.

[28] Angel A. Escobedo, Cristians Auza-Santivanez, Raisa Rumbaut, Maurizio Bonati, and Imti Choonara, "Cuba: Solidarity, Ebola and Covid-19," *Bmj Paediatrics Open* 5, no. 1 (2021): e001089.

[29] Robert Huish, "Why Does Cuba 'Care' So Much? Understanding the Epistemology of Solidarity in Global Health Outreach," *Public Health Ethics* 7, no. 3 (2014): 261–76.

empires collapsed, the US and USSR emerged as influential international figures alongside China's Maoist revolution.

The formation of the United Nations in 1945 and the rise of Cold War factions between the US and USSR precipitated the founding of the Non-Aligned Movement in 1956. This movement sought a platform for the countries not aligned with these significant power blocs to discuss battles over national self-determination against all forms of colonialism and imperialism. Cuba's Cold War alliance with the Soviet Union was also influential in importing the language of Soviet-style Marxist-Leninism into Cuba's political discourses (e.g., proletariat internationalism). However, throughout the 1960s, 1970s, and early 1980s, the anti-imperialist and anticolonial leanings of Cuba's active involvement in liberation struggles were evident in the military, technical, and medical realms. Participation in campaigns in Angola, Algeria, Bolivia, Congo, Grenada, and Nicaragua, among others, provides ample instances. Fidel Castro argued in the Second Declaration of Havana (1962) that these formative acts of solidarity, both military and medical, could not be reduced to the idea that "revolutions can be bought, sold, rented, loaned, exported and imported like some piece of merchandise."[30] The revolution is not a commodity, Castro affirmed. Instead, it was a worldview centered on cultivating an ethics of humanity committed to ending exploitation and cycles of structural violence. Early political discourses of solidarity as struggle were present in the Tricontinental Conference hosted in Havana in 1966. With representatives from eighty-two countries spanning three continents, Castro asserted internationalism was about "strengthening the bonds of revolutionary and anti-imperialist solidarity in the battle against the imperialist, colonialist and neocolonialist system of exploitation, against which we declared a fight to the death."[31]

From medical brigades (e.g., Henry Reeves) to vaccines (e.g., Abdala Covid vaccine), the resignification of the transformative properties of biomedicine signals a complex, entangled history of solidarity in liberation struggles for self-determination. In Cuba's post-Soviet era, solidarity humanitarianism moves beyond crisis as an exceptional event or emergency to an approach to crisis defined by the quotidian experience of multiple forms of structural violence. This new page of humanitarian intervention is focused more on capacity-building and strengthening primary healthcare infrastructure, training health professionals, and developing extensive South–South cooperation, concentrating on health, social welfare, and biotechnology. Solidarity, then, rather

---

[30] Fidel Castro Ruz, "Second Declaration of Havana, 1962," in James Nelson Goodsell (ed.), *From Fidel Castro's Personal Revolution in Cuba* (New York, NY: Knopf), 1975), 264–68.

[31] Fidel Castro Ruz, "Declaración General de la Primera Conferencia de Solidaridad de Los Pueblos de Asia, África y América Latina," Speech delivered in Havana, January 15, 1966, accessed July 21, 2021, at: http://constitucionweb.blogspot.com/2014/06/declaracion-continental-de-la-primera.html.

than an identarian project, is an activity that emerges when working together on a common task, cutting across presumed attributes such as class, nationality, or ethnicity, thus destabilizing the "reductive binarity of similarity and dissimilarity, as Fertherstone asserts."[32]

The postcolonial anxieties of Latin America reflect a unique set of historical concerns, incorporating the demographic richness and conflicts of the region. Yet it is clear from historical events – such as the emergence of the Non-Alignment Movement and centuries of liberation battles for self-determination, political sovereignty, and an end to exploitative economic relations – that Cuba's approach to humanitarian solidarity crystallizes and addresses a shared set of geopolitical tensions. For an increasing number of populations, some even within the Global North, everyday life has become unlivable and shaped by exceptional poverty and the abandonment of care. As a form of solidarity, Cuba's medical brigades are an experiment in "actually building new social relations that are more survivable," following Dean Spade's work on mutual aid.[33] This gesture is a form of *restitution as care*, acknowledging cumulative injuries of histories in the present and attempting to remediate the structural conditions that cyclically enact bodily harm.

For Cuban officials, developing an ethics of care as solidarity, as an ethos of cooperation, is part of the broader resignification of medicine in the country's development of humanitarian biomedicine. Such strategies of care need to be adapted to confront the liberation struggles of the present day. The twenty-first century has given rise to unprecedented levels of global inequality, reordering previous colonial mappings. The increase of indirect and insidious forms of economic accumulation and dispossession, through neoliberalism, for instance, has hollowed out the social welfare state, resulting in unprecedented global inequity. How does Cuba's approach to social medicine, as mobile technology, transform discursively and materially from a domestic to an international context through different social-economic and political contexts? What configurations of care are envisioned through Cuba's explicitly politicized variant of solidarity humanitarianism? To demonstrate this, I turn for a moment to the historic agreement between the government of Venezuela (and President Hugo Chávez, d. 2013) and President Fidel Castro (d. 2016) to form the program "Inside the Neighborhood" in March 2003. This program, known as Missions, not in the religious sense but as a social justice project, was at the heart of Chávez's Bolivarian Revolution (named after anti-imperialist fighter Simon Bolivar). To do so, however, also requires that we contend with

---

[32] David Featherstone, *Solidarity: Hidden Histories and Geographies of Internationalism.* London and New York: Zed Books, 2012, 23.

[33] Dean Spade, *Mutual Aid: Building Solidarity during This Crisis (and the Next)* (New York, NY, and London: Verso, 2020), 6.

political contingencies, or, I will discuss, constraint, that is, on the one hand, an act or force that restrains and on the other, a condition, sense of the state of being restricted, or kept in check to avoid or perform some action, thought or way of life. It is an Otherwise, kept at bay.

Between Constraint and Possibility

After Hugo Chávez was elected president of Venezuela in 1998, a new alliance with Cuba gave birth to several bilateral and subsidized trade agreements (e.g., subsidized oil) between the two countries. Chávez's populist political movement amended the constitutionality of access to health(care) as a priority for the newly formed Bolivarian government. However, this plan proved challenging to put into practice. After failing to secure Venezuelan doctors willing to live and work in underserved communities nationwide, with minimal healthcare infrastructure, the Chávez government turned to Cuba for support.

In March 2003, Plan Barrio Adentro, renamed Misión Barrio Adentro (MBA) in 2005, emerged from an agreement between Chávez's government and Cuba as part of the larger project of redesigning the welfare state in Venezuela, funded petro-capital and formation of a hemispheric alliance known as ALBA, or the Bolivarian Alliance for the Peoples of Our America. ALBA was created as a decisive turning away from the Free Trade Area of the Americas, as a new day in politics, defined by an anti-imperialist, regional, and hemispheric united front against US interventionism and the logic of capitalist development. Moving against the 1990s trend of other Latin American countries, where neoliberal reforms and loan conditions of international financial institutions had curtailed state investments in healthcare, Barrio Adentro (Inside the Neighborhood) proposed a radically different model of care. With access to healthcare a constitutional right, the MBA model would seek the assistance of 20,000 Cuban physicians and auxiliary health professionals stationed in primarily poor neighborhoods in Venezuela to provide free medical care. In this context, "missions" (*misiones*), typically associated with Catholic or evangelical projects of conversion or with civilian or militarized mobilizations, take on new meaning within programs centered on antipoverty, social welfare, education, and social justice.

Since MBA's emergence, the program has been subject to vigorous discussions, from declarations of it as a striking example of Latin American social medicine to criticisms of the oil-for-aid deal as a totalitarian form of humanitarian business For example, the summer of 2013 witnessed mass protests staged by private medical associations in Brazil over the intent of former President Dilma Rousseff's government, which committed to a program of universal health coverage, to subcontract 4,000 Cuban physicians (with the hopes of obtaining 20,000) to work in rural, underserved outposts, through a program known as Mais Médicos. Rousseff's impeachment and removal from office in 2016, and the subsequent election of Jair Bolsanaro in 2018, who espoused a tough stance against Cuba, labeling the socialist government a "troika of tyranny" (alongside Venezuela and Nicaragua) resulted in the Cuban government later recalling all of its doctors in protest, which had grown to over 10,000 by that time. Still facing gaping holes in healthcare access for large swaths of the population precipitated by the closure of Mais Médicos in May 2020, surging Covid cases led the Brazil government to license and rehire 157 Cuban doctors who had remained in the country.[34]

Cuba's cooperative missions form a biopolitical project working to fill in the gaps of state-sponsored social welfare programs, where rights discourses, such as the constitutionality of health, break down at the level of quotidian access. Such an endeavor is never apolitical and the Cuban government, its solidarity missions, and individual Cubans must traverse these overlapping histories and controversies. In so doing, they must face conflictual world-making strategies engendered through enacting definitions of what constitutes health(care) vis-à-vis the state. Cuban solidarity missions, caught in this nexus, have thus also become the target of aggressive foreign policies. For over sixty years, and throughout thirteen US presidents, Cuba has navigated the contours of the ongoing obstacles of the US economic embargo. From this enforced position, and because of it, Cuban socialism, and its variant of solidarity humanitarianism, is a history of antagonism. The country has hit brick walls, thwarted, and persisted *beyond* and *in the face of* existing normative and regulatory logics (dominated mainly by US interests) operating in concert with the forces of liberal states and laissez-faire capitalist markets – markets designed by Bretton Woods agreements, the World Trade Organization, World Bank, and International Monetary Fund. For example, Cuban political cartoonist Alfredo Martirena compellingly visualizes Cuba's solidarity missions within a context of political contingency (see Figure 15.3).

Examining political contingency and Cuba's solidarity humanitarianism must also confront what José Quiroga asserts: "that there are at least two histories" of the Cuban Revolution, divided into categories of the "official and the dissident."[35] Quiroga's insistence on the multivocality of Cuba's historiography problematizes, as other scholars have noted, that no shared neutral vocabulary exists to discuss the Cuban Revolution of 1959.[36] The revolution is a utopic dream for some and a nightmare for others. For instance, as Misión Barrio Adentro expanded in Venezuela, the U.S. Department of Homeland Security

[34] Shasta Darlington and Letícia Casado, "Brazil Fails to Replace Cuban Doctors," *New York Times*, June 11, 2019.
[35] José Quiroga, *Cuban Palimpsests*. Minneapolis: University of Minnesota Press, 2005, 22.
[36] See Michael J. Bustamante and Jennifer L. Lambe (eds.), *The Revolution from Within: Cuba, 1959–1980* (Durham, NC: Duke University Press, 2019).

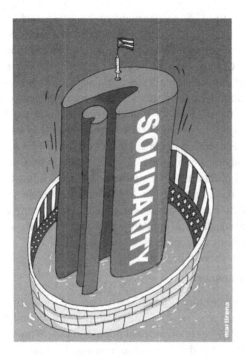

Figure 15.3 "Cuba solidarity blocked, October 5, 2014" ©Alfredo Martirena.

(DHS) and the Department of State instituted the Cuban Medical Professional Parole Program (CMPP) under President George W. Bush's administration. The CMPP, created in 2006, allowed Cuban medical personnel, and in some cases, their family, working in third-party countries to apply for "parole" in the United States. Cuban physicians were given a legal path to seek resident status in the United States. US senators argued that the rationale for the CMPP is to rescue Cuban doctors living in impoverished conditions without necessities, such as food and electricity, and a small salary. The Obama Administration suspended the CMPP program in January 2017. By then, the United States had approved parole for 7,117 Cuban medical professionals, mainly from missions in Venezuela. However, the suspension of the program prompted a concerned group of senators and representatives to urge the DHS to reinstate it, claiming that the Cuban government exploited medical workers in return for as much as $8 billion in payments a year, drawing heavily on the language of human trafficking and the "doctor-as-slave" discourse.[37]

---

[37] Ernesto Londoño, "Cuban Doctors Revolt: 'You Get Tired of Being a Slave,'" *New York Times*, September 29, 2017.

In 2020, an official for the U.S. Department of State asserted in a statement to the *Washington Post*, "Cuba's deployment of medical missions overseas, while cloaked in altruism, is a scheme to generate income that exploits Cuban medical workers. Cuba's medical missions program is not inherently humanitarian; the regime earns income by retaining up to 90 percent of the doctors' salaries."[38] Yet, eclipsed from this selective framing is why altruism is the universal benchmark for defining humanitarianism as a practice. For instance, why does the insertion of any form of economic value intrinsically change the nature of the relationship of care? Historically, Western humanitarianism, which includes much of mainstream global health, is tied, sometimes obliquely, to disaster and philanthropy capitalism, structural adjustment programs and conditional trade agreements, and blossoming industries of NGOs and for-profit voluntourism in health and development. These complex entanglements suggest that the marriage of humanitarianism to explicit or implicit (or both) economic and political agendas is not unique to Cuba.

Social Medicine, *Otherwise*

At the end of the twentieth century, global health became the dominant narrative and organizing logic for a "new regime of representation and intervention" into the health and well-being of targeted populations.[39] What is needed, then, is a critical analysis of the dominant discourses and practices of global health as a particular kind of problem space. The concept of "problem-space," introduced by David Scott, examines an "ensemble of questions and answers around which a horizon of identifiable stakes (conceptual as well as political stakes) hangs."[40] This approach provides critical conceptual resources to explore the discursive historical context that generates questions that may be vibrant and urgent for a period but sometimes lose traction and stop being relevant over time. Still, as Scott notes, other questions persist in relevance and importance. He argues that the task at hand is in recognizing at what moment a problem-space of questions *about* the past *from* the past is "no longer in sync with the world they were meant to describe and normatively criticize."[41]

As the ravages wrought by the Covid-19 epidemic lay bare, globally divergent histories of colonialism and racism, redlining, and institutionalized forms of structural violence and modern-day extractive capitalism negatively and

---

[38] Anthony Faiolo, and Kimberly Brown, "U.S. Allies, Encouraged by Washington, Said Goodbye to Their Cuban Doctors." *The Washington Post*, April 10, 2020.

[39] Vincanne Adams, Dominique Behague, Carlo Caduff, Ilana Lowy, and Francisco Ortega, "Re-imagining Global Health through Social Medicine," *Global Public Health* 14, no. 10 (2019): 1383–400, at 1384.

[40] David Scott, *Conscripts of Modernity: The Tragedy of Colonial Enlightenment* (Durham, NC: Duke University Press, 2004). 2.

[41] Scott, *Conscripts of Modernity*, 2.

disproportionately impact the health of Black, Indigenous, and People of Color. Yet, these complex and often violent entanglements contributing to health and well-being are often excised out of view, bracketed as questions of a different order outside interventions targeting health in the problem space of global health. This demands questions: What constitutes health or well-being, or the notion of a healthy subject, why, and to whom? Within the dominant global health discourses, some answers to these questions are illegible "because [they defy] the terms under which the questions are phrased."[42] What is needed is to question the stable, timeless, and transparent concepts that establish the political conditions for "unthinkability." This interrogation requires confronting paradigm paralysis: the inability, epistemic blindness, or political refusal to see beyond the current models that structure the logic and practice of contemporary global health.

For example, in mid 2020, calls to decolonize global health, bolstered by ongoing social movements such as Black Lives Matter, Standing Rock, Idle No More, and the People's Health Movement, challenged the pervasive logics of intervention defining global health. Consider the work of Hi'ilei Hobart and Tamara Kneese, who advocate for radical care as "a set of vital but underappreciated strategies for enduring precarious worlds."[43] Such strategies, they argue, are attentive to the plurality of care and differential objectives and aims. Solidarity, not aid or charity, they note, drawing on the work of Dean Spade, offers a strategy for "working with communities and asking them what they need rather than making paternalistic assumptions. Instead of following neoliberal, colonialist development models around innovation and the mining of hope, mutual aid offers a space of collaboration."[44]

Chávez died in 2013 and Castro in 2016. In 2025, Misión Barrio Adentro continues to persist, even as the socioeconomic conditions in Venezuela deteriorate under US sanctions, dropping global oil prices, and political factionalism within the country. What, then, of the future of solidarity as care? With the dominant script of global health, there is a tendency to rapidly skim over programs like Barrio Adentro or Mais Medicos as transparent forms of political theater, as radical or socialist dystopic fantasies, and thus dismissible without much consideration. *What if* we examined Barrio Adentro with the same critical scrutiny and serious engagement as past and current global health ambitions, such as the Sustainable Development Goals by the United Nations in 2016, defined as: "A blueprint to achieve a better and more sustainable future for all people and the world by 2030." This latest UN program, following a similar

---

[42] Trouillot, "North Atlantic Universals," 847.
[43] Hi'ilei Julia Kawehipuaakahaopulani Hobart and Tamara Kneese, "Radical Care," *Social Text* 38, no. 1 (2020): 1–16, at 2.
[44] Hobart and Kneese, "Radical Care," 10.

trajectory of other multilateral, transnational global health programs sponsored by the WHO, among other leading institutional actors, will undoubtedly join the growing archive of past-tense promises, populating growing lists of elusive target goals (e.g., WHO's "Health for All by 2000"). Despite repeated failures, such promissory campaigns generate a distinct genre of futurity, defined by speculative and political stakes of health equity. This genre, essential to the liberal imaginary, prescribes, reinforces, and calcifies a limited political vocabulary for defining the present and expanding future possibilities for constructing economies of care.

Like all the promissory targets of mainstream global health programs, social medicine projects such as Mais Medicos and Barrio Adentro have political stakes and they all stake political claims as an investment in futurity. Most global health discussions of Cuba's humanitarian solidarity programs are relegated to Cuban or Latin American studies or bracketed as South–South collaboration models in development studies literature. As a result, different iterations of a "single story" – that is, Cuba's solidarity humanitarian missions as *a case study* of global health *from the South* – continue to be the only narrative framing available.[45] My argument goes in a slightly different direction. Cuba's solidarity programs envision radically different health(care) geographies through institutional practices, producing innovative arrangements of capital, labor, commodities/goods, and services. Such programs generate critical optics to redact and annotate the dominant script of global health.

Writing about futurity amidst debates focused on anti-relationality and the impossibility of a queer political collectivity, the late queer theorist José Muñoz argues, "We must strive in the face of the here and now's totalizing rendering of reality, to think, and feel a *then and there.*"[46] Queerness, rather than anti-relational, he suggested, is a "performance because it is not simply a being but a doing for and toward the future."[47] Queerness is not yet here but an ideality, Muñoz asserted. His insistence on queer futurity challenges the normative responses to the fear of hope and utopia as affective projects of disappointment and failure. The history of global health is an archive of broken promises as health inequities continue to rise, sediment, and become institutionalized. Interventions necessitate interventions that necessitate further interventions in perpetuity. The queering of care in global health interventions may offer another framework to theorize care as an ideality, not-yet-here, as anticipatory.

[45] The question of narrative framing draws on the work of Nolwazi Mkhwanazi, "Medical Anthropology in Africa: The Trouble with a Single Story." *Medical Anthropology* 35 no. 2 (2016): 193–202.

[46] José Esteban Muñoz, *Cruising Utopia: The Then and There of Queer Futurity* (New York, NY: New York University Press, 2009), 1.

[47] Muñoz, *Cruising Utopia*, 1.

This chapter ends with a speculative thought experiment. *What if* capitalism is the disease and rampant economic inequality is the symptom? *What if* global health interventions took the form of sovereign debt alleviation, restitution of land, or reparations for slavery, among other macro-structural targets? Of course, to express such speculative utterances is to adopt the style of a manifesto, bearing uncanny cadence to the opening epigraph outlining Breton's surrealist ambitions for thought, language, and human experience to escape the reductive forces of Enlightenment rationalism. Cuban heath(care) praxis offers a lens to think and theorize an Otherwise, unveiling dominant ideological networks of power but, equally and crucially, creating space to interrupt the so-called canon, explore other modalities of existence, and imagine different speculative futures. I argue that rather than a script of an illogical plot, it sets the stage to repeat Muñoz's words, "to think and feel a *then and there*" of future praxis.

Afterword: Struggling with and for Social Medicine

Anne-Emanuelle Birn

The (re-)making of histories of social medicine across both place and time is a welcome endeavor, for the arena's past, like its present, remains ever in formation (or gestation) amid breakers of remembering and forgetting. This afterword, unabashedly charting scholar-activist tendencies, offers an aspirational call for social medicine as a political endeavor to be articulated at both a grand and quotidian scale, forwarding possibilities of social medicine becoming a social movement, and social movements becoming more entangled with social medicine.

Notwithstanding the volume's titular *global* dalliance, the exercise of revisiting social medicine underscores the overarching importance of the context of – as well as conversations among – the book's fascinating and original accounts. Necessary and deft incorporation of, for example, more women, key players from the Middle East/Arabic-speaking world, sub-Saharan Africa, Asia, and the Pacific, the socialist world, and racialized social medicine thinkers and practitioners from across the Americas, nonetheless begs a query or two regarding how the role of (male) European and white physicians – in this volume mercifully far less dominant than in virtually every other past account – might be further challenged.

Transcending Doctors and Politics

Myth-and-icon-busting might appear to detract from crucial narratives and learnings that continue to inspire the next generations and present alternatives to biomedical triumphalism. Instead, I would argue that constructive challenging of the usual cast of male social medicine icons only heightens the field's potential reaches and repercussions. In India and Sri Lanka, communist and Third World feminist physician-activists played pivotal roles in proffering homegrown, unpretentious approaches to transforming health through redistributive approaches that transcended or even countered European and imperial social medicine understandings.

What might an even deeper focus on medicine's humble rank-and-file practitioners – midwives, nurses, Indigenous healers, community health workers, among others – tell us about the promise and challenges of social medicine in the streets and in the polis, from the two Bandungs to Alma-Ata to Rio? After all, Mozambique's *agentes polivalentes elementares* (sanitary cadres) were a cornerstone of the 1960s–70s revolutionary struggle against Portuguese colonialism.[1] How did this medicine of liberation approach interact with, and especially inform, primary healthcare and social medicine efforts of the day?[2] Exploring such questions might lead us to think through how perennial revivals of social medicine, and historical studies thereof, might propitiously focus on and engage with health workers who are closest to made-marginalized communities that are putatively of most concern to social medicine praxis.

Another illustration from the same era relates more directly to the World Health Organization (WHO)–UNICEF 1978 International Conference on Primary Health Care, considered by many to be a pinnacle of global social medicine approaches articulated through the United Nations (UN). At the conference and in its preparations, physicians, politicians, and physician-politicians (or physician-international bureaucrats) were visibilized over everyday health workers in both speeches and in the crafting of the Alma-Ata Declaration. Moreover, WHO and Western primary healthcare advocates accused Soviet health approaches of being overmedicalized or over-doctored. Yet even as Soviet authorities sought to showcase medical-technological advances, conference participants themselves remained hungry to see social(ist) medicine on the ground, that is, in the (Central Asian) yurt, witnessing through site visits "not only universal, free, equitable healthcare coverage, but health protection writ large, in terms of housing, sanitation, employment, nutrition, education, elimination of poverty, and so on."[3] There, the interlocking roles of ordinary social workers, community health agents, teachers, and others were far more transcendent (and memorable) than politician-physician pronouncements.

Struggling for Health, Backward and Forward

The Fabian approaches of many past (and certain present) social medicine leaders, who tend(ed) to pursue connections to parliaments, philanthropies,

---

[1] Julie Cliff, Najmi Kanji, and Mike Muller, "Mozambique Health Holding the Line," *Review of African Political Economy* no. 36 (September 1986): 7–23.

[2] Stephen Gloyd, James Pfeiffer, and Wendy Johnson, "Cooperantes, Solidarity, and the Fight for Health in Mozambique," in Anne-Emanuelle Birn and Theodore M. Brown (eds.), *Comrades in Health: US Health Internationalists, Abroad and at Home* (New Brunswick, NJ: Rutgers University Press, 2013), 184–99.

[3] Anne-Emanuelle Birn and Nikolai Krementsov, "'Socialising' Primary Care? The Soviet Union, WHO, and the 1978 Alma-Ata Conference," *BMJ Global Health* 3, s. 3 (December 2018): 1–15 at p. 12, 3: e000992. doi:10.1136/bmjgh-2018-000992.

UN agencies, and elite universities, reveal both limits and possibilities. Such associations with "the establishment" certainly portend(ed) political access but also risk(ed) increasing the distance from struggles on the ground. Here, 1930s union activism and people's militancy for bona fide social and working condition improvements, whether in Argentina, Scandinavia, or China, merit being mined for conceivable or realized intersections and routes between mobilized laborites and social medicine acolytes. Likewise, dialogues and solidarity between anti-colonial uprisings and anti-racist resistance may well have incorporated social medicine activists and demands.[4] How did, for instance, radical peasant unionists in Mexico perceive and interact with health advocates, who themselves pushed and shaped the progressive physician-advisors to President Lázaro Cárdenas's leftist administration?[5] That agrarian reform and (social) medicine's centrality to the revival of traditional collective landholding communities (*ejidos*) unfolded simultaneously urges us to study far more than the heartfelt and eloquent ideas of physician-activist leaders of the period.[6]

Amplified routes of understanding also emerge via foci on other unexpected social movement–social medicine intertwining, such as between early twentieth-century Tunisian feminist physicians and anti-colonial movements. Similarly, links between theological and medico-political liberation movements in repressive regimes in Brazil, Central America, and elsewhere might lead us to double back on perhaps not-so-strange science–religion bedfellows to glean new insights on social medicine's varied engagements.

Moving forward in time, how might the dynamic accounts of the previous chapters provide perspectives and touchstones for social medicine's current endeavors? In 1935, Uruguayan painter, sculptor, theorist, and parent of Latin American constructivism Joaquin Torres García famously sketched the first of his inverted maps of South America to introduce his text "School of the South," declaring, "the South is our [magnetic] north."[7] So might renewed social medicine histories and calls to action make exciting inversions and incursions, by heeding the compass of social movements and activism in the South.

---

[4] Clayton Vaughn-Roberson "Grassroots Anti-fascism: Ethiopia and the Transnational Origins of the National Negro Congress in Philadelphia, 1935–1936," *American Communist History* 17, no. 1 (2018): 4–15.

[5] Ana María Carrillo, "Salud pública y poder en México durante el Cardenismo, 1934–1940," *Dynamis: Acta Hispanica ad Medicinae Scientiarumque Historiam Illustrandam* 25 (2005): 145–78, at: https://raco.cat/index.php/Dynamis/article/view/114016.

[6] Ana Maria Kapelusz-Poppi, "Physician Activists and the Development of Rural Health in Postrevolutionary Mexico," *Radical History Review* 80 (2001): 35–50.

[7] Joaquín Torres García, "La Escuela del Sur. Lección 30. 1935," in *Universalismo Constructivo* (Buenos Aires: Poseidón, 1944), 213–19, at 213, AEB's translation from Spanish.

Cuban "social medicine across borders," perhaps the most obvious contemporary exemplar, may be more fraught than meets the (romanticized) eye. Still, the last half-century-plus of South–South medical cooperation remains a crucial starting point, not least because it brings to the surface to-be-further-unpacked dimensions of how social medicine grapples with "the biological and the social."[8] Latin American social medicine studies that highlight tensions of the technical versus the political serve several guises: certainly as a hiding place for leftist radicals but also as a place of contestation amid claims of horizontal international South–South health cooperation.[9]

The involvement of social medicine in progressive, so-called Pink Tide administrations that have ebbed and flowed across Latin America since the turn of the millennium offers a cautionary tale. Transformative social redistribution in the name of health has long been a fundamental social medicine ambition. But what happens when such redistribution is extractivism-based and leads to widespread destruction of Indigenous communities, lands, and livelihoods, not to mention further driving the climate crisis and jeopardizing the planet's very survival?[10] Clearly historians of social medicine should play a role in examining such dilemmas. Analogous moments of crisis worthy of a historian's analytic gaze might be evidenced in health movements that challenge capitalist and imperialist hegemony yet fail to confront patriarchy in their own practices.

In sum, here's hoping that the volume invites (history of) social medicine's more sustained focus on social movements, comprising sociopolitical incorporation of made-marginalized people(s) and struggles around political/policy transformations and revolutions related to health justice, Indigenous rights, workers' rights, racial justice, gender justice, and environmental justice, to name but a sextet of movements. A solidifying handle on institutional dimensions of social medicine involving the state, academe, the medical profession, and the medical complex enables such an expanded focus on people's health struggles. The reflections emerging from these chapters herald an exciting, productive, and much needed wave of novel approaches and insights on social medicine's pasts and futures. Such a storied field, certainly needs (to make) more stories.

---

[8] María Isabel Rodríguez (ed.), *Lo biológico y lo social: Su articulación en la formación del personal de salud* (Washington, DC: PAHO, 1994).

[9] See, for example, Alila Brossard Antonielli, "How Do Experts Resist a Development Cooperation Project? The Case of the Mozambique–Brazil Generic Medicine Factory," *Contexto Internacional* 44 (2022): 1–24.

[10] People's Health Movement (PHM)-Canada, PHM-Ecuador, and PHM Ecosystems and Health Thematic Circle, *Beyond an Extractivist World: Why Imagining and Acting upon Alternative Modes of Living Are Crucial to Saving the Planet from Capitalism*, January 2023, at: https://phm-na.org/2023/03/beyond-an-extractivist-world/.

Afterword: The Future(s) of Social Medicine

Helena Hansen

The collection in this book represents the most wide-ranging critical reviews of the history of social medicine globally to date, both in terms of its historical reach – over two centuries – and its geographic reach spanning every continent, including the "Global South," Eastern Europe, and the Middle East. The collection pays homage to social movements outside of organized biomedicine that have profoundly shaped social medicine as developed by biomedical practitioners. Its authors carefully excavate the multiple origins of "social" in academic and organized professional medicine, including a critical examination of colonial and racial-eugenic impulses including concepts of hygiene and development, as well as later responses to external Black power, feminist, Indigenous rights movements. The collection examines social medicine as a product of state-making, including the uses of social medicine in advancing of broader socialist (Nordic), democratic (Brazil), international diplomatic (*à la* Cuban medical diplomacy) political structures. It tracks the imperial and globalizing strands of social medicine including colonial and developmentalist health policies, in tension with critical resistance from reformist to revolutionary political groups. It also tracks socially based healthcare outside of biomedicine as it interfaces with organized biomedicine, health social welfare policy, such as midwifery and migrant mutual aid. Finally, it takes up movements to decolonize social medicine that reorient healthcare to be critical, self-reflexive, and health justice oriented.

What is evident throughout the collection is that social medicine is a strategic term, usually denoting a context-bound political project, and it is not a stable entity. The term "social medicine" serves as a boundary object; a concept that is plastic enough to adapt to local needs and constraints of local sites, yet with enough of a common identity across sites that it is recognizable and translatable across sites.[1] The most important question answered by this collection in relation to social medicine is therefore not "what is it?" but rather "who has used it, what has it accomplished, and what can be done with it?"

---

[1] Susan Star and James Griesemer, "Institutional Ecology, 'Translations' and Boundary Objects: Amateurs and Professionals in Berkeley's Museum of Vertebrate Zoology, 1907–39," *Social Studies of Science* 19, no. 3 (1989): 387–420, PDF.

Because this collection does such a thorough job of illuminating who has used social medicine and what that has accomplished, I will turn for a moment to what can be done with social medicine in the future. The present and future force us to reconsider what is "social" and what is "medicine." The right to health equity currently has more gravity than the right to social equity or human rights internationally – that is, it is easier to mobilize political intervention in response to healthcare needs and disease than it is to mobilize political intervention in response to social needs, such as housing and food deprivation to violence and discrimination. This has led healthcare to inhabit a special role as a leading edge for consensus and cooperation among politically distinct groups within and among nations. The present and future of social medicine also lead us to reconsider the "local" in sites of social medicine practice. Here is a brief sketch of the timeliness of social medicine as a concept with promise as a corrective to a number of contemporary social ills.

Trans-national projects. In the introduction to this volume, the editors point to Planetary Health as a more recent development and could be counted among social medicine movements but with a more global scale of focus. Planetary Health exemplifies the ways that human health is dependent on international agreements to intervene on climate change, and that the practices of multiple nations, in relation to environmental degradation, affect global trends that affect human health transnationally. Food shortages, climate refugees, accelerating pandemics, and natural disasters are but a few sequelae of environmental degradation that require multinational cooperation to address. This will demand international movements, multistate cooperative agreements and new organizations and methods for enforcing those agreements. As is also evident from the political struggle to make essential pharmaceuticals such as HIV ARVs affordable to low income countries through international agreements allowing exceptions to patent restrictions on local manufacture, the locus of action for social medicine must not only be local and national but also transnational, coordinating the efforts of locally rooted leaders animated by common concerns.

The reimagined and evolving techniques of social justice movements. As one example, Black Lives Matter (BLM) protests erupted internationally in the summer of 2020 in the setting of not only racially motivated police violence, but also of disproportionate Covid deaths by race and class among frontline workers with little access to protective gear, medical care, or vaccines. Outside of the US, groups not identified as Black but which identified with similar experiences of extreme marginalization and exposure to violence and infection, adopted similar slogans and strategies of protest, including robust social media platforms and digital organizing techniques. White Coats for Black Lives, a group of multiracial health professionals that held "die-ins" at medical schools, hospitals, and clinics in support of BLM protesters, used similar techniques to organize practitioners around racial justice in healthcare. This example provides a window on what future cross-pollinations of social justice with health justice movements in future social medicine interventions might be like.

Biosocial knowledge and health interventions. Life science discoveries in areas such as lifelong neuroplasticity in response to social exposures, the role of the gut microbiome in immune function and brain development, and the strong influence of social environments in epigenetics – the regulation of gene expression, which can in many cases be inherited intergenerationally – are potential fuel for a biologically grounded social medicine. While these areas of biosocial inquiry are also fraught with the risk of molecularizing and reducing social environments, in the hands of collaborating social scholars and social medicine practitioners they might be harnessed to usher in a new life science paradigm to accompany time-tested social medicine commitments to intervening on social environments, in addition to individual bodies or minds. Another danger is that life scientists would use their enormous symbolic capital to silence and speak over grassroots community organizations in defining the nature of health problems and their solutions, so one role for social medicine practitioners would be to instruct their life science colleagues in the principles of community participatory research, which has to date been constrained to public health and clinical research, rather than permeating laboratory research. This potential for social medicine to play these bridging roles has yet to be realized but would be represent a new and contemporary chapter among the rich and varied forms of social medicine presented in this collection.

It is the very agility of social medicine as a set of concepts and approaches that will keep it relevant moving forward and that agility is enhanced by the rich histories and political landscapes traced by this collection. The more social medicine practitioners see the depth of the well from which they can draw, the more they can remedy the evolving forms of our social pathologies and enhance our collective adaptations.

Index

Note: Page numbers in *italics* refer to figures; those followed by 'n' refer to the footnotes.

AAMC (American Association of Medical Colleges), 156, 157
al-Abhath (journal), 48
Abi-Rached, Joelle M., 7, 40
Aboriginal health care, 238, 251, 252, 252n56
abortion laws, 52, 68, 126, 134
Abrasco (Associação Brasileira de Pós-Graduação em Saúde Coletiva), 7, 230
academic institutions. *See also* research
Australia, 244, 246n31, 253, 253n63
India, 291–2, 294
Latin America, 171n18, 178–9, 221, 225, 226, 227–32, 236
Scandinavia, 135, 141
US, 154–6, 161–3, 161n89, 164, 165n112, 165n115
academic journals, 45, 77, 111, 118, 142, 153, 164, 224, 233
Ackerknecht, Erwin, 22n4, 63
Advisory Committee on Medical Research (ACMR), 175, 179
Africa, 110, 271. *See also* Ghana; Pholela Community Health Centre (PCHC), South Africa
agrarian reforms, 110, 117, 201, 202, 205, 206, 320. *See also* rural health
ALAMES. *See* Latin American Social Medicine Association (ALAMES)
ALBA (Bolivarian Alliance for the Peoples of Our America), 311
Algeria, 44, 58
Allende, Salvador, president of Chile, 64, *67*, 68, 70, 75
Alliance for Progress, US, 71, *72*, 174
Alma-Ata Declaration (1978), 11, 116, 251, 267, 286
Ambedkar, Babasaheb Bhimrao, 281, 282
AMECH (Chilean Medical Association), 66, 70

America. *See* United States (US)
American Association of Medical Colleges (AAMC), 156, 157
American Medical Association (AMA), 120, 156
AMI (Assistance Médicale Indigène), 87–9
Amrith, Sunil, 280
Anderson, Warwick, 12, 237, 246n31
anthropology, and social medicine, 21, 161n89, 164, 197, 244
Arab world
Arabic term for "social medicine," 7, 40, 45, 46
Ben Cheikh, Tawhida, 50–3, *52*
El-Saadawi, Nawal, 56–7
Halim, Abdel Halim Mohamed, 53–5
Khairallah, Amin A., 40, 45, 47–9
Nahda movement, 45, 47
Shumayyil, Shibli, 40, 45–7, 48
social justice movements, 52, 58
women's health, 50, 52
Argentina, social medicine in, 70, 236
Arogya Swaraj ("people's health in people's hands"), India, 281, 285, 285n16
Arole, Raj and Mabelle (CRPH), 288
Arouca, Antônio Sérgio da Silva, 75, 170, 227
ash-Shifa' (journal), 45
Assistance Médicale Indigène (AMI), 87–9
Atiyah, Edward, *An Arab Tells His Story*, 55
Australia
academic institutions, 244, 246n31, 253, 253n63
Cilento, Raphael, 239–41, 239n1
community health, 12, 249–54
growth of social medicine, 12, 237
leftist scholars, 241–2
McMichael, A. J. "Tony," 247–9
racist policies, 237
stigma of socialist medicine, 255n70

bacteriology, and medicine, 35
Baehr, George, 147
Bandung (Asian-African) Conference
    (1955), 308
Bandung Conference on Rural Hygiene (1937)
    colonialism and, 8, 99–103, 104–5
    delegates, 81n1, 97–9, 99, 103–4
    location, 81–2, 82, 83, 100n56, 102
    outcomes, 82–4, 101, 103–4
    Primary Health Care and, 289
    and Rockefeller Foundation, 149
Banerji, D., 291
Bang, Abhay and Rani (SEARCH), 289
Bannister, David, 13, 217, 257, 276, 277
barefoot doctors, China, 202
    establishment of, 201, 202–4, 205,
        208–9, 216
    international influence of, 11, 116, 215–16,
        217, 269, 285
    and rural community, 204, 207, 210, 211,
        212, 216
Baru, Rama V., 13, 278, 278n2, 318
Basaglia, Franco, 76
Basic Health services, Scandinavia, 137
Beaumont, William, 36
Ben Cheikh, Tawhida, 50–3, 52
Berkeley Center for Social Medicine, US, 323,
    165n112
Bhore Committee, India, 13, 147, 150, 279–80
Bibilie, Seneka, 290
Biomedicalization project, Scandinavia,
    1n*, 122n*
biomedicine
    community health and, 216, 253, 305–6
    Eastern Europe, 115, 121
    Gandhi on, 287
    plasticity of, 302–6
    and social justice, 14, 309
    Virchow on, 21
biopolitics, 42, 43, 128, 166, 318
biosocial aspects of medicine, 17, 63,
    163–4, 324
Birn, Anne-Emanuelle, 18, 149–50, 215, 318
birth attendants (Ba mu), French
    Indochina, 89, 92
Black Lives Matter protests, 166, 315, 323
Black Panther Party, 158–9, 215
Black social theorists, US, 151–3, 160
Bluestone, Ephraim (Montefiore), 155–6
Boas, Ernest, 155n62
Bolivar Country Farming Cooperative, 199
Bolivarian Alliance for the Peoples of Our
    America (ALBA), 311
Bolsanaro, Jair, president of Brazil, 312
Bombay Plan, India, 280, 281
Bonnevie, Paul, 134
Borowy, Iris, 84, 140

Boston Medical and Surgical Journal
    (BMSJ), 145
bota abaixo riots, Brazil, 225
Bourdieu, Pierre, 218, 235
Bowditch, Henry Ingersoll, 144
Brazil
    Abrasco, 7, 230
    academic institutions, 227–32
    health equity, 220, 221, 223, 233
    historiography of public health, 219–26
    IMS, 12, 219, 232, 233, 236
    industrialization, 220
    Mais Médicos program, 312
    saúde coletiva, 63, 76, 219, 226–7, 230,
        233, 234–6
    social security organizations, 233
    SUS, 224, 232–4
Brimnes, Niels, 122n*
Britain, 37, 55, 251n53, 266, 270, 272
British Gold Coast. See Ghana
Brotherton, P. Sean, 14, 297
Brown, Theodore, 83, 109n10
Brundtland, Gro Harlem, prime minister of
    Norway, 139–40
Buda, Béla, "The sociology of medicine and
    healthcare," 118–19
Bugri, Sam, 270

Cabot, Richard, on social medicine, 144
Camargo, Kenneth Rochel de, 12, 218
Canguilhem, Georges, 42, 235
CAPES, Brazil, 231
capitalism. See racial capitalism
Cárdenas, Lázaro, president of Mexico, 320
Carter, Eric D., 1n*, 7, 8, 60
Cassel, John, 162
Castro, Fidel, president of Cuba, 307, 309,
    310, 315
Castro, Josué de, The Geography of
    Hunger, 74
CEBES (Centro Brasileiro de Estudos de
    Saúde), 230, 233
CENDES, Venezuela, 71
Centre of Social Medicine and Community
    Health, India, 291–2
CEPAL (Economic Commission for Latin
    America and the Caribbean), 71, 227
Chakrabarti, Pratik, "Health as
    Activism," 284–5
Chávez, Hugo, president of Venezuela,
    310, 311, 315
Chesneau, Pierre, 91–3, 92n34, 93, 98
Chile, 66–9, 67
Chilean Medical Association
    (AMECH), 66, 70
China. See also barefoot doctors, China
    African missions, 110

Communist Party, 201, 206, 216, 217
Cultural Revolution, 205, 208
medicines, 203, 204, 207, 208, 213
People's Commune, 202–3, 209, 212
Rockefeller Foundation in, 150
CHPS (Community-Based Health Planning
     and Services), Ghana, 266, 267
Christian Medical College, India, 283, 284
Cilento, Raphael W., 239–41, 239n1
Civil Medical Service, Dutch East Indies, 90–1
civil rights. *See* social justice movements
CMPP (Cuban Medical Professional Parole
     Program), 313
Cold War era
     China and, 214
     Latin America, 70–4
     socialized medicine in, 106, 118
     US and socialized medicine, 9, 120, 143,
          144, 153–7
Colegio Médico, Chile, 70
Colombia, US missions in, 169, 175, 176
colonial health policies. *See also* Bandung
     Conference on Rural Hygiene (1937)
     Africa, 44–5, 258, 264, 266–7, 308
     AMI, 87–9
     Australia, 237, 239–40
     Cuban anti-colonialism, 214, 309
     decolonization, 44, 167, 308
     Dutch East Indies, 89–90, 102n60
     Indian subcontinent, 278–9
     NAM, 289
     Portugal, 319
Colonial Welfare and Development Acts,
     Britain, 266
communism, in Cold War era, 70, 71, 175.
     See also specific countries
community health, 322. *See also* barefoot
     doctors, China; Pholela Community Health
     Centre (PCHC), South Africa; public health
     China, 204, 212, 213
     CHPS, Ghana, 266, 267, 275–6
     community health program, Australia, 12,
          249–54
     community health workers, 189–90, 287, 288
     COPC, South Africa, 10, 186, 187, 197–8
     definition (Opit), 254
     Indian subcontinent, 285, 287–9,
          288n19, 291–2
     Latin America, 185n84, 302, 303–4
     and medicine, Australia, 239, 252, 255, 256
     Scandinavia, 137
     and universal health care, 116
     US, 157–60, 288
Comprehensive Rural Health (CRPH)
     project, India, 288
Convention People's Party (CPP), Ghana,
     267–8, 269

Cordeiro, Hesio de Albuquerque, 183,
     227–8, 229, 232, 233
Covid-19, 60–1, 142, 165, 295–6, 297–8,
     298, 300
Crenshaw, Kimberlé, on intersectionality, 163
Cruz, Oswaldo, 225
Cruz-Coke, Eduardo, 68
Cuba, 321
     CMPP, 313
     community health, 302, 303–4, 305
     Covid-19, 297, 300
     ELAM, 300
     international missions, 110, 298, 299,
          306–11, 312, 314, 316
     Soviet Union alliance, 309
     Venezuela alliance, 310, 311, 315, 316
Cuban Revolution (1959), 14, 75, 299, 312
Cuenca I meeting, Ecuador, 77, 178–9, 183
Cultural Revolution, China, 203, 205, 208
CUNY Medical School, US, 165
Czechoslovakia, 108, 111, 113, 117, 119

Dark, Eleanor, 241
Dark, Eric P., 241–2
de Vogel, W. T., 90
Denmark, 125, 126, 133, 134, 136
dependency theory, 8, 74, 79, 167
Deuschle, Kurt (Many Farms), 155, 160
Diepgen, Paul, 36
Diretas Já movement, Brazil, 223
disability benefits, Scandinavia, 135
diseases. *See* epidemiology
Division of Social Medicine, US, 155–6
doctors. *See* physicians
Donnangelo, Maria Cecília Ferro, 76, 229
Du Bois, W. E. B., 9, 151–3
Dubos, Jean, 153
Dubos, René, 153–4
Dunham, Francis Lee, *An Approach to
     Social Medicine*, 145
Dunk, James, 1n*, 12, 237
Dutch East Indies. *See also* Bandung
     Conference on Rural Hygiene (1937)
     Civil Medical Service, 90–1
     economy, 94–5
     health policies, 87, 95, 96–7
     Sangkuriang Legend (Bandung), 82

Eastern Europe
     and Cuba, 109–13
     health policies, 112, 113–18
     social medicine in, 107–10
     Weinermans on, 119
Ebert, Robert, 161
ecology, and health, 6, 141, 247, 248, 323
Economic Commission for Latin America and
     the Caribbean (CEPAL), 71, 227

Ecuador, 60, 77, 176, 178–9, 183
Educación Médica y Salud (journal), 10
Egypt, revolutionary doctors, 45, 52, 57
El Salvador, 178, 183
ELAS (Latin American School of
    Sociology), 171n18
Ellery, Reg, 242
El-Saadawi, Nawal, 56–7
Engh, Sunniva, 122n*
environmental health, 139, 247. See
    also ecology, and health
epidemiology
    control programs, 210–11, 293
    dispensarización (Cuban
        classification system), 305
    ecology and, 248
    rural diseases, 209–10, 304
    socioeconomic factors and, 125
equality. See health equity
eugenics, 15–16, 16n13, 126–8, 144n3, 241
Evang, Karl
    health policies, 131, 132, 137, 138
    views, 125, 127
    and WHO, 128–9, 137, 138n80

Faculdade de Saúde Pública, Brazil, 226
Fadl, Farouk, 55
Family Medicine Programme, Australia, 253
Fang, Xiaoping, 11, 201
Fanon, Franz, 159
Far Eastern Association for Tropical
    Medicine (FEATM), 86, 87
Farmer, Paul E., 17, 64, 163–4
fascism, 15
Fassler, Clara, 76
Fee, Elizabeth, 35, 64, 83, 109n10, 149
feminist physicians, Arab world, 50–3,
    52, 56–7
Fiocruz (Fundação Oswaldo Cruz),
    Brazil, 225
Fiori, José Luis, 233
first-wave social medicine, Latin America,
    7, 8, 61, 62, 64, 65–9, 76, 167
FLACSO (Faculty of Social Sciences), Latin
    America, 171, 171n18, 172, 173
Floyd, George, 166
Fog, Mogens, 125
Fonseca, Sebastian, 10, 167
Foucault, Michel, 42, 66, 229
Franco, Saul, 177
Frank, Andre Gunder, 74
Freire, Paulo, 74, 79
French Indochina. See also Bandung
    Conference on Rural Hygiene (1937)
    AMI, 87–8
    Ba mu (birth attendants), 89, 92

Great Depression, 91
    rural health, 87, 91–3, 92n34, 93
Fugelli, Per, 141
Fundação Oswaldo Cruz (Fiocruz),
    Brazil, 225

Galdston, Iago, 147, 148
Galeano, Eduardo, 74
Gandhi, Mahatma, 280, 281, 285, 285n16, 287
García, Carlota Rios, 172
García, Joaquin Torres, 320
García, Juan César
    ALAMES, 169–73, 174, 177, 181, 184
    MMF survey, 175–9, 183
    US on, 176n45
    work with PAHO, 75, 168, 226–7
Geiger, H. Jack, 157–8, 199–200
Germany, 25, 26, 27, 30, 36n36, 107
Ghana
    CHPS program, 274–6
    Medical Field Units (MFUs), 13, 257–8,
        263–7, 268, 269–74
    Native Authorities, 257, 259–63, 275–76
    and socialist countries, 272
Ghetto Medicine Law (1968), US, 159
Gibson, Count, 158
global health
    analysis of, 103, 299n5, 314–17
    Cuba and, 298, 300–2, 306
    future of, 16–19
    US and, 148–51, 164
    WHO and, 140
Gordon, Douglas, Health, Sickness, and
    Society, 254–6
Goschler, Constantin, 22n4
Grant, John, 13, 150, 157, 162, 280
Great Depression, 85, 91, 242
Greene, Jeremy A., 9, 143
Gregg, Alan, 147
Grotjahn, Alfred, 16, 38, 125, 127
Grunfeld, Berthold, 134
Guérin, Jules, 41–5, 48
Guevara, Che, 65, 74, 159, 307
Guimarães, Reinaldo, 232, 233
Guimarães, Ulysses, 223

Haave, Per, 9, 122
Haitian Revolution, 301
Halim, Abdel Halim Mohamed, 53–5
Hansen, Helena, structural competency,
    164, 322
Haroun, Georges, "Šiblī Šumayyil," 46
Harsch, Donna, "medicalized social
    hygiene," 114
Harvard School of Public Health (HSE), 283
Health Action International, 290

health equity
  Brazil, 220
  China, 205–9
  in global health, 306
  India, 281, 295
  intersectionality, 163
  rural areas, 163–4
  Scandinavia, 130, 132, 142
  structural inequality, 305
  US, 151–3
  WHO report (2005), 18
  women, 56, 57
Heiser, Victor (RD), 86, 87, 148
Helou, Lidia, 7, 40
Heni, Gogo (PCHC health worker), 189–90,
  189n11, 200
Henry Reeve Medical Brigade (HRIMB),
  Cuba, 297, 307, 308
herbal medicine. *See* traditional medicine
Hermant, Pierre, 94
Hetzel, Basil, 238, 245–6
Hindu caste system, 281
Hirak movement, Algeria, 58
Höjer, Axel, 127, 138
Horton, Richard, "Health in the Arab
  World," 59
Horwitz, Abraham, 72
Hospital Act (1969), Norway, 131
HRIMB (Henry Reeve Medical Brigade),
  Cuba, 297, 307, 308
Hubbard, John Perry, 143, 156
Hübener, Carl Wilhelm, *The Silesian
  Weavers*, 27
humanitarianism
  Cuban missions, 299, 306–11, *313*,
    314, 316
  from Global South, 298
  and social medicine, 43
  South–South aid, 10, 321
Hungary, 112, 114, 117, 118–19
Hurricane Katrina, US, 307
Hydrick, J. L. (IHD), 94–5, 99, 148
hygiene policies. *See* social hygiene policies

IAPs (*Institutos de Aposentadoria e Pensão*),
  Brazil, 220, 222
IHD. *See* International Health Division (IHD)
Illich, Ivan, 76
IMF (International Monetary Fund), 273–4
IMS (Instituto de Medicina Social), Brazil, 12,
  219, 224, 228–30, 232, 236
INAMPS (Instituto de Assistência Médica da
  Previdência Social), 233
Indian subcontinent
  academic institutions, 291–2
  Arogya Swaraj, 281, 285, 285n16

Bhore Committee, 13, 147, 150, 279–80
  community health workers, 287–9
  health equity, 285, 287, 289, 295
  international influences, 138, 285
  Khanna and Narangwal studies, 283–5
  NRHM, 293
  postcolonialism, 278, 283
  reproductive health policies, 293n23
  SAP, 292
  women's health, 289, 318
Indigenous communities
  Aboriginal communities, 238, 251, 252,
    252n56
  AMI, 87–9
  Bandung Conference (1937), 101–3
  Navajo Reservation, 154, 160
Indochina. *See* French Indochina
Indonesia. *See* Dutch East Indies
inequality. *See* health equity
Inghe, Gunnar, 126, 134, 135
Instituto de Medicina Social (IMS), Brazil, 12,
  219, 224, 228–30, 232, 236
International Federation of Socialist
  Physicians, 124, 127
international health, 9, 11, 70–3, 74, 78,
  271–2. *See also* Bandung Conference on
  Rural Hygiene (1937)
International Health Board (IHB), 86, 86n12
International Health Division (IHD), 148–50,
  151, 284
International Labor Organization (ILO), 69
International Monetary
  Fund (IMF), 273–4
Italy, 297, *298*
Iyengar, Sudarshan, "Health Care: The
  Gandhian Way," 287

Jali, Amelia, 187
Jali, Edward, 187, 189
Jan Swasthya Abhiyan (JSA), India,
  286–7, 292
Johns Hopkins University, 73, 165, 283
Jones, David S., 9, 143
Jones, W. J. A., 262
Joseph Bhore Committee. *See* Bhore
  Committee, India
Journal of the American Medical Association
  (*JAMA*), 145, 156

Kark, Emily (PCHC), 157, 187–9, 189n10,
  196–7, 200
Kark, Sidney (PCHC), 10, 157, 186–9, 187n5,
  189n10, 198, 200
Kaufman, Jay S., 64
Kennedy, Edward, Senator, 158
Kennedy, John F., president of US, 307

Khairallah, Amin A., 40, 45, 47–9
Khanna project, India, 284–5
Kleinman, Arthur, 1n*
Knorr-Cetina, Karin D., 218, 235
Kreuder-Sonnen, Katharina, 108
Krieger, Nancy, 64
Kuhn, Thomas S., 218, 235
Kullerberg, Patricia, on Hungary, 115
Kveim Lie, Anne, 9, 122

labor unions, 70
    Chile, 66
Latin America. *See also*
    specific countries
    academic institutions, 70, 174–84
    anti-communism in, 183
    Cold War era, 70–4
    Covid-19, 60–1
    first-wave social medicine, 7, 8, 61, 62,
        64, 65–9, 76, 167
    "health in adversity," 61
    higienismo policies, 66
    journals, 77
    MMF surveys, 171, 175–9
    OPS/CENDES method, 71–3
    PALTEX/BIREME medical library,
        174, 179–84
    "Pink Tide" governments, 64, 78
    postcolonialism, 310
    second-wave social medicine, 7, 8, 61, 62,
        63, 74–7, 168
    Western influences on, 78
Latin American Faculty of Social Sciences
    (FLACSO), 171, 171n18, 172
Latin American School of Medicine (ELAM),
    Cuba, 300
Latin American Social Medicine Association
    (ALAMES)
    and community health, 185n84
    formation of, 7, 77, 168
    García, Juan César, 169–70, 171,
        177, 184–5
    and PAHO, 10, 178, 179, 182
League of Nations Health
    Organization (LNHO), 4, 69, 81,
    83, 85–7, 97
Lebanon, White Coats movement, 58
Lecomte, Dr. A., 88
leftist scholars, 64, 124–5, 173–9, 184
Leunbach, Jonathan, 126
liberation theology, 8, 77, 79, 164, 167
López, Raúl Necochea, 215
Lorde, Audre, on intersectionality, 163
Loureiro, Sebastião, 227
Loyolla, Maria Andrea, 232
Luz, Madel, 230

Maalouf, Nicola, 55
Machado, Francisco de Assis, 75, 231
Machado, Roberto, 230
Mæland, Gunnar, 122n*
Mahanand, Jadumani, 282
Mahler, Halfdan T., 84, 116, 138
Mais Médicos program, 316
Malabou, Catherine, on plasticity, 306
Malhamé, Syrian, 55
Many Farms experiment, US, 154
Mao Zedong, 116–17, 159, 206
Marcel, Henri, 88
Marquez, Miguel, 176–7, 183
Marshall, Carter, 160
Martirena, Alfredo, *313*
Marxism, and social medicine, 7, 9, 75, 172,
    177, 226, 285
MBA (Misión Barrio Adentro), Cuba–
    Venezuela, 310, 312, 316
McCarthyism, US, 71
McDermott, Walsh, 154–5
McKeown, Thomas, 243
McMichael, A. J. Tony, 238, 247–9
Medibank, Australia, 243
medical education surveys, Latin
    America, 174–9
Medical Field Units (MFUs), Ghana, 13,
    257–8, 263–7, *268*, 269–74, 276
Medical Journal of Australia (journal), 241
medical schools. *See* academic institutions
medicalization of health, 1, 42, 66, 114
Medico Friends Circle (MFC), India, 292
Medicinische Reform, Die (journal), 20, 24,
    24n5, 30, 31, 32
MEF (Family Physician and Nurse Program),
    Cuba, 303, 304
Mello, Carlos Gentile de, 222
Menéndez, Eduardo, 76
mental health, 15n12, 96
Metzl, Jonathan, structural competency, 164
Mexico, 75, 320
MFC (Medico Friends Circle), India, 292
MFUs. *See* Medical Field Units (MFUs), Ghana
Milbank Memorial Fund (MMF) project,
    Latin America, 171, 173, 175
Miller, Kelly, sociology of racism, 152
MINSAP (Cuban Ministry of Public
    Health), 304
Misión Barrio Adentro (MBA), Cuba–
    Venezuela, 310, 312, 316
Molina Guzmán, Gustavo, 64, 76, 183
Møller, Anker, 126
Monash University, Australia, 245
Monnais, Laurence, 8, 81
Montefiore Hospital, US, 155–6, 160, 164
Montes Claros, Brazil, 231

Moraes, Nelson Luiz de Araújo, 228
Morman, Edward T., 35
Moser, Gabriele, 114
Mount Sinai Hospital, US, 160
Movimento de Reforma Sanitária (MRS),
    Brazil, 222, 224, 233, 234
Mozambique, 319
Mudaliar, Sir Arcot Lakshmanaswami, 138
Muñoz, José, 316
Mūsā, Salāma, 45
Musolino, Connie, 12, 237
al-Mustakbal (journal), 45

Nahḍa movement, Ottoman Empire, 45, 47
Narangwal study, India, 284
National Health Service (NHS),
    Britain, 37, 110
National Planning Committee, India, 280–2
National Rural Health Mission (NRHM), 293
nationalism, and social medicine, 15, 238,
    240, 241
nation-state, and social medicine, 241, 252
Native Authorities (NAs), Ghana, 257,
    259–63, 275–6
Navajo Reservation, US, 154, 160
Navarro, Vicente, 64, 76, 76n39, 138n80
Navrongo Experiment, Ghana, 275, 276
Neely, Abigail H., 10, 157, 186
Nehru, Jawaharlal, 281
Nelson, Alondra, Body and Soul, 159
New England Journal of Medicine, 144
New York Academy of Medicine (NYAM),
    37, 147
New York Hospital, 154
Newsholme, Arthur, 108, 242
Ngcobo, Gogo (PCHC community), 200
Ngcobo, Gogo (PCHC resident), 190, 194
Nkrumah, Kwame, president of Ghana,
    267–8, 272
Non-Aligned Movement (NAM), 289, 309
Nordic countries. See Scandinavia
Nordic Journal of Social Medicine
    (journal), 142
Noronha, José Carvalho de, 232
North Carolina University (UNC), 162–3,
    199, 200
Norway
    academic institutions, 135, 141
    Brundtland, Gro Harlem, 139–40
    eugenics and sterilization laws, 127
    health policies, 124, 126, 133, 134, 138
    public health system, 130–2
Norwegian Research Council, 122n*
Nunes, Nina Vivina Pereira, 227, 232
NYAM. See New York Academy of Medicine
    (NYAM)

occupational therapy, Dutch East Indies, 96–7
Office of Economic Opportunity (OEO), 158
Offringa, J., 90, 91, 95, 99, 101
Opit, Lou, 254, 254n66
OPS/CENDES program, Latin America, 71, 75
Orvosi Hetilap, journal, 111
Ottesen-Jensen, Elise, 126

Packard, Randall, 84
PALTEX/BIREME library (PAHO), 169,
    174, 179–84
Pan-American Health Organization (PAHO),
    10, 71, 75, 168, 170, 173–9, 183, 225
Papua New Guinea, Cilentro in, 239, 245
Park, Robert, 153
participatory action research, 167
Partido Comunista Brasileiro (PCB), 221
Partners in Health (PIH), 164
pathologies, and social medicine, 48
Pavlov, Ivan, 112, 113
PCHC. See Pholela Community Health
    Centre (PCHC), South Africa
peasants. See agrarian reforms
People's Commune, China, 202–3, 209, 212
People's Free Medical Clinics (PFMCs),
    159, 215
People's Plan, India, 280, 281
People's Republic of China. See China
Peru, 215
Petrov, Boris Dmitrievich, 112
pharmaceuticals, 207, 208, 210, 213, 290–1
Philippines, 100
Pholela Community Health Centre (PCHC),
    South Africa, 186–200
    background, 191–2
    community health workers, 189, 192, 200
    Kark, Sidney and Emily, 10, 157, 186–9,
        187n5, 189n10, 196–7, 198, 200
    seed cooperatives, 195–7
    vegetable gardens, 194–5, 199
physicians
    Arab women, 50–3, 52, 56–7
    IMS, 228
    Latin America, 66, 227
    leftist, 64, 173–9, 184
    postcolonial movement, 84, 86, 87, 278
    training of, 304
Physis (journal), 232
PIH (Partners in Health), 164
Pink Tide governments, Latin America, 78
Pioneer Health Centre, Britain, 251n53
planetary health, 6, 141, 249, 323
plasticity in biomedicine, 306
Podolsky, Scott H., 9, 143
Poland, 112, 119
Pols, Hans, 8, 81

Popular Journal for Sex Education
    (journal), 126
Porter, Dorothy, 16n13, 65, 151
poverty. *See* social determinants of health
Powles, John W., 246–7, 247n32
preventive medicine
    China, 210
    Ghana, 261, 265
    India, 150, 280, 287
    Latin America, 73, 170, 177
    Pavlov on, 112
    US, 144, 156, 161
primary health care. *See* Alma-Ata
    Declaration (1978)
Prussia, *25*, 26, *27*, 29, *30*
public health
    Alma-Ata Declaration (1978), 11, 83,
        116, 251, 267, 286
    Indian subcontinent, 286–7
    Latin America, 12, 311
    as preferred term, 142
    in socialist countries, 111
    state and, 31, 35
Public Health Care (PHC) conference
    (WHO), 319
Public Health Foundation of India, 294

queerness, and global health, 316
Quiroga, José, 312

racial capitalism, 188, 188n7, 192, 195
racism, 151–3, 160, 188, 191–2, 237, 239, 240
Rajchman, Ludwik, 84, 85
Rasyid, Abdul, 95
Reagan, Ronald, president of US, 120
Reeve, Brigadier General Henry, 307
Reform and Opening-Up period, China, 208–9
religion, and social medicine, 77, 292
Renault, Emmanuel, "Biopolitique," 42, 44
reproductive health, 16, 51, 126, 134, 137,
        138n80, 293n23. *See also* eugenics
research. *See also* academic institutions
    importance of, 133
    journals, 45, 118, 145, 153, 164, 224, 233
    PALTEX/BIREME library, 174, 179–84
    scientific development of, 218
revolutions, and social medicine
    Egypt, 45, 52, 57
    Haiti, 301
    Latin America, 14, 75, 299, 312
    Prussia, 26, 29–33
Rio de Janeiro, Brazil, 219, 225
Robinson, Cecil, "racial capitalism," 188n7
Rockefeller Foundation, 9, 86, 94–5, 143, 147,
        148–51, 155n62, 226, 283
Rockefeller Institute, 153

Rodriguez, Maria Isabel, 178, 179, 182–3
Roemer, Milton, 64, 132, 138n80, 279
Rose, Gillian, 197
Rosen, George
    and historiography of social medicine, 3,
        22, 35–8, 122–3
    NYAM conference, 147
    and Virchow, 34, 39, 63
Rosenau, Milton, 144, 144n3, 162
Rosenberg, Charles, 1n*
Rosenstam, Ida, 130
Rousseff, Dilma, president of Brazil, 311
Rovere, Mario, 170, 177
Roy, M. N, People's Plan, India, 281
RSFU (Swedish Association for Sexuality
    Education), 126
Ruiz, Dr. (Cuban *consultorios*), 302–3,
    302n17, 304
rural health. *See also* barefoot doctors, China;
    social hygiene policies; *specific countries*
    China, 116–17, 208, 209–11, 214
    CRPH, India, 288
    Eastern Europe, 117–18
    French Indochina, 87, 91–3, *93*
    and rural community, 207
Russia. *See* Soviet Union
Ryle, John, 13, 146, 147, 150, 280

Saint, Eric, 244–5
SAIRR (South African Institute for Race
    Relations), 188, 188n9
Sand, René, 63, 150
São Paulo, University of (USP), 221
Sardell, Alice, 158
Sarney, José, president of Brazil, 223
saúde coletiva, Brazil, 63, 76, 219, 226–7,
    230, 233, 234–6
Saúde em Debate (journal), 233
Savelli, Mat, 106
Sax, Sidney, 242–4, 250, 253
Scandinavia. *See also* Denmark; Norway;
    Sweden
    basic health services, 131
    development of social medicine, 122, 135–7
    eugenics and sterilization laws,
        16n13, 126–8
    "social medicine" term, 142
    socialism, 124–5
    welfare model, 9, 129
Scandinavian Journal of Public Health
    (journal), 142
Schedule Tribe communities, India, 289
Scheper-Hughes, Nancy, 164
Schipperges, Heinrich, 22n4, 32
Schumaker, Lynn, 197
Scott, David, 'problem-space', 314

SDOH (structural determinants of health), 305, 314
second-wave social medicine, Latin America, 7, 8, 61, 62, 63, 74–7, 168
seed cooperatives (PCHC), 195, 199
Servicio Nacional de Salud (SNS), Chile, 68, 69, 70, 73
Sesia, Paola, 79
sexual health, 58, 126, 134
Sheps, Cecil, 162
Shumayyil, Shibli, 40, 45–7, 48
Sigerist, Henry, *34*, 145–8
  Bhore Committee, 13, 280
  and Black social theorists, 153
  and historiography of social medicine, 22
  influence of, 36, 64, 157, 242, 243, 266
  and Rockefeller Foundation, 148, 150, 155n62
  on socialized medicine, 108
  on Virchow, 34, 63, 64
Silesia. *See* Upper Silesia
Silva, Rodrigues da, 227
Simonovits, István, 113, 117
Sindicato de Médicos (labor union), Chile, 66
Sistema Único de Saúde (SUS), Brazil, 224, 232–4
Sithole, Gogo (PCHC community), 192–3, 200
Škovránek, Vilém, 115
SMC (Social Medicine Consortium), 164
Smythurst, B. A., 252–3
SNS (Servicio Nacional de Salud), Chile, 68, 69, 70, 73
social determinants of health
  biological, 17, 324
  ecological, 6, 141, 247, 248, 323
  economic, 188, 192, 255
  racial, 152, 160
  rural areas, 148, 163–4, 205
social hygiene policies
  Eastern Europe, 113–18
  eugenics, 15–16, 16n13, 126–8, 144n3
  Indian subcontinent, 290
  Latin America, 66, 78, 225
  Scandinavia, 133
  and social medicine, 86
  Southeast Asia, 88, 92, 94–5, *95*
  Soviet Union, 107–9
  in twentieth century, 114
social justice movements
  Africa, 51, 52, 54, 55, 58–9, 189n10
  Latin America, 310
  US, 158–60, 166, 215, 315, 323
social medicine
  definition, 1–2, 3, 21, 42–4, 48, 322
  future of, 3, 19, 323

historical context, 3–4, 13, 122, 278
  India, 285
  international terms for, 7, 45, 142, 278n2
  postcolonial role in, 4–5
  and socialized medicine, 109–13, 118–19, 120, 121, 125, 154–6
Social Medicine (journal), 123, 164
Social Medicine Consortium (SMC), 164
socialist countries, 8. *See also specific countries*
Socialist Medical Association, 110
socialist scholars, 173–9
Socialistisk Medisinsk Tidsskrift (journal), 125
socialized medicine
  definition, 43, 106–7
  health policies, 116
  hygiene policies, 113–14
  Latin America, 66–8, 69, 74–5, 173–9, 184, 226
  Scandinavia, 124–5, 133
  and social medicine, 109–13, 118–19, 120, 121, 125, 154–6
  as statist, 111
  US and, 143
  Western medicine and, 118–19
socioeconomic factors, 125, 127, 134, 163, 188, 305
solidarity humanitarianism
  China, 110
  Latin America, 74–7, 76n39, 78, 306–11, *313*
  Scandinavia, 140
Solomon, Susan, 108
South Africa, 188, 188n7, 192, 195. *See also* Pholela Community Health Centre (PCHC), South Africa
  African Reserves, 191–2
  Community-Oriented Primary Care, 10, 157, 186, 187, 197–8
  Rockefeller Foundation and, 150
South African Institute for Race Relations (SAIRR), 188, 188n9
Southeast Asia, 85, 91. *See also* Bandung Conference on Rural Hygiene (1937); *specific countries*
South–South humanitarianism, 10, 321
Soviet Union
  Cuban alliance, 309
  Dark, Eric P. on, 242
  health policies, 106, 107–9, 111, 319
  US relationship, 147
  views of Alma-Ata Conference, 116
Spinelli, Hugo, 172
Sri Lanka, 282–3, 290–1, 295, 318
Štampar, Andrija, 109, 131, 137, 138n80, 148, 150, 151, 266

sterilization laws, Scandinavia, 127
Strathern, Marilyn, 197
Strøm, Axel, 133, 135
Structural Adjustment Program (SAP), World
    Bank, 293, 294
structural competency (Hansen and Metzl), 164
structural determinants of health (SDOHs),
    305, 314
structural violence, 152
Sudan, 53–5
Sundby, Per, 134
Sustainable Development Goals (SDGs), 315
Sweden
    academic institutions, 136, 141
    eugenics and sterilization laws, 127
    "folkhälsan"/"folkehelse," 123–4
    health policies, 133, 138
    welfare state, 130, 132
Swedish Association for Sexuality
    Education (RFSU), 126
Symon, Karel, 117
Syria, medical professionals in, 53

Taylor, Carl, Rockefeller Foundation, 284
Ten-Year Public Health Program, Latin
    America, 174
Terris, Milton, 64
Testa, Mario, 75
the 1930s. Since 1999, Ghana's Community-
    Based Health Planning (CHPS), 274–6
Theunissen, W. F., 96–7, 99
Timmermann, Carsten, 6, 20, 122
tobacco policies (WHO), 140
Toverud, Kirsten Utheim, 124
traditional medicine, 49, 203, 204, 207,
    208, 281
transepistemic arenas (Knorr-Cetina),
    218, 222, 235
Tricontinental Conference (1966), Cuba, 309
Trouillot, Michel-Rolph, 301, 302
tuberculosis in Black communities, US, 154
Tunisia, 50, 51, 52
typhus epidemic, Upper Silesia, 24

UCLA, US, 165
UCSF, US, 161n89, 165
UK. See Britain
UNC (University of North Carolina), 162–3,
    199, 200
United Nations (UN), 139, 227, 309, 315
United Progressive Alliance, 293
United States (US)
    academic institutions, 156, 161–3, 161n89,
        164, 165n112, 165n115
    Alliance for Progress, 71, 72, 174

AMA, 120, 156
Black social theorists, 151–3, 160
Cold War era and socialized medicine, 9,
    120, 143, 153–7, 156
community health care, 157–60
Cuban aid to, 307–8, 314
historiography of social medicine, 62–3,
    144, 145
international projects, 169, 215, 283–5, 288,
    313, 314
Navajo Reservation, 154, 160
PAHO, 10, 71, 168, 170, 173–9, 183, 225
preventive medicine, 144–8, 156, 161
social justice movements, 158, 159, 215, 315
and Soviet Union, 147
Universidade do Estado do Rio de Janeiro
    (UERJ), 219
Upper Silesia, 22n4, 23, 24–9, 25, 27
urban health, Australia, 246
USSR. See Soviet Union

vaccines, 210–11
Valóság, journal, 118
Vanguardia Médica, Chile, 66, 67, 68, 69
Vargas dictatorship, Brazil, 220
Vargha, Dora, 8, 106
Venezuela, 71, 310, 311, 315, 316
Vieira-da-Silva, Ligia Maria "Jules Guérin,"
    41–2, 219, 235
Viel, Benjamin, 73
Vietnam. See French Indochina
Vilakazi, Mkhulu (PCHC community),
    190–1, 200
village doctors. See barefoot doctors, China
Villareal, Ramon (PALTEX/BIREME), 183
Virchow, Rudolf
    "decentred," 4, 6, 21, 39
    influence of, 33, 63–5, 147, 157
    and Pavlov, 112, 113
    political career, 21, 23–4, 26, 29–33,
        36, 38
    portraits of, 23, 33
    social medicine views, 3–4, 5, 20, 35, 47
    and typhus epidemic, Upper Silesia,
        24, 26–9
Virchows Archiv (journal), 23, 32
Volta Redonda steel mill, Brazil, 220
von Behring, Emil, 35

Waddy, B. B. (MFUs), 265
Waitzkin, Howard, 64
Weindling, Paul, 16n13
Weinerman, Richard and Shirley, Social
    Medicine in Eastern Europe, 119
Welch, William Henry, 145

white, 240
Whitlam, Gough, prime minister of Australia, 251, 253
WHO. *See* World Health Organization (WHO)
Williams, David, Detroit Area Study, 160
Williams, Rebecca, 284
Winter, Kurt, 22n4
Witwaterswand University, South Africa, 187n5
women physicians, 50–3, *52*, 56–7, 304
women's health
    Arab world, 50, 52, 56, 57
    Australia, 252
    Indian subcontinent, 286, 289
    Scandinavia, 123, 124, 134, 137
workers' rights, Brazil, 221
World Bank, 273–4, 293, 294

World Commission on Environment and Development (UN), 139–40
World Health Assembly, 215
World Health Organization (WHO)
    creation of, 128, 137, 151
    global health programs, 4, 138n80, 251, 316, 319
    policies, 140
    reports, 17, 215
World War II (WWII), impact on Eastern Europe, 107–9, 114

Young Lords, activist group, 159

Zanele (PCHC health worker), 190
Zuckerberg San Francisco General Hospital, US, 165, 165n115
Zylberman, Patrick, 107

Printed in the United States
by Baker & Taylor Publisher Services